P9-BYW-228

CHILDREN with CEREBRAL PALSY

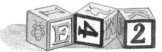

A Parents' Guide

Edited by Elaine Geralis

Foreword by Tom Ritter

WOODBINE HOUSE • 1991

Published by Woodbine House, 6510 Bells Mill Road, Bethesda, MD 20817. 800/843-7323.

Copyright © 1991 Woodbine House, Inc.

All rights reserved under International and Pan-American Copyright Conventions. Published in the United States of America by Woodbine House, Inc.

Figure 3 in Chapter Six reprinted by permission of Pro-Ed, Inc.

Photo credits: pp. 232, 266, 278, 346 courtesy of United Cerebral Palsy Associations, Inc.; pp. 50, 68, 126, 202, 246, 256, 285, 301 courtesy of Sparks Center for Developmental and Learning Disorders, University of Alabama at Birmingham; pp. 29, 75, 288, 298, courtesy of UCP of Philadelphia (Ken Seibert, photographer); p. 205 courtesy of UCP of Central Arkansas; pp. 22, 342 courtesy of UCP of Nassau County, N.Y.; pp. 106 (fig. 14, 15), 107 (fig. 17), 111 (fig. 26, 29) courtesy of J.A. Preston © 1990 Bissell Healthcare Corporation and authorized Preston dealers; pp. 106 (fig. 13), 110 (fig. 22), 111 (fig. 27, 28) courtesy of Kaye Products; pp. 107 (fig. 18, 20), 111 (fig. 30) courtesy of Ortho-Kinetics.

Cover design and illustration: Lili Robins
Illustrations (Chapter 4): Gary A. Mohrmann
Illustration (Chapter 1): Elliot S. Gersh, M.D.
Book design and typography: Robin Dhawan, Woodbine House

Library of Congress Cataloging-in-Publication Data

Children with cerebral palsy : a parents' guide / edited by Elaine Geralis
      p.   cm.
   Includes bibliographical references and index.
   ISBN 0–933149–15–8 : $14.95
     1. Cerebral palsied children. 2. Cerebral palsy—Popular works.
I. Geralis, Elaine
RJ496.C4C49 1991   88-40660
618.92'836—dc20   CIP

Manufactured in the United States of America

This book is printed on acid-free paper.

6 7 8 9 10

TABLE OF CONTENTS

ACKNOWLEDGEMENTS

There is a long list of people who have contributed in one way or another to this book. I would like to thank each and every one of them with a personalized acknowledgement, but that might be a book in itself. Instead, I'll express my appreciation in as few words as possible.

First, I want to thank my son, Robert, without whom I would never have been privileged to understand the world of those with special needs. A very special thanks also goes to Susan Stokes, Robin Dhawan, and the rest of the staff of Woodbine House. They had the patience and perseverance to see this book through. Tom Ritter, thanks for supporting us and for saying "yes." I am especially indebted to the chapter authors—all of whom generously contributed their time, energy, and knowledge out of nothing more than devotion to the well-being of children with cerebral palsy. United Cerebral Palsy Associations, Inc., also supplied valuable information as well as photographs. Thanks also to all the families who opened up their lives to me and to the readers of this book. Last of all, I would like to thank my husband, whose love and support has been immeasurable and unwavering every step of the way.

FOREWORD

Tom Ritter*

The best advice parents of children with cerebral palsy could receive is to treat your child like a person. This may sound trite, but it is too easy to focus on the disabling condition and not the whole person. I am a person with cerebral palsy *but* I am also a person who likes baseball. I am a person who likes to dance. I am a person who wants to be a parent. And I am a person.

There are deep and serious concerns both parents and their children with cerebral palsy must face. Whether it be walking with crutches, using a wheelchair, learning to verbalize, or using a word board, a lot of hard work, perseverance, and patience is necessary. You, as parents, will experience anger, frustration, sadness, and joy in seeing your child grow. Don't be afraid to allow your child to experience life. Overprotection, no matter how well-intentioned, is a detriment to a child's growth. Your child needs to know the pain of defeat as well as the joy of success. He or she must learn like everyone else from failures as well as successes.

In some respects, experiencing life will be easier for your child than it was for me. Today, there are United Cerebral Palsy centers and other service agencies that provide programs for families and children with cerebral palsy. In recent years, legislation has been passed mandating accessible transportation, equal employment, and education for people with disabilities. Unfortunately, however, some things remain the same. Many people still view people with disabilities in a patronizing way or avoid the disabled person entirely. Your child may have to confront these responses at times. The experience of successes and failures enables your child to conquer these discriminating perceptions.

---

* Tom Ritter is National Public Relations Chair for United Cerebral Palsy Associations (UCPA) and a national board member of UCPA. He is also a television producer.

I often remember the words my dad used to say to me: "Son, you have to play the cards that you were dealt." My dad helped me to accept myself and to play to win.

INTRODUCTION

Elaine Geralis

My son, Robert, was born nine weeks early. He weighed in at only four pounds, three ounces, and had such immature lungs that he needed a respirator and ventilator to help him breathe. Robert also developed many other problems related to his premature birth, and this is where our lives took a turn.

While Robert was in the neonatal intensive care nursery, I spent hours each day with him, and when I was home, called the hospital frequently. Finally, after ten long, emotional weeks, Robert was released from the hospital. I thought I was going home with a perfect miracle baby, the son I had longed for during my thirty-one week pregnancy. I had no reason to doubt the doctors' assurances that Robert's "mild delays" were typical of a premature baby. I was told "not to worry. . . . He will catch up by two."

Despite what the doctors said, Robert's progress seemed very slow. In fact, as the months went by, I found more and more that his delays were becoming as obvious to the outside world as they were to me. Why wasn't he rolling over? Why wasn't he up on his knees? Why did he keep his hands in such tight fists? Why did his eyes sometimes cross? My routine answer, "He was born prematurely and is expected to catch up by two," no longer satisfied others' curiosity . . . or mine.

Finally, when Robert was nine months old, our assessment team recommended that he start a physical therapy program twice a week. At the time, I thought we were dealing with a temporary or very mild disability of his left hand. But as the weeks and months passed and Robert's progress remained extremely slow, I began to realize that this was no mild disability. I began to question Robert's doctors more, only to find that nobody really knew the extent of his disability. They told me that only time could tell us what we were dealing with.

This period of uncertainty was an incredibly emotional time for me. Why and how could this happen to such a precious child, and how could this happen to me? Why should I have to answer to

vii

everyone else's curiosity when no one was satisfying mine? I was very angry, very confused, very worried, and very much in love with Robert.

When my son was around fifteen months old, I finally asked my developmental pediatrician to label the delays. He was hesitant to do so, but explained that Robert had some brain damage. He also said that with early intervention, some children with cerebral palsy actually can overcome these early obstacles and end up with only a mild disability. At about twenty-four months, Robert entered an early intervention program and began receiving speech and occupational therapy in addition to his physical therapy.

Robert is now a delightful, intelligent seven-year-old who is mainstreamed in a second-grade class at a public school. He is still going to physical therapy, but is walking with the aid of calf-length braces (AFOs) and a walker. Last summer, he graduated from three years of speech therapy with flying colors. He has risen above the turmoil of his parents' divorce and has joyously accepted each of our remarriages. I am extremely proud of his daily accomplishments. I see his will and stamina prevail when mine have long since gone. He is a constant reminder of how precious life is and of how important it is never to take anything for granted. He is my strength . . . not my weakness.

When I was asked to edit this book, it brought back a lot of memories. In particular, I remembered how starved I was for information after Robert was finally diagnosed with cerebral palsy. I recalled how I used to attend support group meetings, as much for the exchange of information as the emotional support. I also remembered how I combed the public libraries and bookstores, but found little or no up-to-date literature on cerebral palsy. And I realized that there really is a need for a book that speaks just to parents of children with cerebral palsy. Woodbine House has published an extraordinary series of such books for parents of children with special needs. So, together, we now give you *Children with Cerebral Palsy: A Parents' Guide.*

This is a book to help you understand your child's condition so that you can help your child reach his or her full potential. This is also a book to help you enjoy what your child has to offer. We are not talking about making your child an Olympic athlete. We are talking about understanding your child's life and understanding how your life has changed. We are talking about loving and accepting your child and the challenges you will face together.

To help you put your own and your child's life into perspective right from the start, this book provides Parent Statements at the end of each chapter. In these statements, other parents share their feelings, thoughts, and advice about raising a child with cerebral palsy. I think you will find that nothing helps soothe the frustration and hurt of having a child with special needs more than knowing that other people have gone through what you are experiencing now.

Children with Cerebral Palsy covers a wide range of subjects you need to know about during your child's first five years or so. It is not, however, intended to answer all of your questions. I think of it more as a primer for further self-education. Therefore, I have included a glossary to help you understand the new language that goes along with being the parent of a child with cerebral palsy. Additionally, the Reading List at the back of the book will direct you to books and magazines recommended for further reading. Finally, I have compiled a Resource Guide that lists addresses of parent and professional groups, as well as of federal, state, and local government agencies that can give you the support and information you need.

Throughout this book, I use the personal pronouns alternately by chapter. I did not want to imply that all children with cerebral palsy are either boys or girls, and it can be cumbersome to constantly use "he or she" to refer to children with cerebral palsy. I think this arrangement will be clear.

I can only hope that the dedicated professionals and parents who wrote this book can supply you with some much-needed answers—and encouragement. I wish all of you lots of love and success with your child.

Children w/ Cerebral Palsy:
A Parents Guide
Edited by Elaine Geralis 1991

ONE

❦

What Is Cerebral Palsy?

ELLIOT S. GERSH, M.D.*

Your child is special. Like every child, she was born with a highly distinctive set of strengths and weaknesses and a personality all her own.

Now that your child has been diagnosed as having cerebral palsy or a movement disorder, you may have begun to hear the word "special" used in different ways. Medical specialists, therapists, and teachers may tell you that you have a "special child" with "special needs." Each of these professionals may explain some of the ways cerebral palsy makes your child special, and may offer suggestions about treatment and care of her special needs. Yet you probably still have many questions about what to expect for your child.

This chapter presents some basic information parents often want to know about cerebral palsy. It explains what cerebral palsy is, discusses causes and treatments, and describes conditions that may be associated with the disability. To help you communicate with the medical professionals who care for your child, this chapter also clarifies some of the medical terminology you will likely encounter. In addition, the glossary at the back of this book defines other terms commonly used by special-needs professionals.

Some information in this chapter may be helpful to you immediately, but other information may not apply to your child until later,

---

* Dr. Elliot S. Gersh is Director of Developmental Pediatrics at the Georgetown University Child Development Center in Washington, D.C. He has extensive experience working with babies, children, and adults who have cerebral palsy and other special needs, as well as with their families.

if ever. You can sort out the information that is useful to you now and reread this chapter for additional information as needed. In general, you will find that the better informed you are as a parent, the better prepared you will be to get the best services from medical, educational, and community programs. Armed with accurate information and realistic expectations, you and your family will be able to develop unique ways to help your child succeed in the world.

What Is Cerebral Palsy?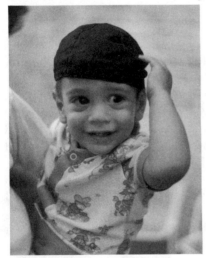

"Cerebral palsy" is a catchall term for a variety of disorders that affect a child's ability to move and to maintain posture and balance. These disorders are caused by a brain injury that occurs before birth, during birth, or within the first few years after birth. The injury does not damage the child's muscles or the nerves connecting them to the spinal cord—only the brain's ability to control the muscles. Depending on its location and severity, the brain injury that causes a child's movement disorders may also cause other problems. These problems include mental retardation, seizures, language disorders, learning disabilities, and vision and hearing problems.

Because cerebral palsy influences the way children develop, it is known as a *developmental disability*. In the United States today, more people have cerebral palsy than any other developmental disability, including Down syndrome, epilepsy, and autism. About two children out of every thousand born in this country have some type of cerebral palsy.

Although children with very mild cerebral palsy occasionally recover by the time they are school-aged, cerebral palsy is usually a lifelong disability. In most cases, the movement and other problems associated with cerebral palsy affect what a child is able to learn and do to varying degrees throughout her life. Exactly how cerebral palsy will affect your child's life will depend on a variety of factors. Many factors—such as your child's attitude toward her disability, the support you provide her, and the medical, educational, and therapeutic care she receives—are under your control. Although you cannot predict what your child's potential may be any more than you can predict any other child's, you certainly can help your child to achieve her potential and the highest quality of life possible.

Types of Cerebral Palsy

Understanding the Labels

As mentioned above, cerebral palsy is a broad term which encompasses many different disorders of movement and posture. To describe particular types of movement disorders covered by the term, pediatricians, neurologists, and therapists use several classification systems and many labels. To understand these labels and classification systems, you must first understand what professionals mean by one key term: *muscle tone*.

Muscle tone refers to the amount of tension or resistance to movement in a muscle. Muscle tone is what enables us to keep our bodies in a certain position or *posture*—for example, to sit with our backs straight and our heads up. Muscle tone, or more precisely, changes in muscle tone, is also what enables us to move. For example, to bend your arm to bring your hand up to your face, you must shorten, or increase the tone of, the biceps muscles on the front of your arm at the same time you are lengthening, or reducing the tone of, the triceps muscles on the back of your arm. To complete a movement smoothly, the tone in all muscle groups involved must be balanced—the brain must send messages to each muscle group to actively change its resistance.

All children with cerebral palsy have damage to the area of the brain that controls muscle tone. As a result, they may have increased muscle tone, reduced muscle tone, or a combination of the two (variable or fluctuating tone). Which parts of their bodies are affected by the abnormal muscle tone depends upon where the brain damage occurs.

High Tone (Spasticity). Children with increased tone are said to have *high tone, hypertonia,* or *spasticity.* If your child has high muscle

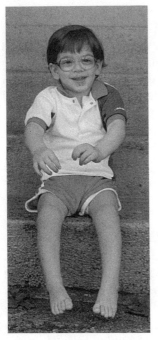

tone, her movements will be stiff and awkward because her muscles are too "tight" and their tone is not balanced. Babies with high muscle tone can be recognized by the way they arch their backs and stiffly extend their legs. Instead of rolling over in smooth, fluid movements, they move their trunks as one solid unit and flip over. Frequently, babies with increased tone roll over very early—for instance, at one month of age instead of the usual three to five months. They also love to stand on their stiff legs, but stand on their toes or scissor (cross) their legs tightly together when held upright.

Low Tone. Children with decreased tone are said to have *low tone, hypotonia,* or *floppiness.* If your child has low muscle tone, she has trouble maintaining positions without support because her muscles do not contract enough and are too relaxed. Babies with low tone like to lie on their backs (supine) with their head, trunk, arms, and legs limply resting on the floor or other surface. It is difficult for children with low tone to remain upright against the pull of gravity in positions such as sitting and standing. As a result, a child with low tone usually sits leaning forward with a rounded back. Low tone also affects a child's ability to keep her trunk stable enough so that she can use her arms to reach and grasp. And when low tone affects a child's abdominal and respiratory muscles, it can hinder the development of speech.

Fluctuating Tone. Children who have a combination of high and low tone are said to have *fluctuating* or *variable* muscle tone. If your child has fluctuating tone, her muscle tone may be low when she is at rest but then increase to high tone with active movement. Her tone increases to help stabilize a position such as sitting with a straight back, but may end up making movements such as reaching impossible because too many muscle groups in the shoulders and arms tighten.

Classifying Types of Cerebral Palsy

To understand how and why cerebral palsy affects your child as it does, it helps to understand how and why medical professionals classify cerebral palsy into different types. But before you can understand their classification systems, you may need to review how the human nervous system works.

The nervous system is made up of two parts: the central nervous system and the peripheral nervous system. The central nervous system consists of the brain and spinal cord. The peripheral nervous system consists of two sets of *nerves* which transmit information between the central nervous system and other body parts. These sets of nerves are known as sensory nerves and motor nerves. Sensory nerves carry information about senses such as pain, touch, position, and muscle tension from other parts of the body to the central nervous system. Motor nerves carry information from the central nervous system to the muscles.

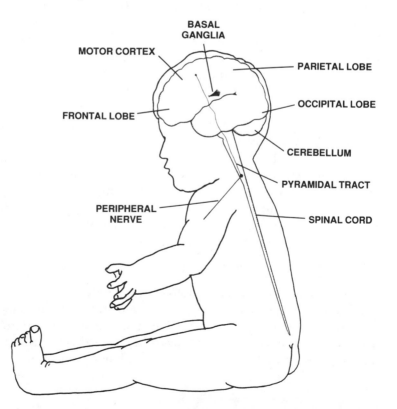

For voluntary movement to occur, each element within the nervous system must work in harmony. Movement begins in the area of the brain known as the *motor cortex*, which is shown at the top of the diagram on page 5. From here, the brain sends the initial signals to start a particular movement. The signals are then interpreted and modified by two other areas of the brain: the *cerebellum* and *basal ganglia*. The cerebellum helps coordinate muscle activity, maintains muscle tone, and controls balance. The basal ganglia control adjustments in posture needed during movement.

After these areas of the brain have processed the movement impulses, they travel to the spinal cord. The spinal cord, in turn, transmits the movement information to the peripheral nerves, which carry the impulses to the appropriate muscles. Upon receiving the impulses, the muscles contract and make the intended movement.

That, in a nutshell, is how people *without* motor disabilities move. Because children with cerebral palsy have injuries to the brain, they cannot control their movements normally. Exactly how their movement is affected depends on the location of the injury in their nervous system and the resulting type of muscle tone problem. Medical professionals sometimes classify types of cerebral palsy based on these two factors—the type of muscle tone problem and the location of the injury. Another way they classify types is according to the parts of the body that are affected by movement problems.

If your child's early signs of cerebral palsy were quite clear-cut, you may already have been told what type she has. But if the exact nature and extent of your child's movement problems are still not clear, professionals may not yet have determined the type of cerebral palsy your child has. In either case, you may be able to recognize some of your child's symptoms among the many types of cerebral palsy described below.

¥ Classification Based on the Location of Brain Injury

When using the classification system based on the location of the brain injury, doctors identify three broad types of cerebral palsy: 1) *pyramidal (spastic)* cerebral palsy; 2) *extrapyramidal (choreoathetoid)* cerebral palsy; and 3) *mixed-type* cerebral palsy. Sometimes a child with cerebral palsy is diagnosed as having one of these types when she is young, and a different type when she is older. This is not because the extent and location of brain injuries change with time, but rather because differences in muscle tone and control may become noticeable as a child grows.

⟨ **Pyramidal (Spastic) Cerebral Palsy.** Spastic cerebral palsy is the most common type of cerebral palsy. It affects about half of all children with cerebral palsy. Children with this type of cerebral palsy have one or more tight muscle groups which limit movement. They may also have these symptoms:

1. *Exaggerated stretch reflexes*—When the doctor taps the tendons over the elbow, knee, ankle, etc., with a reflex hammer, the limb extends with a jerk that is much stronger and faster than normal.
2. *Ankle clonus*—When the calf muscles in the leg are quickly stretched by flexing and holding the foot upward, muscles in the calf and foot rapidly and rhythmically contract. The rhythmic beats in the foot and calf can be clearly seen and felt. Clonus may occur when the foot is deliberately flexed upward or when the child is placed in a standing position.
3. *Positive Babinski*—When the foot is stroked from heel to toes, the toes extend and fan out rather than flex. This is considered abnormal only in children over a year old.
4. A tendency to develop *contractures* or abnormal shortening of the muscles and tendons around a joint. Contractures limit movement around the joint, and are caused by tight muscles and lack of full movement. Chapter 3 discusses prevention and treatment of contractures.
5. *Persistent primitive reflexes*—early reflexes (involuntary movements in response to stimulation such as touch, pressure, or joint movement) which persist for months or years longer than usual. See Chapter 6 for more information on persistent primitive reflexes.

If your child has spastic cerebral palsy, it is because she has damage to the part of the brain that controls voluntary movements (the motor cortex). She may also have damage to the pyramidal tracts, the pathways that link the motor cortex with the nerves in the spinal cord that relay motor signals to the muscles. In the illustration on page 5, the motor cortex is at the top of the brain, with the pyramidal tracts leading downward from it.

When the motor cortex or pyramidal tracts are damaged, the brain has trouble communicating with the muscles on either or both sides of the body. Damage to the motor cortex on the left side of the brain makes it difficult to control movements on the right side of the body, and damage to the motor cortex on the right side makes it difficult to control movements on the left side of the body. This is because the tracts from the right side of the cortex cross over to the left side of the spinal cord at the base of the brain, and vice versa.

Extrapyramidal (Choreo-athetoid) Cerebral Palsy. Roughly one quarter of children with cerebral palsy have this type of cerebral palsy. It is caused by damage to the cerebellum or basal ganglia. As mentioned earlier, these areas of the brain normally process the signals from the motor cortex, enabling smooth, coordinated movements and maintaining posture. In the illustration on page 5, the cerebellum is at the base of the brain and the basal ganglia at the center.

Damage to these areas may cause a child to develop involuntary, purposeless movements, especially in the face, arms, and trunk. These abnormal movements often interfere with speaking, feeding, reaching, grasping, and other skills requiring coordinated movements. For example, involuntary grimacing and tongue thrusting may lead to swallowing problems, drooling, and slurred speech. Involuntary *flexion* (bending) of the wrist and *splaying* (spreading) of the fingers may make reaching for objects difficult. In addition, children with extrapyramidal cerebral palsy often have low muscle tone and have problems maintaining posture for sitting and walking.

Medical professionals use a variety of terms to describe the types of involuntary movements that can be associated with extrapyramidal cerebral palsy. Here are some common terms:

- *dystonia*—slow, rhythmic, twisting movements of the trunk or an entire arm or leg. Dystonia may also involve abnormal postures such as severe rotation of the trunk.
- *athetosis*—slow, writhing movements, especially in the wrists, fingers, and face.
- *chorea*—abrupt, quick, jerky movements of the head, neck, arms, or legs.

- *ataxia*—unsteadiness and lack of coordination in standing and walking and problems with balance. Children with ataxia have damage to the cerebellum.
- *rigidity*—extremely high muscle tone in any position, combined with very limited movements.
- *dyskinesia*—a general term for involuntary movements, used when the exact type of movement is difficult to classify.

Parents do not usually notice involuntary movements until after nine months of age. Usually the first symptoms appear in the face, tongue, and arms. Involuntary movements may become worse with voluntary activities such as reaching, walking, and talking. Emotional stress, fear, or anxiety may also make involuntary movements more pronounced. For example, a child's speech may become more slurred if she has to speak up in a group. Before abnormal movements appear, children often have low muscle tone. Frequently, involuntary movements go away while children are sleeping.

Mixed-Type Cerebral Palsy. About one quarter of children with cerebral palsy have what is known as mixed-type cerebral palsy. These children have both the spastic muscle tone of pyramidal cerebral palsy and the involuntary movements of extrapyramidal cerebral palsy. This is because they have injuries to both the pyramidal and extrapyramidal areas of the brain. Usually the spasticity is more obvious at first, with involuntary movements increasing when the child is between nine months and three years old.

Classification Based on
Location of Movement Problems

To classify your child's cerebral palsy as pyramidal, extrapyramidal, or mixed-type, doctors look at how cerebral palsy affects your child's nervous system. But doctors will also classify her cerebral palsy based on how it affects her face, arms, trunk, and legs. For example, some children have movement problems primarily on the right or left side of their body, or with their legs but not their arms. Depending on which parts of your child's body are affected by movement problems, her cerebral palsy may be classified as *monoplegia, diplegia, hemiplegia, quadriplegia,* or *double hemiplegia.*

Monoplegia. In monoplegia, cerebral palsy affects only one limb (arm or leg) on one side of the child's body. Movement impairments are usually mild and often disappear with time. Monoplegia is very rare.

Diplegia. Diplegia means that cerebral palsy mainly affects a child's legs. Due to spastic leg muscles, children with diplegia tend to stand on their toes and scissor their legs—that is, to bring their legs and feet strongly together in a crossed position when upright. Children with diplegia may also have subtle or mild muscle tone problems in the upper part of the body, but they have adequate control of their trunk, arms, and head for most daily activities.

Hemiplegia. In hemiplegia, one side of the child's body is affected by cerebral palsy. The arm is usually more affected than the legs, trunk, or face, and is typically held in flexion—flexed or bent at the hand, wrist, and elbow. The arm or leg on the affected side may be shorter or less developed than the arm or leg on the other side. The child may or may not be able to use her affected hand, depending on the degree of impairment and how much sensation she has in her hand. For example, children with little sense of touch or position in their arm tend to ignore it. Fifty percent of children with hemiplegia have some loss of sensation.

Quadriplegia. When cerebral palsy affects a child's whole body—face, trunk, arms, and legs—she is said to have quadriplegia. In quadriplegia, a child's legs and feet are generally more affected by abnormal muscle tone and involuntary movements than are her arms and hands. Children with quadriplegia may also have significant impairment of the facial muscles used in feeding and speaking. Because of the extent of their motor disabilities, children with quadriplegia have difficulty with most activities of daily living.

Double Hemiplegia. Like quadriplegia, double hemiplegia affects a child's whole body. The difference is that the child's arms, not legs, are most affected by cerebral palsy. Children with double hemiplegia, too, may have major feeding and speech impairments.

What Causes Cerebral Palsy?

Why does your child have cerebral palsy?

The simplest answer to this question—because your child has brain damage—leads naturally to another question:

Why does your child have brain damage?

There are many possible answers to this second question, because there are many reasons children can suffer brain damage. To try to pinpoint the cause of your child's brain damage, your physician needs to carefully review your child's health history and conduct a variety of medical and neurological tests. In general, however, there are two problems that can cause cerebral palsy:

1. failure of the brain to develop properly (developmental brain malformation);
2. neurological damage to the child's developing brain.

Developmental Malformations. In the first and second trimesters of pregnancy, a human embryo's brain cells (*neurons*) rapidly multiply and grow near the inner layers of the brain. Later, the brain cells migrate to specific areas within the developing brain, according to the function they will serve. For example, in the typical infant's brain, several million brain cells eventually end up in the part of the brain which controls movement.

Occasionally, something may disrupt the brain's normal development process. A fetus's brain may fail to develop the normal number of brain cells, communication between brain cells may be impaired, or brain cells may not migrate to the areas they are supposed to. Causes of these malformations are frequently unknown, but can include genetic disorders, chromosome abnormalities with either too much or too little genetic material, or faulty blood supply to the brain. Developmental brain malformations in the areas of the brain which control voluntary movement may cause cerebral palsy.

Neurological Damage. If your child does not have a developmental brain malformation, then her cerebral palsy may be the result of an injury to her brain before, during, or after birth. These injuries are most often caused by problems associated with premature births, difficult deliveries, neonatal medical complications, or trauma to the brain.

Types of problems that can lead to brain injuries include:

1. lack of oxygen before, during, or after birth;
2. bleeding in the brain;

3. toxic injuries, or poisoning, from alcohol or drugs used by the mother during pregnancy;
4. head trauma resulting from a birth injury, fall, car accident, or other cause;
5. severe jaundice, very low glucose levels, or other metabolic disorders (disorders which usually impair the body's use of energy or impede the breakdown or production of the body's building blocks);
6. infections of the nervous system such as encephalitis or meningitis.

Table 1 shows other common *risk factors*, or conditions that increase the likelihood that a child will have a neurological problem.

Table 1

Pregnancy Risk Factors

- Maternal diabetes or hyperthyroidism
- Maternal high blood pressure
- Poor maternal nutrition
- Maternal seizures or mental retardation
- Incompetent cervix (premature dilation) leading to premature delivery
- Maternal bleeding from *placenta previa* (a condition in which the placenta covers a portion of the cervix and leads to bleeding as the cervix dilates) or *abruptio placenta* (premature separation of the placenta from the uterine wall)

Delivery Risk Factors

- Premature delivery (less than 37 weeks gestation)
- Prolonged rupture of the amniotic membranes for more than 24 hours leading to fetal infection
- Severely depressed (slow) fetal heart rate during labor, indicating fetal distress
- Abnormal presentation such as breech, face, or transverse lie, which makes for a difficult delivery

Neonatal Risk Factors

- Premature birth—the earlier in gestation a baby is delivered, the more likely she is to have brain damage
- Asphyxia—insufficient oxygen to the brain due to breathing problems or poor blood flow in the brain
- Meningitis—infection over the surface of the brain
- Seizures caused by abnormal electrical activity of the brain
- Interventricular hemorrhage (I.V.H.)—bleeding into the interior spaces of the brain or into the brain tissue
- Periventricular encephalomalacia (P.V.L.)—damage to the brain tissue located around the ventricles (fluid spaces) due to lack of oxygen or problems with blood flow

Whatever the cause of your child's cerebral palsy, the severity of the brain damage generally depends on the type and timing of the injury. For example, in very premature babies, bleeding into the brain (interventricular hemorrhage) can cause extensive damage. This is because the brain is still producing and organizing brain cells even after birth. Sometimes, too, a brain injury may be the result of several risk factors, each of which may not have been sufficient to cause damage on its own.

The presence of one or more risk factors does not necessarily mean that a child *will* have cerebral palsy. In fact, most children who have these problems do *not* develop cerebral palsy. For example, 70 to 90 percent of children born prematurely—depending on gestational age—don't have cerebral palsy or other developmental problems. Even in children who do have cerebral palsy, it is often

difficult to say which, if any, of these risk factors caused their brain injury. It can be frustrating to be told that the cause of your child's cerebral palsy is "unknown," but unfortunately, this is the case for about 20 percent of children with cerebral palsy.

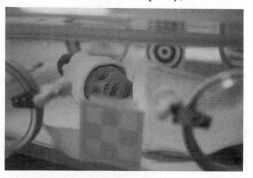

Other Conditions Associated with Cerebral Palsy

In addition to having movement impairments, children with cerebral palsy frequently have other conditions that may impede their growth and learning. This is because the same brain injury that causes muscle tone problems or involuntary movements can also cause or contribute to problems in other areas. For example, a brain injury can cause mental retardation, seizures, learning problems, and vision and hearing problems. Just as movement problems do, many of these conditions make learning intellectual, speech and language, and other skills more difficult. This section gives a brief overview of some of the problems that may be associated with cerebral palsy. The chapters on medical problems, development, and therapy later in this book discuss these problems and their treatment in more detail.

Mental Retardation

Intelligence is a tricky concept to define. Most people, however, use the term to refer to the ability to reason, conceptualize, solve problems, and think. Intelligence also reflects the ability to get along in the real world, to take care of oneself, and to behave in ways society considers appropriate.

To measure a child's intelligence, professionals most often use standardized tests known as IQ tests. The results of these tests are computed into a score called an Intelligence Quotient or IQ. People who score in a certain range—generally between 70–130—are said to have normal intelligence. People who score below 70 are said to have *mental retardation*. In the U.S., roughly 3 percent of all children and 25 percent of children with cerebral palsy have some mental retardation. Estimates vary because children with cerebral palsy sometimes cannot talk or control their bodies well enough to answer questions on an IQ test. To ensure that a child's IQ is accurately measured, the psychologist must carefully select the most appropriate tests for a child with motor or speech impairments.

You should be aware that an IQ score is only one measure of intelligence. The psychologist will also measure your child's *adaptive level*, or ability to manage common daily activities such as feeding, dressing, toileting, and social interaction. Because of motor problems, children with cerebral palsy may be delayed in these areas. Again, the accuracy of these tests depends upon the expertise and experience of the test administrator. Your child needs to be assessed by professionals from many different fields so that many observers can work together to give an accurate picture of your child's potential.

If your child has mental retardation, how the condition affects her will depend somewhat on the degree of her retardation. Just as there is a wide range of intelligence among children with "normal" intelligence, there is also a wide range among children with mental retardation. Children who are least affected by mental retardation are said to have mild retardation (55 to 69 IQ); those with greater cognitive delays are classified as having moderate (40 to 54), severe (25 to 39), or profound (below 25) retardation.

In general, children with mental retardation learn new skills more slowly than other children and find it harder to learn advanced skills such as reading, math, and complex problem solving. Children with mental retardation also may not be as motivated to learn new skills as are other children. This does not mean than children with mental retardation *can't* learn, however. Given a good educational program and support from family and friends, all children can make important, steady progress in intellectual abilities. See Chapter 8 for information on helping your child get the most from her education.

Seizures

About 50 percent of children with cerebral palsy have *seizures*—episodes in which abnormal nerve activity disturbs the functioning of the brain. Children with quadriplegia or hemiplegia are most likely to have seizures.

Seizures are common among children with cerebral palsy because brain injuries provide a focus for abnormal nerve impulses to occur. Depending on where the abnormal activity occurs in the brain, seizures may affect children in a variety of ways. A child may have staring episodes; minor involuntary movements such as eye blinking, lip smacking, or arm jerking; or major convulsions with unconsciousness, stiffening of the body, and then violent spasmodic jerking of the whole body. When seizures occur repeatedly, they are diagnosed as epilepsy. As Chapter 3 explains, many medications are used to treat seizures. These medications can often reduce or prevent seizures.

Learning Problems

Children with cerebral palsy frequently develop learning disabilities. A child with a learning disability has normal intelligence, but has difficulty processing certain types of information. For example, she may have trouble following spoken instructions or distinguishing certain letters from others. She has the ability to do advanced academic work, but needs a great deal of educational support to achieve her potential.

Learning problems usually become evident in the preschool or early school years. Often they are the result of two other problems common in children with cerebral palsy: visual-perceptual disorders or developmental language disorders. Sometimes young children with mild or minimal cerebral palsy outgrow their cerebral palsy, but then develop learning disabilities later. Chapter 8 explains how a special education program individually tailored to a child's learning needs can help her minimize her learning disabilities.

Attention Deficit Hyperactivity Disorder (ADHD)

Roughly 20 percent of children with cerebral palsy have some kind of attention deficit hyperactivity disorder. Children with an attention deficit disorder may be distractible and have difficulty focusing their attention and concentrating. They may move from one activity to another before fully grasping a concept. They have a hard time listening to and following directions, and, because they have trouble controlling their impulses, may frequently act before thinking. Children with ADHD may find it difficult to sit still without fidgeting or squirming. Additionally, they may have *labile* (unstable) emotions or frequent mood swings. For example, they may be easily frustrated when doing difficult tasks or overly excited by stimulating activities or environments. Because of their behavior, children with these disorders can have problems with social adjustment, academic performance, and self-esteem.

ADHD is treated by: 1) changing the environment to decrease distractions and help the child focus on appropriate activities; 2) behavioral approaches to reinforce and improve attention to tasks and concentration, as well as social interaction and self-esteem; 3) medicine such as Ritalin™ to help the child concentrate on appropriate activities and to decrease her distractibility and impulsiveness. All three alternatives should be considered to maximize the child's academic performance, social interaction, and self-esteem. When medication is prescribed, however, its effects on the child should be carefully monitored for a trial period to determine if its benefits outweigh possible side effects such as sleep problems, irritability, or loss of appetite.

Vision Problems

Due to problems with muscle tone, children with cerebral palsy are more likely than other children to have certain vision problems. For example, half of all children with cerebral palsy have eye muscle imbalance or *strabismus* (crossed eyes) and *refractive errors* (nearsightedness or farsightedness). In fact, strabismus occurring in the first few months of life is sometimes the clue that first alerts medical professionals to the presence of cerebral palsy. Children with cerebral palsy are also more likely to develop *amblyopia*, the condition known as "lazy eye" in which the brain suppresses vision in one eye because of problems caused by strabismus or cataracts. Amblyopia can be corrected if discovered early in life. A few children are partially or totally blind due to brain injury in the visual pathways *(cortical blindness)*. Chapter 3 provides more information about the diagnosis and treatment of vision problems.

Hearing Impairment

Approximately 5 to 15 percent of children with cerebral palsy have some degree of *sensorineural* hearing loss. Sensorineural hearing loss is due to damage to the inner ear where the sound is picked up by the cochlea or the auditory nerve. This type of hearing loss is frequently caused by an injury to the brain, excess jaundice in the newborn period, or by meningitis, and can be mild to severe. Chapter 3 discusses the diagnosis and treatment of hearing impairment in children with cerebral palsy.

Speech Impairment

Children with cerebral palsy often have speech impairments. This is because the same muscle tone problems that make it difficult for children to control other body movements also make it

difficult for them to control *oral-motor* movements—movements of
the jaw, lips, tongue, and facial muscles used in speaking. Because
of problems with trunk muscles, they may also have insufficient
breath control to speak loudly or clearly enough to be understood.
Children with major speech impairments who cannot fully control
their oral-motor movements are said to have *dysarthria*. The section
on speech and language therapy in Chapter 7 explains the techniques most often used to treat speech impairments.

Sensory Impairments. Children with cerebral palsy often
have injuries to the *parietal lobe*—the areas of the brain responsible
for interpreting and using information from the senses. (See
diagram, page 5.) As a result, they may have a variety of *sensory
impairments*, or problems handling information relayed to the brain
from the senses. (You may also hear sensory impairments referred
to as *agnosia.)* The senses that children with cerebral palsy most
often have trouble with are touch, position (*proprioception*), movement (*vestibular*), and balance.

Children with cerebral palsy may have two types of sensory
impairments related to touch: *tactile hypersensitivity (tactile defensiveness)* and *tactile hyposensitivity*. Children with tactile hypersensitivity
are abnormally sensitive to being touched, and find certain kinds of
touch intolerable or quite disagreeable. For example, a light caress
to the cheek may cause a child to withdraw or cry. Children with
tactile hyposensitivity, on the other hand, are less sensitive to touch
than normal, and may appear insensitive to pain.

About half of the children with hemiplegia have sensory impairments on the affected side of their body. This combination of a
motor impairment with a sensory impairment can make movement
doubly hard. For example, a child with both motor and sensory
problems in her hand not only has difficulty physically manipulating
objects, but also cannot tell whether her grasp is too loose or too
tight. A child with sensory problems in her legs has trouble feeling
where her feet are and how much pressure they exert on the ground,
and is therefore insecure in her movements.

Frequently, children with sensory impairments have difficulty
using their senses to help them plan their movements. The term for
this problem is *dyspraxia*. Because they can only plan one movement
at a time, children with dyspraxia have a great deal of trouble
smoothly connecting the many smaller movements that make up a

more complex movement. For example, to put on her clothes, a child with dyspraxia has to do each movement involved separately, taking time between each movement to plan the next. This makes dressing very time-consuming and laborious.

Chapter 7 explains how occupational and other therapists work to help children with cerebral palsy overcome their sensory impairments.

Your Child's Diagnosis

When an infant or child has brain damage, a variety of symptoms can lead doctors and parents to suspect that something is wrong. In the first few months of life, an infant with brain damage may have some or all of these symptoms:

- lack of alertness; lethargy;
- general irritability or fussiness;
- jitteriness or trembling of the arms and legs;
- abnormal, high-pitched cry;
- *apnea* (altered breathing patterns or periods when the child stops breathing);
- *bradycardia* (very slow heart rate). Apnea and bradycardia are very common in prematurely born infants;
- poor feeding abilities due to problems sucking and swallowing;
- abnormal primitive reflexes (involuntary responses to certain kinds of stimulation from the environment). For example, a very exaggerated startle response to a loud noise or sudden movement;
- low muscle tone;
- seizures (staring spells, eye fluttering, changes in consciousness, body twitching).

During the first six months of life, telltale signs of a brain injury may also appear in an infant's muscle tone and posture. These signs include:

- Muscle tone may change gradually from low tone to high tone. For example, a baby may go from floppy to very stiff.

- The infant may hold her arms and shoulders back and retracted and her hands in tight fists.
- There may be *asymmetries* of movement—that is, one side of the body may move more easily and freely than the other side.
- The infant feeds poorly and her tongue pushes her food out of her mouth very forcefully rather than carrying food to the back of her mouth.
- The infant may have advanced head control and roll over earlier than normal by arching her back instead of by smoothly rotating her trunk.
- Primitive reflexes persist longer than normal. For example, the reflex called *asymmetric tonic neck reflex* (ATNR) may persist after the infant reaches six months—the age at which the reflex usually fades away. This reflex occurs when a child's head is turned to one side. It causes the arm and leg on the side the child is facing to straighten and extend due to increased tone, at the same time the arm and leg on the other side bend or flex. When ATNR persists longer than usual, a child may have trouble overcoming this position in order to roll over.

Once a baby with brain damage reaches six months of age, it usually becomes quite apparent that she is picking up movement skills slower than normal. Additionally, the baby often starts developing unusual *motor patterns*—or sequences of movements. For example, because the baby cannot easily sit upright, she sits with a rounded back or she arches her back and tends to fall backward. She may arch her back when rolling over, show a strong tendency to stand on her toes, or use only one of her hands in reaching.

Parents and grandparents are frequently the first to notice these signs in their children. Sometimes when they express their concerns to their physicians, their child is immediately diagnosed as having cerebral palsy. More often, however, medical professionals hesitate to use the term "cerebral palsy" at first. Instead, they may use broader terms, including:

1. *motor delay*, which means that a child is slower than normal to develop movement skills such as rolling and sitting;
2. *neuromotor dysfunction* or delay in the maturation of the nervous system;
3. *motor disability*, indicating a long-term movement problem;
4. *central nervous system dysfunction*, which is a very general term to indicate the brain's improper functioning; or
5. *static encephalopathy*, meaning abnormal brain function that is not getting worse.

Initially, doctors also usually shy away from making predictions about a child's *prognosis*, or the long-term effects her disability is likely to have on her life.

Why do doctors so frequently delay making a final diagnosis and prognosis when a child may have cerebral palsy?

Part of the answer lies in the *plasticity* of a child's central nervous system—its ability to recover completely or partially after an injury. The brains of very young children have a much greater capacity to repair themselves than do adult brains. This is because a child's central nervous system produces many more brains cells and connections than are eventually used for complex motor tasks. If a brain injury occurs early, the undamaged areas of a child's brain can sometimes take over some of the functions of the damaged areas. Although the child may still have some motor impairment, she can often make great progress in other motor skills.

Because of the plasticity of children's brains, doctors are usually reluctant to make a firm diagnosis of cerebral palsy when a child is very young, especially when she is under six months of age. As long as a child's nervous system has not yet matured, there is still a chance that the child may make at least a partial recovery from early movement problems.

As mentioned earlier, there is another reason doctors may delay in diagnosing cerebral palsy. As your child's nervous system organizes over time, damage to the brain may affect your child's motor abilities differently. For example, tone can go from low to high or vice versa, or involuntary movements can become more obvious. Generally, however, a child's motor symptoms stabilize by two to three years of age. After this age, tone is probably not going to change dramatically and abnormal movements such as athetosis are apparent. Given appropriate therapy, the child's motor impairments will gradually improve during her remaining childhood years. Occasionally, a rapidly growing child may temporarily become more awkward as her muscles and tendons adjust to the new bone growth. And as Chapter 3 discusses, the older child, adolescent, and adult may have additional problems because of orthopedic deformities.

Getting an Interdisciplinary Assessment

Since the extent of your child's problems will probably not be clear for some time, her symptoms need to be monitored by an *interdisciplinary team*—a group of professionals with specialties in different areas. These professionals can gather information on her accomplishments and make comparisons over the months and years. They will keep you up to date on your child's current needs and problems, as well as the medical reasons for these problems, if known.

To develop an initial picture of your child's special problems, the interdisciplinary team must first conduct an *assessment*, or evaluation of her strengths and needs in all areas. As your child grows older, additional assessments will periodically be necessary—especially when she is ready to enter school. Some of the professionals who are likely to examine your child are introduced below.

Developmental Pediatrician. The developmental pediatrician is a physician who has specialized training in working with children with disabilities in addition to general pediatric training. He works as part of an interdisciplinary team and is able to diagnose and assess children with disabilities. The developmental pediatrician is also

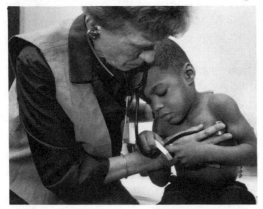

very familiar with the types of therapy that can benefit children with cerebral palsy and can help coordinate services.

The developmental pediatrician will carefully review your child's health history and medical records. He will do a thorough physical exam and developmental assessment to determine whether any medical factors are affecting your child's health and development. He may order medical tests such as urine and blood tests or X-rays and also check for genetic disorders. The developmental pediatrician will want your child to be seen by other members of the interdisciplinary team and by other medical consultants to determine your child's areas of strengths and needs and to help develop diagnoses and treatment plans.

Neurologist. A neurologist is a medical doctor who specializes in diseases of the nervous system. In assessing your child, the neurologist will probably use one or more neurological tests to determine the location and extent of your child's brain damage. Commonly used tests include: 1) head sonograms, which use sound waves to visualize the structures of the brain; 2) CAT scans—sophisticated computer X-ray images; 3) magnetic resonance imaging (MRI), which uses magnetic fields to provide detailed pictures of the brain and spine; and 4) electroencephalograms (EEGs)—tests that measure the electrical activity of the brain and help identify seizure activity. The neurologist might also use a specialized EEG known as an *evoked potential* to assess the condition of the visual and auditory pathways in your child's nervous system.

Orthopedic Surgeon. The orthopedic surgeon specializes in medical treatment and surgery of the bones, tendons, ligaments, and joints. During an evaluation, the surgeon assesses the condition and alignment of these structures, and may order X-rays, especially of the hips, back, and legs. Chapter 3 discusses ways orthopedic surgeons treat problems they diagnose.

Therapists. Several therapists, including an occupational therapist, a physical therapist, and a speech-language pathologist may assess your child. Physical therapists (PTs) specialize in evaluating motor abilities. They treat movement problems such as high or low muscle tone or weak muscles, and facilitate the development of movement skills—rolling, sitting, crawling, pulling up to stand—requiring the use of larger muscles. Occupational therapists (OTs) evaluate motor and sensory impairments and treat these problems to help develop skills which involve the small muscles of the body—grasping an object or fastening a zipper, for example. Speech-language pathologists (SLPs) are trained in diagnosing and treating problems with speech and language skills, as well as with other skills such as breathing and feeding which involve the muscles in and around the face, mouth, throat, and chest. Chapter 7 explains the techniques these therapists use to assess and treat children with cerebral palsy.

Physiatrist. A physiatrist is a physician who specializes in evaluation and treatment of physical impairments. He has special expertise in rehabilitation and works closely with OTs and PTs, helping direct the therapeutic program.

Audiologist. The audiologist evaluates hearing and corrects hearing impairments. To assess the frequencies, intensities, and types of sound your child can and cannot hear, the audiologist may use a sound booth or headphones. She will observe your child's behavior to determine how well your child hears the different types of sounds. The audiologist will also use an instrument called a tympanometer to determine whether your child has fluid behind the eardrum due to a cold, allergy, or ear infection. If necessary, she will recommend a hearing aid for your child.

Nutritionist. The nutritionist will assess the adequacy of your child's diet as well as her physical growth (weight, height, and body fat). He will also evaluate your child's feeding skills and provide therapeutic help for oral-motor disorders that affect chewing or swallowing.

Ideally, all the professionals who assess your child will work together as part of the interdisciplinary team. Information will be shared within the team and with your child's pediatrician. At the conclusion of the assessment, a family *interpretive session* will be held. During this meeting, team members will review your child's areas of strengths and needs with you, and with your input, will begin developing treatment goals and approaches. This is an excellent opportunity for you to get information and answers to the many questions you have about your child and her cerebral palsy. Many parents find it helpful to prepare a list of written questions to ensure that all their questions are answered.

¥ Treatment

Following your child's interdisciplinary assessment, the professionals on your child's team will develop recommendations for her treatment. If your child is under two, one of their chief recommendations will likely be that your child begin receiving *early intervention* (infant stimulation) services. Early intervention services are intended to minimize the effects of any neurological conditions that might make it harder for an infant or toddler to learn and acquire developmental skills. For instance, early intervention services can reduce the effects of mental retardation or a learning impairment on the development of a child's thinking or communication skills or reduce the effects of muscle tone or sensory problems on the development of movement skills.

Early intervention services are provided by a variety of professionals, including medical specialists, education specialists, occupational and physical therapists, speech-language pathologists, nutritionists, audiologists, and social workers. Chapters 7 and 8 discuss how and where each of these professionals work with children with cerebral palsy; Chapter 9 explains the laws that may entitle your child to receive the services she needs at public expense.

Since no two children are affected by cerebral palsy in exactly the same way, individual treatment programs vary widely. But because all children with cerebral palsy have movement problems, you can expect that an important component of your child's treatment will be a therapeutic exercise program. Depending on your child's needs, a physical therapist, an occupational therapist, and a speech-language pathologist will work with your child to help her improve posture and movement. These therapists may also recommend special equipment to make it easier for your child to move, speak, or feed herself independently. Additionally, the physical therapist will develop an exercise program to prevent potential complications such as hip dislocation, curvature of the spine, or further tightening or contractures of your child's musculoskeletal

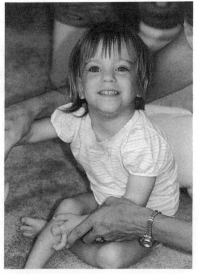

system. Chapter 3 provides more information on these complications.

At first, your child will likely see her therapists quite often, sometimes at least twice a week. As your child grows, she may need a less intensive program. Her therapists will probably expect you to work on her movement skills at home, and will train you in special exercises and handling techniques. Because the time commitment to a therapy program is tremendous, it is wise for both parents, and possibly grandparents and other caretakers, to be involved.

At present, there is some controversy about how early children with cerebral palsy should begin therapy. Some medical researchers feel that newborns may be too ill or may not have enough stamina to benefit from treatment, while other researchers believe it is never too early to lay the foundation for later learning. In general, it is considered very early intervention if a baby begins therapy before six months of age. Most infants are not referred until later in the first year or sometime in the second year of life. Of course, the age at which *your* child is referred will depend to some extent on how quickly your physician diagnoses a motor delay or other problem requiring therapy.

Researchers are still studying the long-term benefits therapy can offer. But it is generally agreed that children who receive good treatment not only have fewer movement limitations, but also have better postures, better balanced muscle development, and better abilities in toileting, feeding, and dressing themselves. Furthermore, therapy programs enrich children's lives by enabling them to explore and experience activities that they might not otherwise be able to do independently. For example, a therapist might make special adaptations to a toy to allow a child with limited hand control to operate it with head movements, or teach a child with severe speech impairments to communicate with sign language. Therapy programs also foster social interaction for children and their family and community. For instance, by helping a child develop better communication skills, therapy enables her to interact with other children and make her needs known. Last, but not least, therapy programs give parents and family members valuable information about ways to help the child with cerebral palsy make the most of her abilities. And therapists themselves can be a wonderful support system for parents who are struggling to understand and cope with their child's special needs.

Because therapy will be the keystone of your child's treatment program, this book devotes an entire chapter—Chapter 7—to physical, occupational, and speech and language therapy. In addition, Chapter 3 discusses several other treatment methods sometimes used in conjunction with therapy. These include surgery and *orthotics*—devices that stabilize joints or stretch the muscles.

What about Future Babies?

Although the chances of having a second child with cerebral palsy are very small, there are a few conditions that can reoccur. This means that before planning to have another child, it is critical that you know what caused your child's neurological injury so that you can take steps to prevent this complication again.

If your child is among the 35 to 40 percent of children with cerebral palsy born prematurely, the reason for her early delivery should definitely be evaluated. About 50 percent of premature births can now be prevented with thorough and comprehensive prenatal care. For example, obstetric procedures can sometimes prevent an incompetent cervix from dilating early in pregnancy so that the baby can make it to full term. Prematurity or other neonatal problems linked to maternal problems such as diabetes, seizures, drug and alcohol use, and infections such as herpes can also frequently be prevented.

Many parents find that having another child has a very positive effect on their family. Other parents decide against having additional children, even though the possibility of having another child with cerebral palsy is very, very low and the risk factors are known. Because of the large commitment of energy needed to raise a child with cerebral palsy, some parents feel they could not adequately care for another child. Whatever your feelings, the professionals on your child's team can help you to explore your questions and concerns and to make the family planning decision that is right for you.

🎇 The History of Cerebral Palsy

Cerebral palsy is not a new disorder. There have probably been children with cerebral palsy as long as there have been children. But the medical profession did not begin to study cerebral palsy as a distinct medical condition until 1861. In that year, an English orthopedic surgeon, Dr. William John Little, published the first paper describing the neurological problems of children with spastic diplegia. Spastic diplegia is still sometimes called Little's Disease.

The term "cerebral palsy" came into use in the late 1800s. Sir William Osler, a British medical doctor, is believed to have coined the term. Dr. Sigmund Freud, the Austrian neurologist better known for his work in psychiatry, published some of the earliest medical papers on cerebral palsy.

Today it is believed that prenatal risk factors play at least some role in most cases of cerebral palsy, but in the early years most cases were thought to be caused by obstetrical complications at birth. Until recently, many medical and educational professionals had similarly erroneous ideas about the physical and mental abilities of children with cerebral palsy. Children were frequently separated from their families at an early age and placed in residential institutions, where they had little if any opportunity for education, employment, or even socialization.

Fortunately, in the past few decades, information on the many facets of cerebral palsy has significantly increased. Today, the medical community has great interest in studying cerebral palsy to determine its causes and the most effective ways to treat it. As knowledge and treatment techniques have expanded and improved, so too have the prospects of all children with cerebral palsy.

🎇 The Future of Children with Cerebral Palsy

The outlook for children with cerebral palsy has never been brighter. Not only are advanced therapeutic and surgical techniques helping to minimize the effects of cerebral palsy and its complications, but new treatment methods are helping to control problems such as seizures that are often associated with cerebral palsy. In addition, special equipment is helping children with cerebral palsy to unlock their potential as never before. For example, computers are giving voices to children who might not otherwise be able to speak, and orthotics and mobility devices made from lightweight plastics and metals are granting new freedom of movement to children with limited motor skills.

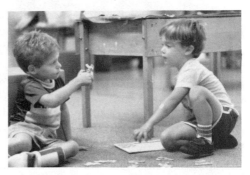

Advances in medicine and technology are not the only reasons things are looking up for children with cerebral palsy and their families. Increased opportunities in education are also helping children with cerebral palsy make giant steps toward conquering the effects of their disabilities. Thanks to several important federal laws which are explained in Chapter 9, children with cerebral palsy are now guaranteed the right to a free appropriate public education specially designed to help them overcome problems that might otherwise impede their learning. This education is provided at no cost to the parents and may be in a "normal" school with "normal" classmates, or in a school that is equipped to deal with children with more serious disabilities.

Yet another reason the future is getting brighter for children with cerebral palsy is that parents are taking on increasingly larger roles in helping their children reach their potential. Therapists, for example, now routinely train parents to reinforce their child's movement and speech skills at home. And teachers rely on parents' input in deciding how and what children with cerebral palsy should learn in school. Because most professionals recognize that parents are *the* experts on their child and her special needs, you will often be able to help your child receive the services that are best for her. You can also pitch in and work side by side with teachers and therapists to help your child grow and learn. These kinds of parent-professional partnerships naturally help children with cerebral palsy make better progress.

How much progress *your* child will eventually make depends on many factors, including her intellectual abilities and the type and severity of her movement problems. Some children with cerebral palsy graduate from regular "academic" high school programs and then go on to college; others succeed in completing vocational high school programs; and still others spend their school years in programs designed to help them become as self-sufficient as possible. Likewise, some children with cerebral palsy grow up to hold jobs that enable them to support themselves, while others need varying amounts of financial help throughout their adult lives.

Today, all children with cerebral palsy have the potential to live rich, fulfilling lives—to enjoy good health, good friends, and good feelings about themselves and their accomplishments. The right therapeutic and educational programs will help get your child started on the road to a rewarding future; your motivation and support will help to keep her on track.

Parent Statements

The neurosurgeon who saw our daughter when she was two weeks old said that nine chances out of ten she would be a vegetable. He said we should consider discontinuing the treatment and taking her off the respirator. The next day, when a second neurosurgeon saw her, he said that she did not look so bad. He thought he saw signs of brain activity and that she probably would be pretty much like her identical twin sister, except that she would obviously have motor problems. In reality she is somewhere in between.

❊❊❊

No one wanted to say she had cerebral palsy. The doctors didn't know any more than we did.

❊❊❊

I had no idea that premature babies could have neurological problems.

❊❊❊

We knew she had brain damage and "cerebral palsy" was just a name they threw on several months later. The word itself doesn't have any meaning for me.

❊❊❊

It doesn't matter how it's defined. They can call it brain damage, brain dysfunction, brain injuries, cerebral palsy. I just want to talk about functioning.

❧❧❧

When our son was born the hospital was wonderful. It was staffed by wonderful people. But once we checked out with all of our problems, there was no follow-up. We could have had our son home for four years and would not have known anything. We just happened to know enough to call a neurosurgeon who pointed us in the right direction.

❧❧❧

Before my daughter was diagnosed with cerebral palsy, I had never even heard of muscle tone. Now it rules our lives.

❧❧❧

Emma had her first developmental evaluation at four months. The developmental specialist said, "At this point, she is developmentally delayed, but hang in there, she might catch up." Then at ten months, they requested that she be examined at the hospital because she wasn't responding normally. So we followed through only to have the doctor announce, "This kid has CP. She's not going to walk, talk, or be independent." We were devastated. It took me quite a long time to adjust to the fact that Emma had CP. I never did believe that she would never walk or talk—I kept hoping. Now Emma walks, talks, and is just doing great.

❧❧❧

The doctors told me that "cerebral palsy" was a garbage can term. The label is so broad that it can mean many different things.

❧❧❧

One day an older woman approached me and said, "You are such a good mother not to lock him up." Needless to say, I took great offense, but I suppose in the past, many children with cerebral palsy *were* put in institutions because of their parents' lack of knowledge, if nothing else.

>✻✻✻

It has been so hard to find information that applies directly to my child's specific needs. There are so many variations of cerebral palsy.

>✻✻✻

TWO

Adjusting to Your Child's Disability

RITA BURKE*

Getting the News

"Is there something you call this developmental delay?" I asked my son's kind developmental pediatrician. The question remains etched in my memory.

The doctor paused and said, "Well yes, we call it 'cerebral palsy.'"

And there it was. After seventeen long months of uncertainty and vague terminology, I finally had a diagnosis, a label, something I could pin on my little baby. (Actually, he wasn't so little anymore, but he hadn't progressed in any of the familiar ways that my older three children had.) No longer did I have to try to believe the phrase that everyone kept echoing in my ears: "Don't worry, all preemies catch up by the time they are two."

Now I knew why my son could barely hold up his head, and didn't sit, crawl, or try to stand. I knew why his fists were clenched and why one was held tightly to his chest. I knew why his body was a stiff rod that looked like a log rolling if he turned over, and why he couldn't get back to the other side. And I knew why my son screamed all the time and could only be comforted if we held him—which we did twenty-four hours a day. What I didn't know then was how my new knowledge would affect me, and what I

---

* Rita Burke is the mother of four children, one of whom has cerebral palsy. She has a master's degree in social work and currently teaches first grade.

would have to go through before I could adjust to my son's cerebral palsy. At the time, though, there was some relief in the knowledge that I now had something to work with—something defined that I could try to do something about.

As parents of children with cerebral palsy, we all have our stories as to how and when we received the diagnosis. Most parents learn 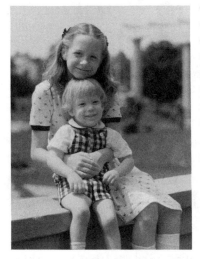 of their child's disability before his or her first birthday, but when cerebral palsy stems from an accident or illness, parents may not find out until much later on. Some parents get a diagnosis almost immediately, but others remain in diagnostic limbo for months while medical professionals bandy around such frightening-sounding terms as "developmentally delayed," "brain injured," "abnormal tone," or "central nervous system disorder." Occasionally, parents hear the diagnosis only because their insurance company demands a specific label. They may never have realized that this is what their child's condition is called.

However and whenever you are first faced with the news, the initial period after diagnosis is highly stressful. Not only must you cope with a variety of painful and conflicting emotions, but you must also help your family cope with their reactions. This chapter offers suggestions to help you understand and come to terms with your feelings so that you can then turn your attention to your child and your family.

Your Emotions

Whether you learn of your child's disability all at once or in bits and pieces, nothing can prepare you for the moment when the reality of his condition sinks in. You may be overwhelmed by intense feelings of rage, rejection, guilt, or grief. One moment you may feel like hugging your child and never letting go, and the next like running away. You may also be flooded with so many emotions at once that you aren't quite sure what you are feeling. In fact, these responses are *all* perfectly normal reactions to the news that your child has cerebral palsy. You have just learned that your life—and your child's life—will never be the same. How could any reaction be too extreme? You, like all parents of children with cerebral palsy, will pass through a range of emotions in your struggle toward acceptance of your child's disability. Although it may seem incredible to you right now, it is possible to come to grips with these feelings—on your own terms, in your own time. Most parents do. To help you sort out what you might be feeling, this section describes some of the emotions parents of children with cerebral palsy often experience.

Shock

Many parents go into a state of shock when they learn that their child has cerebral palsy. They may feel completely numb inside, and detached from everything going on around them. I experienced a feeling of disbelief as if I was part of a movie, or in a dream, and the words the doctor was saying weren't really meant for me. I remember telling myself that these sorts of things happened to other people, and that I would soon wake up and life would seem normal again. I didn't feel much emotion at all, although the words "cerebral palsy" conjured up visions of pathetic children and adults that people stare at or turn away from and then thank God for the normalcy of their own loved ones. The next day, my son's doctor called me up to see how I was doing. I must still have been in shock, because I recall thinking only, "Now wasn't that nice of him to call?" I still couldn't grasp the reality of my son's condition.

Denial

Denial is another common early reaction, especially if your child is still a baby when you get the news. Your baby may seem fine to you, just a little slow. The doctor or therapist uses the word "tone" to explain what is wrong, but you can't see tone. You can feel tone, but maybe that tone can go away just like it came. Maybe the professionals are wrong. . . .

I experienced the kind of denial known as "wishful thinking." I thought that if I got Chris started on an intensive exercise program, then his tone would improve or he would outgrow his problems in time. My husband, too, felt that cerebral palsy just wouldn't be that much of a problem. No one wants to believe that their child is going to have a handicapping condition for life. But you have to believe it before you can put your heart and soul into helping your child make the most of his abilities.

Grief

After the shock and denial wear off, grief is often the strongest emotion to emerge. Parents grieve for the child they have and for the child that might have been. They grieve for their families and for relationships that will be permanently changed. And they grieve for themselves and for the ideal life they imagined that now will never be. Even if you don't recognize this tremendous grief reaction, you may experience an overwhelming feeling of sadness. In my own case, I imagined my son's growing-up years spanning before me, and visualized all the normal, everyday activities he would never be able to do. I worried that this sadness would permeate our whole family, and we would never feel happy or lighthearted again.

If your depression is at its darkest now, my words are probably of little consolation. But one day you will see that these intense feelings of grief are actually an expression of your love and concern for your child—and of your fierce desire that his life be lived to the fullest. In time, the very same love and concern that feeds your despair will fuel your drive to help your child achieve the highest quality of life possible.

Guilt

To complicate your feelings of grief, you may feel as if you are somehow to blame for your child's cerebral palsy. But as Chapter 1 explains, there are several reasons why your child may have damage to the part of the brain that controls movement. And in many cases it is virtually impossible to pinpoint the exact moment when the brain damage occurred. In the long run, your energies are better spent in helping your child achieve his fullest potential than in agonizing over something you did or did not do.

I was fortunate enough to have a wonderfully wise obstetrician who immediately told me there was nothing I did to cause the cerebral palsy, nor was there anything I could have done to prevent it. It was "an accident of pregnancy." No matter what your situation, do not allow yourself to be blamed. Guilt is an ugly, dangerous emotion that can only come between you and your child. We should be busy adjusting and not blaming.

Anger

Sometimes the causes of a child's cerebral palsy can be fixed squarely on faulty care. In parent support groups, you may hear about pending or resolved lawsuits. In these cases, it is common for parents to be blinded by rage. By rights, their child should have been born physically and mentally perfect, but fate, or circumstances beyond their control, have robbed their child of his some of his potential. Monetary compensation may ease the pain to some degree; at best it will help cover the unusual expenses of caring for their child throughout their lifetime.

Even if your child has received competent medical care from conception on, you may still be overwhelmed by anger at times. You most likely will wonder why this had to happen to your child, to your family, or to yourself. You may immediately target the helping professionals who work with your child for some of this anger. Especially as the irreversibility of the condition sinks in, you may feel that the doctors and therapists are not doing enough to help your child. You could also be furious at God for "choosing" you to have a child with cerebral palsy.

I was angry at the condition itself—at the permanency of it. Initially, I rationalized that if I combined as much therapy as I could do (quantity) with the best therapy I could find (quality), the cerebral palsy would eventually go away. I accepted the reality of the brain damage only after I could feel "it" in his body—feel the tone pulling against me. In time I came to appreciate the tremendous power of the brain and the nervous system.

Whether your anger is rational or irrational, justified or unjustified, it is a perfectly normal reaction to have. But remember, no amount of anger—however valid—will reverse your child's condition. As time goes on, you will be able to help your child most if you can learn to channel the energy your anger generates into fighting your child's cerebral palsy. You can make the choice to do this constructively—through advocacy, education, and hard work—and eventually, maybe even with a sense of humor.

Resentment

Another emotion closely related to anger that parents often feel is resentment. Many parents resent the disruption to family life and future plans that having a child with cerebral palsy can cause. Mothers in particular may experience resentment because they feel an overwhelming responsibility for the care of their child and no one seems to be offering to help. Parents may also begrudge other parents their "normal" children and resent the way they seem to take their children's normalcy for granted. Occasionally, some parents may even resent their child. Even though they know it is not their child's fault that he has cerebral palsy, they cannot help thinking that if only he would try a little harder, he would be able to control his movements better or to speak more clearly.

I always felt a little resentment when I saw other children my son's age who were "normal" and starting to walk—and I was still carrying Chris. It took a few years for me to get used to that. My worst bout of resentment occurred at the second reunion of all the premature babies who had been in the Intensive Care Nursery together. Many of the children at the reunion had been more premature or had weighed less at birth than my son had, and yet they were all running effortlessly around the room. It was a very painful experience. My son had definitely not "caught up" by the age of two, nor did it appear at that time that he ever would. I was devastated.

Although you, too, have a perfect right to feel resentment, recognize it for what it is and let it go. Belaboring negative feelings will eventually drive away the very people you need for support. Simply put, avoid comparing; try to dwell on the positive, and not the negative.

Beginning the Adjustment

Adjusting to having a child with cerebral palsy does not happen magically. It is a complicated, lifelong process. Along the way, you will need to learn many new and difficult skills. At times you may feel that you must call upon superhuman reserves of patience and discipline. You may also feel the added burden that you are expected to possess special qualities that enable you to care for a child with cerebral palsy.

Difficult as the adjustment process may seem, it is not impossible. Many parents of children with cerebral palsy successfully manage the tricky passage from diagnosis to a different, but rewarding life for their family. Although right now the focus of your life may be your child's cerebral palsy, with time you will be able to view it as only a part—not the center—of your life. Before you will be able to do this, however, you must first address your emotions and then take time to adjust.

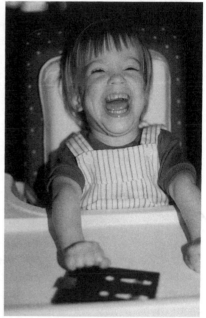

Address Your Emotions

Unbelievably enough, your life does not stop once you find out that your child has cerebral palsy. Your home and job responsibilities continue and your family keeps counting on you just as they always have. Yet right now you may feel too hopeless and helpless to make even the smallest decision. This is completely normal. Give yourself time to feel these painful emotions. You need to come to grips with what you are feeling now so that later you can make clearheaded decisions in your child's best interest.

No two people cope with the diagnosis of cerebral palsy in exactly the same way. Some grieve openly—crying and sharing their misery with anyone who will listen. Others withdraw to lick their wounds in private. Still others seek out a mental health professional to reassure themselves that their feelings are justified and for help learning coping skills. I was very verbal. I needed to ask a lot of questions, do a lot of reading, and rehash everything over and over. My husband ingested information very quietly and needed time to sort it out privately. Your way of dealing with your child's diagnosis may not be your spouse's. Try to be aware of this and do not impose your way as the only way. Remember, there are just as many valid coping strategies as there are valid reactions to the diagnosis of cerebral palsy. Do whatever works for *you*.

Take Your Time

When your child is first diagnosed with cerebral palsy, health care providers may pressure you to make quick decisions about therapies and special treatment programs. But perhaps you are not quite convinced that your child needs these therapies. Or perhaps your decisions are complicated by work or family schedules, or by insurance, transportation, or financial issues. You may want to start trying to help your child immediately, but are overwhelmed by the many programs available and do not know where to begin. What should you do?

Take your time deciding what is best for your child and your family. Early intervention *is* important, but waiting a few weeks or even a month could be in everyone's best interest. It is often better to wait and do your homework, to visit several programs, and to adjust to the idea that your child really needs these services. You will feel more confident when you have found just the right program and therapist. Your life may be changing before your eyes, but remember: you are still the one in charge of your child's life and your own.

What You Should Do

Accept Your Child

You began bonding with your child from the moment of his birth. By now, you are the biggest expert on him. You know just how he likes to be held, how to make him smile, and when he needs to sleep. But suddenly, this diagnosis seems to put everything in a different light. Your baby has a label. You need to ask yourself whether this makes a difference in how you see and relate to your child.

Like many parents of children with cerebral palsy, you must learn to separate your child from his disability. You must accept your child for who he is—a person who just happens to have cerebral palsy—not a cerebral palsied child. I am not suggesting you deny the disability, but that you be careful about your perception of your child's identity. In these early days and months it is typical to let the words "cerebral palsy" overshadow the little person inside. And if your child has other conditions related to his cerebral palsy such as mental retardation or seizures, your acceptance may be complicated even further. You may become so overwhelmed by your child's doctor and therapy appointments, home and school programs, medical bills, and nonstop daily needs that you forget there is a little kid in there. You may become so obsessed with your child mastering a certain skill—be it walking, talking, eating with a spoon—that you overlook how your child is feeling. You may even feel so frustrated and sorry for yourself that you are unable to enjoy your child and open doors for him.

With time, most parents have little trouble seeing their child once again as a child and not as a condition. Common sense tells them that it is not their child who has changed, but only their perceptions of him. They learn to view the cerebral palsy as just one acceptable part of their child, and to help their child understand that he is fine just the way he is. Because you will want to help your child appreciate his own uniqueness and worth, Chapter 5 provides some tips on helping to build self-esteem—one of our primary goals as parents.

Unfortunately, even after you have accepted your child, you may still have trouble accepting the cerebral palsy and the limits it imposes on your child. It is especially hard to accept that your child's progress is not always under your control, nor is it always directly related to the amount of effort you put forth on his behalf. As I mentioned earlier, this was a particularly hard realization for me. Cerebral palsy, as I came to see and feel, is a force much greater than we first realize. Cerebral palsy never goes away. Cerebral palsy is brain damage. When my son was three, and had received therapies for about a year and a half, I was finally able to say these words out loud. This was a day of personal growth and self-realization for me. I reached another milestone when Chris was five. He asked me if he would have cerebral palsy when he was a teenager, and I heard myself telling him that yes, he would always have it—even though his mobility would improve, the tone in his muscles would never go away. Over the years, I've found that answering questions like these from your child and others in the simplest, most straightforward manner helps ease you slowly along the road to acceptance. Chapter 5 offers some additional guidance in reaching this goal.

Get the Facts

When your child was first diagnosed, it is likely that the physician or pediatrician gave you relatively sketchy information about your child's condition. He or she probably gave you a little information about medical concerns, and concentrated on what was going on with your child at the moment. Because cerebral palsy is largely a developmental condition and you don't always see right away what you will get later, physicians often hesitate to predict what the future holds for a child with cerebral palsy.

At the time of diagnosis, you may have been immobilized by denial or despair, and so were content with whatever explanation your physician gave you. And even if you wanted to know everything right from the start as I did, you probably had no idea what questions to ask. For example, when Chris was diagnosed, I remember that it was very important for me to know if he would ever kick a soccer ball. In retrospect, this seems a ridiculous concern given the total picture. At that time, I needed to visualize Chris as a 'normal' kid and then go on from there. Whenever I would see older children with cerebral palsy come to therapy, I really checked them out—sort of comparing—then asked all kinds of questions to see if their "involvement" was similar to my son's. I was always trying to picture what Chris would be like in the next few years so that I could be prepared.

Once you begin the adjustment process, it is important that you gather more information. You will want to be able to answer questions from family members and friends, and also to begin making informed decisions about educational, medical, and legal matters. As a start, you might contact your local chapter of the United Cerebral Palsy Association, Association of Retarded Citizens, or Easter Seals. These groups can supply you with brochures and information packets, and also suggest helpful, up-to-date books and magazines to read. Certainly a must and my most valuable resource has been my yearly subscription to *Exceptional Parent Magazine*. The Reading List at the back of this book lists this and other helpful resources.

Helping Your Family Adjust

Children with cerebral palsy are not just sons and daughters. They are also brothers, sisters, grandchildren, nieces, and nephews. How other family members adjust to your child and his disability will be critical not only to your child's well-being, but also to your family's. Family attitudes are essential in helping your child realize that he is not the center of the family, but rather one small, but important part. How your family treats your child's disability will also help to determine your child's attitude toward his cerebral palsy.

Over the years, my family has learned slowly but surely to treat Chris as an equal. Although we try to be sensitive to his particular needs, we also try to treat him the same as his siblings. Whenever we have to make some special allowance for his cerebral palsy, we make sure that nobody in the family suffers. For example, it would be easiest just to make everyone stay home if Chris can't go along on a family outing that requires a lot of hiking. Instead, if we can't figure out a way that Chris can come, one of us stays behind with Chris and picks another activity to share especially with him.

Most families eventually mobilize well to meet the challenge of having a child with special needs. But because your family is unique, the ways in which your family will learn to adjust to the stresses of having a member with cerebral palsy will also be unique. You cannot expect that what has worked in one family will work in yours, nor should you let others unduly influence you in deciding what you should or should not be doing. You are, after all, the best judge of what will work for your family. Still, there are certain ways in which all families of children with cerebral palsy are similar. First, members of all families generally experience the same range of emotions in coming to terms with a child's cerebral palsy. Second, all family members need to summon up tremendous amounts of love and determination to make the adjustment. The following sections offer some general guidelines to help you understand and assist specific family members during the initial coping process.

Grandparents

There is no textbook formula for breaking the news of your child's cerebral palsy to your parents. How you tell them will depend in large part on your relationship with them and on their prior knowledge of any worries you may have had about your child's development. But however you tell your parents, you should be prepared to deal with a gamut of reactions. Like you, your parents may feel shock, grief, denial, and anger. They may attempt to pin the blame on you, your spouse, or the medical profession, or to fault themselves for defective genes. Later on, your child's grandparents may overwhelm you with "cures" they have read about or the names of specialists you should see. Many have no idea that most of the information they come across is not applicable to your situation. Then again, they may choose to stay away from you and your child and seem completely unsupportive. Bear in mind that this is a trying time for everyone. Give your parents what you think they need most—be it information and support, or time to come around.

Your Children

In the short run, having other children may complicate your family's adjustment to your child with cerebral palsy. You will have to help your other children cope with their emotions and will need

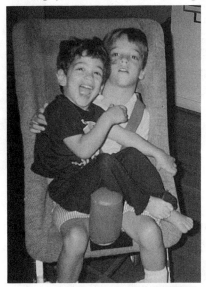

to balance many competing demands on your attention. But in the long run, families with more than one child sometimes have an easier time adjusting. To begin with, brothers and sisters can help your child develop normal social skills. Having siblings helps the child with cerebral palsy to be himself and takes off some of the pressure on him to perform. On the other side of the coin, studies have shown that having a child with a disability has a positive influence on the lives of other children in the family. Children who are actively involved with a brother or sister with a disability have a better sense of themselves and better relationships with others. They are also more sensitive and aware of the world around them. Furthermore, having a child with cerebral palsy in the family can result in new perspectives and a tolerance that might never occur otherwise.

But how do you get your children started along the path to adjustment so that they can eventually reap all these benefits? You must begin, of course, by telling your other children about their sibling's cerebral palsy.

If a baby with special needs is born into the family, all members immediately feel the stress, just as they would any change. As this baby is given special care and taken to many different doctors and therapists, the other children will quickly sense that something is wrong. As in any stressful situation, hiding information is never a good idea.

Since the unknown is always worse than the known, you must give all your children enough information to ease their fears. Don't get overly technical; just give your children information appropriate to their age levels. You might say something like: "Chris needs some extra special exercises to help his legs get stronger," or "Chris's muscles don't work the same as yours; he can't move around as well as you, and might not for a long time, so we need to help him a little more." Try not to tell your children half-truths, even if it seems easiest at the time. For instance, if a sibling asks why the baby cries so much, don't answer that it's because he is sad. Instead, you might say, "Danny's body doesn't handle sounds or touch the same as yours. Small little things really bother him."

To assure your children that their sibling will not die from cerebral palsy is also important. And don't forget to let your children know that it is normal to have strong emotions about their sibling's disability. You can say, for example, "It's OK to feel mad or sad about this—I feel that way too—but it wasn't anyone's fault." To help explain your child's condition, you might also want to use some of the excellent books written about different disabilities for children of different age levels. The Reading List describes some that parents have found most helpful. Remember, a straightforward approach defuses fear and helps your children feel important and a vital part of the care-giving.

Once you have explained your child's disability to your other children, do not assume that they understand how their brother or sister acquired cerebral palsy. Also do not assume that they are completely knowledgeable about what their sibling can or cannot do. Over time, you need to re-explain this information, in increasing detail, especially as your children go through different developmental stages. It often helps if you can periodically point out the small victories of your child with cerebral palsy to his brothers and sisters. For instance, "Remember when Chris couldn't walk? Now he runs on his crutches." Or, "Isn't it amazing how Sally uses her communication board? She's faster than all of us!" This will give your other children added encouragement and positive feelings toward their sibling.

Above all, try to keep in mind that your grief about your child's cerebral palsy is not a private matter. Each member of your family may experience it to different degrees at different times. I remember, for example, the twelfth birthday party of one of my older children. After my son had blown out the candles, I asked what he had wished for. His answer took me by complete surprise. He said he didn't know why he even bothered to wish any more because none of his wishes ever came true. My heart sank as I repeated the question. "I wish on every candle and every star that Chris will be able to walk, but it has never happened," my son replied with a quiver in his voice and a trace of anger. Immediately, I tried to reassure him and to help him see all the progress that Chris had made over his five and a half years. Hearing my own voice say the words helped me to reassure myself. At the same time, I realized that I needed to re-discuss Chris's cerebral palsy with everyone from time to time to see how everyone was feeling.

Incidentally, we all got our wish several months later when Christopher walked for the first time (outside of therapy) out of Christmas Eve Mass and our pastor waited for him to lead the Recessional. Christopher was six years old. He had just recovered from his first surgery, had been fitted with long leg braces, was beginning to use a walker for short distances, and had benefitted from uncountable hours of physical therapy. To add a footnote to this "Christmas miracle," a woman met me outside of church and said, "Now, why didn't you buy one of those gadgets (walkers) sooner? It certainly did the trick!" I just smiled and nodded. There was nothing else to say!

Your Friends

Having a child with a disability doesn't change how you feel about your friends. But it may change how they act or your perception of how they act. It can be a very lonely time for you. Your friends may stay away because they feel uncomfortable—not knowing what to do or say. Or they may say too much, coming up with all kinds of unsolicited help and advice. It may appear to you that people feel sorry for you or your child. You may withdraw, so they do too. You need them, but do not know what to say or do. As many different scenarios can occur as there are different types of people and personalities.

You may become close to the most unlikely people—often people who can listen without giving advice, because they are usually the most supportive. Your parent support group may become invaluable in this in-between time. In any case, time is the healer. Eventually you and many of your old friends will come around if they weren't there all along. Keep the doors open so you can renew your old friendships when you become more self-confident about the situation. This is a time when you need friendship and should not withdraw too much within yourself. You will quickly realize who is able to really listen to your fears and who is too uncomfortable. Be on guard not to monopolize the relationship with talk about your problems, though; remember that your friends have problems, too. The old adage fits well here; to have a friend is to be a friend.

Reaching Out

You will soon become aware that the care your child requires and the decisions that need to be made cause a tremendous drain on your family's energy. Whether it be from a financial, personal, physical, or emotional standpoint, none of us can honestly say that we escape feeling overwhelmed at one time or another. Still, you do not want to fall into the trap of feeling inadequate because you are overwhelmed. The worst thing you can do is to withdraw into a private sorrow. There are others out there who have felt your pain and can help you. How and when you reach out to them is up to you.

Whether you realize it or not, you belong to a whole new world of people—the world of parents who have children with disabilities. At first, you may feel as if you don't really belong. For some parents, it is hard to accept that this little baby who doesn't do too much really won't catch up one day. As yet, the words "physical therapy," "occupational therapy," "infant stim," "wheelchair," "braces," and "surgery" may only seem appropriate for those other children you see in the waiting rooms that will become so familiar to you. Eventually, however, you may feel the urge to chat with and ask questions of the parents of these other children. You will find that no introductions are necessary in this group, for just being there cuts through all the pretensions that strangers normally present to each other. If you let them, these strangers will become your friends, your extended family, your support.

Later, as you get involved in educational, therapeutic, and medical programs, you may have opportunities to join a support group. Or you can make contact directly at any time. Try calling your local chapter of the United Cerebral Palsy Association or Association for Retarded Citizens, or any of the parent groups listed in the Resource Guide at the back of this book. Try one organization out, and if it isn't a good fit, try another.

Remember, your greatest support will almost always come from other parents. Participating in a group and eventually learning how to help others adjust will help you cope with your own feelings. It will also give you the strength and courage to persist. In addition, you will find that other parents are a gold mine of information about the system—about equipment, doctors, therapists, and school programs. Finally, in the best of all scenarios, this new world of people you meet will teach you through humor and common sense how to cope one day at a time with more smiles than tears.

Early Intervention

If your child is not already in an early intervention program, you will likely find that the adjustment process will get a little easier once he begins one. As Chapter 8 explains, the primary goal of these programs is to help children by maximizing their potential in areas that are showing some developmental delay. But they are also designed to help parents by teaching them how best to care for their children.

An early intervention program will focus on the possibilities that your child possesses. It will emphasize what he can do and is trying to do while setting up opportunities for success. Therapists will encourage your child to accomplish the next developmental task by breaking it down into small pieces. These programs look beyond the handicap and attempt to move children along to experience success instead of frustration.

Your child's early intervention program will help you become actively involved in his treatment. The teachers and therapists you meet will teach you how to incorporate handling and positioning techniques into your daily routine and how to build language and cognitive skills. They will also show you how to turn the most ordinary situations into learning experiences. As you gain expertise through hands-on experiences, you will begin to feel an integral part of the team. You will feel empowered because now you can actually do something to help your child learn and develop.

Besides helping you adjust to having a child with cerebral palsy, early intervention programs can have far-reaching benefits for all family members involved. Everyone becomes acutely aware of each step toward progress. Plus, each member becomes personally committed to your child's success and takes great pride in every small accomplishment.

My son's early intervention program combined a home program with center-based instruction. Several times a week we would go to therapy, where I would observe the physical therapist working with my son. I was then shown the various techniques and sent home to practice the exercises with the help of a special book given to me by the therapist. In the book, the P.T. would write what took place at each P.T. visit and what Chris was to work on until his next appointment. We would send the book back with our questions, concerns, and notes on progress. These books came complete with instructions, drawings, and photographs. Occasionally we would even make a video to document each developmental task accomplished. Over the years we have accumulated several of these books—memory books—which chronicle our son's hard work and progress, and what progress he has made!

Don't Be Overprotective

Between the ages of three and five, your child will be ready for instruction in a nursery school setting. By this point you may have become very protective and may feel that you are the only one capable of taking care of your child. You might treat your child as if he is helpless, and not give him the chance to achieve or fail. But sending your child to pre-school will be healthy for both of you. You need a break from caring for your child twenty-four hours a day, and your child needs the social stimulation of other children and other adults. We overprotect out of fear, but it is far better to challenge your child than to deny him opportunities to grow.

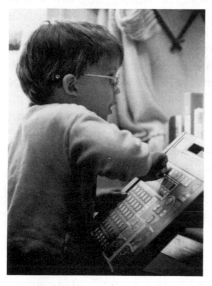

Putting your little child on a school bus can be very difficult, and you just might have to pretend that it isn't until letting go becomes easier. Your child will return, though, and return a happier, more well-rounded person. Be on guard not to pass any of your anxieties on to him. Remember, you always want to impart the message that your child can do it! Although your child will not always succeed, as Chapter 5 discusses, experiencing both success and failure is critical to your child's self-esteem and personal growth.

This brings up an issue that I feel involves the most important but most overlooked adjustment of all. I am speaking about the social adjustment of the child with cerebral palsy—or rather, our tendency as parents to let overprotectiveness get in the way of our children's social adjustment.

The urge to overprotect is strong in all parents, but especially so in parents of children with special needs. Unfortunately, over-protectiveness often makes children insecure, too dependent on the family for socialization, and increasingly isolated. Moreover, overprotected children may not develop the social skills needed to make and keep friendships.

Providing opportunities for your child to socialize may take quite a bit of effort and planning, and safety is always an issue. In addition, you may need to encourage the non-disabled children in your community (as well as their parents) to include your child in their play activities. But in the long run, you are not doing your child any favors by keeping him close all the time. Just as you would with any of your children, you need to encourage your special child's interests while recognizing any real limitations or needs. Adapting bikes, for example, or being creative in mainstreaming your child into outdoor games or recreation department programs is well worth the effort. A sturdy backyard sandbox can help your child attract playmates and also give him a chance to play down on the same level with everyone else. One year my middle son had the idea of taping a street hockey blade to the end of Chris's crutch and lining the bottom with a split piece of rubber tubing to avoid slippage. Chris played indoor gym hockey that year with great determination.

A very wise mother who assisted in my son's preschool perhaps put it best. She shared these words with me when my son was only two and her son was dying of muscular dystrophy at the age of seventeen. What she said was this: "Get him out of the house. Get him away from you all the time. Get him out in the neighborhood with other children, any way you can." This advice from a woman who had been a part of the community of parents and children with disabilities for seventeen years is easier said than done, but crucial to keep in mind. Just remember, the bottom line is that your child should be allowed to participate in community life to the maximum extent of his capabilities.

Conclusion

It is impossible to predict what the future will be like for a young child with cerebral palsy. This is partly because of the nature of cerebral palsy itself. Tests used to measure motor skills and mental abilities in the early years too often provide only a murky or inconclusive picture of your child's eventual potential. Then, too, many children with cerebral palsy exceed all expectations when given time to show what they can do.

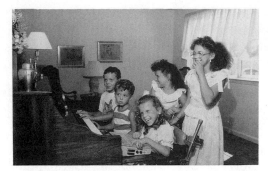

Patience is the key word when dealing with a child with cerebral palsy. I used to describe my son as a flower who would open one petal at a time when he was ready. We found out he had normal intelligence when he was four, he walked with support at six, he printed his name on a line at eight, and so on. Now Chris is ten years old and totally mainstreamed. Although we continue to give him private therapy to improve the quality of his movement and functioning, he has been "dismissed" from physical therapy at school because he is completely independent in his educational setting. He "flies" on crutches, wears AFO's (ankle foot orthoses), and participates in every aspect of playground and P.E. classes (jogging, exercises, kickball, soccer, softball). At school, he performs on grade level in every subject, and is exceptional in any language arts activity because of an incredible vocabulary and memory. His hobby is sports of all types and he carries millions of statistics about every team in his brain. He still needs support in some areas, but he definitely has exceeded all expectations.

As my son has learned and grown, so too has my entire family. And many of the most important lessons we have learned have been provided courtesy of our son. Just by being himself, Christopher has profoundly altered my outlook on life. In a world that puts an inordinate amount of emphasis on perfection, performance, and appearance, he has taught me to treasure the simple things. Having a child with cerebral palsy certainly can put parenting into perspective. It has been said that people like my son are ambassadors of life. If they can do it, then we can too. Every day they put their bodies on the line and their spirits follow. My son's spirit soars, and elevates us all.

I know it can be hard in the beginning to accept your limitations as the parent of a child with cerebral palsy. You'd like to be a physical therapist, occupational therapist, speech/language pathologist, and surgeon all rolled into one, and to work with your child nonstop until his cerebral palsy magically gets "better." But we *are* first of all parents, and that is what our children need us to be. They need us to love them unconditionally. They need to be accepted for who they are, just as they are. They need to be measured for what they can do, not for what they cannot do. All these things are really the heart of the matter.

As unbelievable as it may seem to you right now, there comes a time after the diagnosis has been made, therapies have begun, and programs have started when life continues on. This is the time when your child should be free to be himself. A time when you are not always working on him—when it is OK for him to be a kid who just happens to have cerebral palsy. This is the time when you can feel free enough to let go of what might have been and to accept the reality of the beautiful child who will enrich your life in ways you would never have dreamed possible.

Parent Statements

Our first reactions were devastation, denial, and disbelief. We wondered if it could be "fixed."

>fﬞﬞﬞﬞﬞﬞﬞﬞﬞﬞﬞﬞ<

We wanted our friends to ask questions about our son's disability, but nobody did. They pretended nothing was wrong.

>fﬞﬞ<

We have two children with disabilities. Our second child's handicaps are so much milder that to us he's Bruce Jenner, he's Albert Einstein. When the therapists wring their hands or the doctors look askance at him, I feel like saying, "Are you kidding? This is great, you guys. I know what bad is. I know how difficult it can be. I think this is wonderful."

>fﬞﬞ<

When the doctor first discovered she had CP, I began to cry. He quickly told me I was lucky I had her at all.

>fﬞﬞ<

I read many books and articles when I was trying to come to grips with the diagnosis.

❧❧❧

When Katherine was almost a year old, she started her first program where I met other parents with handicapped children. That helped a lot, but I couldn't help but search for another child like mine. No two kids are alike, but it's always been hard to find anyone close to Katherine.

❧❧❧

The first 18 months were the hardest. Everyone asked, "Is she walking yet?"

❧❧❧

When he diagnosed our son, our doctor told us, "Don't devote your life to this child." It was weird.

❧❧❧

I found myself explaining her disability in medical lingo. No one knew what I was talking about. I was so caught up in it all.

❧❧❧

What's really debilitating is how angry I am at so many people. I am very angry at neurologists for prescribing what I think is the wrong medication, I am very angry at the school professionals for certain oversights. It's so hard being angry, yet I can't not be angry. They should know their jobs.

❧❧❧

Support groups were hard for me. I was looking for a positive attitude and was surrounded by whiners.

❧❧❧

I have the most terrific support team—his therapists, doctors, and teachers. We couldn't have come this far without their constant guidance and wisdom.

❧❧❧

Kyle's grandparents on both sides have been wonderful from the start. They're always asking us what they can do to help out with Kyle.

❧❧❧

He takes up my entire day. It's like having an infant who will never grow up.

❧❧❧

My daughter is seven years old now. I keep thinking the adjustment period should be over. I know I've accepted her limitations, but I will always have to adjust my life to meet her needs.

❧❧❧

The first year after Terry's diagnosis, I was very emotional. I'd be driving in the car and just start crying. I couldn't even deal with talking to my family, let alone friends.

❧❧❧

I just told people she couldn't walk. I never said she had cerebral palsy. Everyone just accepted that it was simply a complication of her prematurity.

❧❧❧

Sometimes I need sympathy, although most of the time it's hard to swallow. I feel Zack has made such great progress—I'm proud of him and I don't need the sympathy.

❧❧❧

Don't ever feel you have an obligation to satisfy other people's curiosity. You don't have to explain.

❧❧❧

THREE

Medical Concerns and Treatments

ELLIOT S. GERSH, M.D.

Today, children with cerebral palsy are growing up much healthier than ever before. Physicians are well aware of the medical problems that may accompany cerebral palsy, and treatments have greatly improved. Although children with cerebral palsy may still develop special medical problems because of motor impairments and injury to the nervous system, many problems can now be prevented or effectively treated. Thanks to early detection of seizures and of respiratory and nutritional problems and treatment of resulting complications, most children with cerebral palsy can have normal life expectancies.

Because good health is paramount to your child's optimum development, this chapter explains the medical problems that children with cerebral palsy may develop. Bear in mind that these are just conditions that children with cerebral palsy are more likely to develop than other children are; your child may have none, some, or many of these problems. Whatever your child's health, however, it is important to know what to expect. Learning the basic facts about medical conditions can help you recognize problems, get proper care for your child, and discuss your concerns with doctors.

Seizures

About one out of two children with cerebral palsy develop *seizures*—involuntary movements or changes in consciousness or behavior brought on by abnormal bursts of electrical activity in the brain. Seizures interfere with normal brain functioning and may affect children in subtle or dramatic ways. For example, your child may have only a slight change in behavior or consciousness such as a staring episode. Or she may shake or stiffen, lose consciousness, and have increased salivation, drooling, and urinary incontinence followed by a period of confusion. When seizures occur repeatedly, they are diagnosed as epilepsy.

Children with cerebral palsy are at high risk for seizures because brain damage and scarring can spark abnormal electrical activity. Children with quadriplegia and hemiplegia are most likely to have seizures.

Types of Seizures

Seizures are classified according to the type and location of the abnormal electrical discharge in the brain. Broadly, any seizure may be classified as either *partial* or *generalized*. In partial seizures, the electrical discharges occur only in one area of one side of the brain; in generalized seizures, the electrical discharges are initially present in both sides of the brain. Depending on the symptoms they produce, seizures are further subdivided into the following types:

Partial Seizures

- Focal Motor (Simple Partial) Seizures cause a few muscle groups to jerk. For example, they may cause involuntary, repetitive jerking of the right leg. Initially, there is no loss of consciousness.
- Sensory Seizures cause dizziness or disturbances in vision, hearing, taste, smell, or other senses. Auditory or visual hallucinations are common. For instance, a child may hear voices, music, or other sounds, or may see flashes of light, colors, or images.
- Autonomic Seizures produce paleness, sweating, flushing, or dilation of pupils. They are often accompanied by rapid heart beat, fear, or anxiety.

- Psychomotor (Temporal Lobe) Seizures usually cause decreased alertness and changes in behavior. The child can have visual or auditory sensations or hallucinations and inappropriate behaviors such as picking at clothes, lip smacking, chewing, or rising out of a chair. This disordered state of consciousness can last from a few seconds to minutes. Psychomotor seizures are common in children with brain damage, including children with cerebral palsy.

Generalized Seizures

- Absence (Petit Mal) Seizures cause a brief, abrupt loss of consciousness for a few seconds followed by a rapid, complete recovery. These seizures are usually associated with staring or repetitive eye blinking.
- Infantile Myoclonic Seizures (Infantile Seizures) produce sudden, brief, involuntary muscle contractions involving one or several muscle groups. Because these contractions usually produce movements such as dropping the head and flexing the legs, trunk, arms, or legs, myoclonic seizures are also known as jackknife seizures. The episodes last only seconds and can occur many times a day.
- Tonic-Clonic (Grand Mal) Seizures are the most common type of seizure. In the tonic phase, muscles throughout the body may stiffen briefly, with the child falling to the floor unconscious. In the clonic phase which follows, extremities jerk rhythmically. These major spasms last for one to several minutes and become progressively slower and less extensive. Frequently, children have trouble breathing and may drool and have a bluish discoloration around the mouth. They may also lose bladder control. When the seizure stops, the child is confused, usually exhausted, and needs sleep.
- Atonic (Akinetic) Seizures cause a sudden loss of muscle tone. The child falls and may hurt herself.
- Febrile Seizures are generalized tonic-clonic seizures brought on by a sudden rise of temperature to 102

degrees or higher. Seizures last less than five minutes. Febrile seizures are very common in young children with fevers, occurring in 5 to 10 percent of children under age six.

Diagnosis and Treatment of Seizures

The best way to find out if your child has seizures is through a test known as an *electroencephalogram* (EEG). During the test, electrodes are placed over your child's scalp to detect the electrical signals produced by her brain. The neurologist monitors and records the electrical activity of the brain for twenty to thirty minutes (sometimes longer), then reads the EEG to look for abnormalities in the brain waves.

Because the best time to perform an EEG is just before and during sleep, you may be asked to bring your child to her appointment tired. An EEG is painless, but if your child is fearful, she may be mildly sedated. Sedation also helps make a child drowsy or fall asleep.

If your child's EEG confirms that she has seizures, the neurologist will discuss possible treatments with you. Usually anticonvulsant medication is recommended, since medication can reduce or eliminate seizures in about 90 percent of children with epilepsy. Medication might not be necessary if your child has febrile seizures or infrequent or minimal seizures such as brief staring spells occurring only every several weeks.

The type of medication prescribed for your child depends on the type of seizures she has. For grand mal seizures, phenobarbital and phenytoin (Dilantin™) are most often used. Carbamazepine (Tegretol™) is frequently used for psychomotor seizures. Valproic acid (Depakene™) helps control myoclonic, petit mal, and grand mal seizures.

Although these medications are very effective in preventing or reducing seizures when given regularly, they may also produce a variety of side effects. For example, they may cause hyperactive behavior, irritability, sleep problems, growth of body hair, lethargy, depression, or sedation, and can affect liver function or blood counts. Because of these possible side effects, your pediatrician and neurologist must monitor your child closely when she is on medication. Through periodic blood tests, they will determine your child's *therapeutic level*—the amount of drug in the blood which usually controls seizures with a minimum of side effects.

What to Do When Your Child Has a Seizure

Once a seizure has begun, there is nothing you can do to stop it. But if you stay calm, you can make your child more comfortable and keep her from hurting herself. First, help ease your child to the floor and move obstacles out of the way. Turn your child on her side so the saliva can flow out of her mouth. *Don't* put anything between her teeth; no matter what you have heard, a child cannot swallow her own tongue. Also remember that it is usual for a child's breathing to become irregular, so don't be alarmed. After the seizure has run its course, let your child rest and be very supportive. Help her get her bearings and understand what has happened.

If it is not your child's first seizure, it is usually not necessary to call a doctor right away. You should, however, seek emergency care immediately if your child's seizure is very active for more than ten minutes.

Gastrointestinal Problems

Because of their motor disorders, children with cerebral palsy often have gastrointestinal problems. The gastrointestinal (GI) system includes the mouth, esophagus, stomach, and intestines, as well as organs such as the gall bladder, liver, and pancreas that produce digestive enzymes. The GI system enables the body to break down food so that it can be absorbed and used to make body tissues and produce energy. The GI system also eliminates waste products from the body. Gastrointestinal problems may make it difficult for children to chew, suck, and swallow; to digest food; or to eliminate waste. These problems can make mealtimes extremely difficult for you and your child and can also lead to poor nutrition. Consequently, prompt medical attention is very important. This sec-

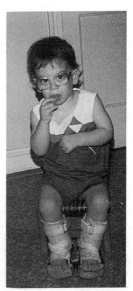

tion describes some of the most common gastrointestinal problems in children with cerebral palsy.

Oral Reflexes

In their first few months of life, children have little voluntary control of their movements. How they react to touch, sound, and other types of stimulation is largely controlled by reflexes. As Chapter 6 discusses, children with cerebral palsy often retain these early reflexes for months or years longer than normal. When these reflexes persist in the face or mouth, children with cerebral palsy can have trouble chewing, sucking, or swallowing.

The oral reflexes most likely to cause problems for children with cerebral palsy are the bite reflex, the gag reflex, and the tongue protrusion reflex. The bite reflex causes a child to close her mouth tightly—for example, when a spoon touches her gums or teeth. The gag reflex causes a child to gag or choke if something touches her palate or tongue. The tongue thrust reaction causes a child to forcefully push food out of her mouth with her tongue when her tongue is stimulated. If these reflexes are too strong, mealtimes become frustrating and time-consuming and food intake is decreased. Strong oral reflexes can also lead to serious problems such as choking, breathing food into the lungs, and malocclusion (see below).

If your child has oral reflex problems, an occupational therapist, speech-language pathologist, physical therapist, or nutritionist can help her by desensitizing her mouth and teaching her how to move food around in her mouth and then swallow it.

Gastroesophageal Reflux

If your child frequently spits up or vomits, she may have *gastroesophageal reflux.* This condition is especially common in children with cerebral palsy. It occurs when the lower esophageal sphincter relaxes, permitting the stomach to eject its contents back up through the esophagus and sometimes into the mouth. The lower esophageal sphincter is an area in the lower portion of the esophagus that normally closes to prevent food from being forced out of the stomach into the esophagus. Relaxation of this sphincter usually allows burping, but when the relaxation is longer and deeper than normal, stomach contents escape into the esophagus.

Gastroesophageal reflux can lead to several complications. For example, stomach acids may irritate the esophagus, causing pain and bleeding, or *esophagitis*. Children with gastroesophageal reflux are also in danger of developing pneumonia if they breathe bits of their stomach contents into their lungs.

Special feeding techniques can usually stop gastroesophageal reflux in children with cerebral palsy. Giving your child more frequent, but smaller portions of food or formula often helps. So, too, does thickening the formula with cereal. It may also help to place your child in a semi-upright infant chair for forty-five minutes to an hour after meals to give her stomach a chance to empty.

Your child's occupational or physical therapist, speech-language pathologist, nutritionist, or pediatrician will initially help you develop appropriate feeding techniques for your child. If these methods do not work, or if your child develops complications or fails to thrive, your child should see a *gastroenterologist*—a specialist in disorders of the GI system. The gastroenterologist can recommend medications or surgery to successfully treat your child's reflux.

Constipation

Most children have periodic bouts of *constipation*, or infrequent, prolonged, or difficult bowel movements. Children with cerebral palsy, however, are more likely to develop this condition. This is because children with spastic abdominal muscles or low muscle tone have difficulty contracting their abdominal muscles to produce the pressure needed to help with elimination. Children with cerebral palsy may also be unable to sense the fullness of the rectum which would ordinarily signal them to contract their muscles. In addition, lack of exercise can contribute to constipation.

If your child has constipation, her symptoms may include: straining with large, hard stools; abdominal pain; rectal bleeding or tearing; soiling underwear; poor appetite; or a swollen or hard abdomen. Constipation may also trigger behavior problems such as fear of toileting, and may make toilet training especially difficult.

Changes in diet can often help children with cerebral palsy who are constipated. Adding certain fruits and vegetables, increasing consumption of fluids, and adding bulk to the diet with whole grains or bran can soften a child's stool, making elimination easier. Reducing consumption of cow's milk may also help if your child has *lactose intolerance,* or lacks the enzyme which breaks down milk sugar. Additionally, your physician may prescribe mineral oil to lubricate your child's bowel, stool softeners such as docusate sodium, or laxatives such as psyllium (Metamucil™). The chronic use of laxatives is usually not recommended, since dietary changes, bulk, and stool softeners are easier on children's bowels. Always check with your child's pediatrician before buying over-the-counter laxatives.

If your child has chronic constipation, she may need further evaluation by your pediatrician or a gastroenterologist. These professionals can determine whether your child's constipation is a side effect of medications she is taking such as anticonvulsants or iron supplements. For particularly stubborn cases of constipation, your child's pediatrician or gastroenterologist may work together with a nutritionist or therapists to design a comprehensive program. Their treatment recommendations may include cleaning your child's bowels with enemas, suppositories, or laxatives; following a regular toileting schedule; and making further diet modifications.

Urinary Infections

Children with cerebral palsy are about three times more likely to have urinary tract infections than other children are. These infections occur when bacteria get into the urine and multiply to great numbers. Urinary infections may cause fever; vomiting; diarrhea; failure to gain weight; abdominal pain; increased frequency or urgency of urination or more toileting accidents; or painful urination. If not properly treated, chronic urinary infections can lead to kidney damage.

In some children with cerebral palsy, chronic constipation may contribute to urinary infections by obstructing the flow of urine. Other children develop urinary infections because of hygiene problems. They may be unable to clean the pelvic area well because of tight hip muscles or hip contractures. Motor impairments, too, may make it difficult for a child to wipe without stool contamination of the bladder area. This contamination can lead to bladder infections.

Your physician can treat urinary infections with antibiotics. You can help your child by giving her extra fluids to help clean the urinary system of bacteria. Especially helpful is cranberry juice, which changes the acidity of urine and impedes growth of bacteria.

You can help prevent urinary infections by giving your child more frequent baths and diaper changes. Careful hygiene after your child has a bowel movement is especially important. If you have a daughter with cerebral palsy, you may also want to limit bubble baths because they can irritate the pelvic area and bladder. Repeated urinary infections should be further investigated by a *urologist*—a specialist in urinary diseases.

Bladder Control Problems

Bladder control requires the coordinated use of many muscles, including the bladder, abdominal wall muscles, diaphragm, pelvic floor muscles, and urinary sphincters. Although learning this control is naturally harder for children with motor problems, most children with cerebral palsy achieve bladder control between three and ten years of age.

If your child is quite delayed in mastering bladder control, she should see a urologist. A urologist can rule out anatomical abnormalities that affect how her bladder works, and can also test bladder and kidney function.

The urologist or pediatrician can also recommend various strategies to help your child overcome her incontinence. For example, you might be advised to try behavioral modification techniques such as rewarding your child for dry days or dry nights with praise or with stickers, stars, or other treats. A conditioning technique involving an alarm system that senses moisture and alerts your child might also be used. Finally, medication is sometimes used in addition to other strategies. The most common medication is Imipramine (Toframil™), which is given one hour before bedtime for nighttime wetting. This medication usually improves bed-wetting in two to three weeks, and then can be tapered off. It may, however, cause nervousness, sleep disturbances, nausea, and heart irregularities.

Respiratory Problems

Most young children have frequent bouts with the common cold. Symptoms such as runny nose and coughing usually are minor and run their course in three to seven days. But in children with cerebral palsy, colds may drag on and on. Some children with cerebral palsy cannot clear the congestion in their upper airway because they do not have the motor coordination to cough adequately. They may also lack the gag reflex needed to prevent mucus and bacteria from entering the lungs.

Sometimes complications of the common cold lead to pneumonia—inflamed and infected lungs. Other problems which cause children to *aspirate* (inhale) mucus, bacteria, or food into the lungs can also result in pneumonia. For example, a child with problems coordinating breathing and swallowing can choke and aspirate. During a seizure, a child can also aspirate, if not positioned correctly on her side. In addition, a child with gastroesophageal reflux (explained above) can sometimes aspirate food from the stomach and esophagus into the lungs.

Pneumonia is very dangerous in infants and young children. It is the most common cause of mortality in children with cerebral palsy. Because pneumonia can be effectively treated if recognized early, it is vital to know the warning signs. Symptoms include fever, deep cough, rapid breathing, increased mucus production, vomiting, and labored breathing with flaring of the nostrils or use of abdominal muscles to aid in breathing.

Pneumonia requires aggressive medical treatment with antibiotics, fluids, and, infrequently, respiratory support such as oxygen or a respirator. In addition, the physical therapist or respiratory therapist (usually a hospital therapist who works with the respirator, mist tents, and oxygen equipment) can teach your child and family *postural drainage* to clear the lungs of mucus. This technique involves positioning your child on her side, back, or stomach, then clapping and tapping her chest to loosen the mucus so she can cough and clear the congestion.

Children who often have pneumonia need a comprehensive evaluation to determine the reason for their recurrent bouts. Medical professionals involved in the evaluation can include a pediatrician, pulmonary specialist (lung specialist), ear, nose, and throat (ENT) specialist, gastroenterologist, nutritionist, and speech-language pathologist. These professionals can treat the reflux and pneumonia and also develop ways to improve problems with swallowing and breathing that lead to pneumonia.

Hearing Problems

Hearing is critical for the full development of language skills. In an infant or young child, even a mild hearing loss can interfere with language development. Because 5 to 15 percent of children with cerebral palsy have hearing impairments, it is important to have your child's hearing checked early and often.

As a parent, you should watch your child for signs of hearing loss. Child with mild to moderate hearing impairment react differently to voices or noises at different times—they seem not to be listening at times. Children with severe to profound hearing impairments usually do not respond to voices or noises. Instead, they respond to touch or to visual or environmental cues. For example, seeing clothes laid out on the bed might tell them that it is time to dress; food on the table might signal them that lunch is ready.

Types of Hearing Loss

Children with cerebral palsy may have two types of hearing impairment: sensorineural or conductive. Both types reduce a child's level of sound perception and make speech sound indistinct to her. In either type, hearing loss may range from mild to profound.

Sensorineural Hearing Loss. Sensorineural losses result from damage to the inner ear (cochlea), the auditory nerve, or both. The impairment can be congenital (present at birth), or acquired later in childhood from meningitis, high fever, or medications such as certain antibiotics. Hereditary sensorineural loss can develop early in infancy or over childhood. About one percent of children with cerebral palsy have this type of hearing loss.

Conductive Hearing Loss. Conductive hearing loss is the more common type of hearing loss in children with cerebral palsy. It is due to middle ear disease (ear infections), anatomic abnormalities such as cleft lip and palate, or malformed ears. A common ear infection that can produce hearing loss is viral or bacterial infection of the middle ear (otitis media). Signs of otitis media are ear pain, fever, ear discharge, or irritability, together with a red, bulging eardrum. Middle ear fluid (serous otitis media), which may accompany colds or allergies, can also cause a conductive hearing loss.

Diagnosis and Treatment of Hearing Loss

Depending on your child's age, the audiologist (hearing specialist) can use a variety of tests to check your child's hearing. For example, to assess the hearing of an infant under six months, the audiologist can use behavioral testing procedures—that is, present a sound, then watch for responses such as a startle, eye blinking, or head turning. An older child might be tested while at

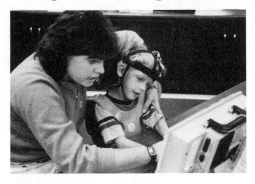

play. The audiologist can then observe whether the child responds to sound by changes in play activity.

To zero in on the type of hearing loss a child has, the audiologist uses a *tympanometer*. The tympanometer is an electrical instrument which measures changes in pressure and mobility of the eardrum and indicates whether middle ear fluid is present. The audiologist might also use *evoked response audiometry*, a type of EEG which detects changes in brain waves when sounds are presented.

If your child has a hearing loss, both an audiologist and an ENT specialist will first look for underlying, treatable causes. All conductive hearing losses are medically treatable. Ear infections, for example, can be cleared up with antibiotics. Middle ear fluid can be treated with decongestant medications, and, if it persists, by surgical placement of tubes in the eardrum (myringotomy tubes). Cleft palate and malformation of the middle ear can be surgically corrected.

Children with a sensorineural hearing loss may need a hearing aid to amplify sounds. To improve a child's responses to sounds, both the audiologist and the speech and language pathologist generally work with her to adjust the hearing aid properly. Language skills can be further enhanced with speech-language therapy and other early intervention or special education services.

Vision Problems

Visual impairments can result from problems with any part of the visual system, including the eyes, eye muscles, optic nerve, or the area of the cerebral cortex that processes visual information. Because cerebral palsy frequently affects the visual system, children with cerebral palsy are more likely to have visual problems than are other children.

The ophthalmologist, a medical doctor who specializes in eyes, is trained to recognize disorders of the visual system and to detect vision problems. During an eye examination, he will measure your child's visual *acuity,* or ability to see clearly. In infants, visual acuity can be assessed by checking their ability to look at and follow a light or an object and to reach for objects. Older children are asked to identify special pictures or charts held at a distance. During the exam, the ophthalmologist will also examine your child's eye, usually after dilating the pupil with eye drops.

Some of the vision problems that may be diagnosed in children with cerebral palsy are described below.

Refractive Errors

About three out of four children with cerebral palsy have refractive errors, or decreased acuity. Most commonly, they have *hyperopia* (farsightedness)—they can see far objects clearly, but nearby objects are blurred. Children with cerebral palsy are also more likely to have *myopia* (nearsightedness)—they can see close objects, but distant objects are blurry. Some children with cerebral palsy have *astigmatism,* or blurry vision caused by abnormal curvature of the cornea. Symptoms of refractive errors you may notice in your child include squinting, crossed eyes, holding objects close to her face, bumping into objects, and problems with fine motor coordination. Your child might also complain of blurred vision or eye fatigue.

Glasses or contact lenses can improve vision for children with refractive errors. While your child is an infant or still quite young, however, she may be able to manage without corrective lenses. For example, a moderate refractive error which makes far objects blurred may not interfere with a young child's daily activities. Deciding whether or not to use glasses in these cases is often up to the parents and the ophthalmologist.

Strabismus

Strabismus or crossed eyes affects half of all children with cerebral palsy, and is especially common in children with diplegia and quadriplegia. In strabismus, both eyes do not focus together. An eye can turn in (*esotropia*) or it can turn out (*exotropia*). Either problem can affect depth perception and cause double vision or amblyopia (see below). The motor problems of children with cerebral palsy can affect eye muscle control and cause this misalignment of the eyes.

Strabismus is often treated by putting a patch over the stronger eye to force the muscles of the weaker eye into proper alignment. Corrective glasses may also be prescribed. In addition, surgery is frequently needed to assure the development of good muscle coordination so that both eyes focus together.

Amblyopia

In amblyopia (lazy eye), the brain turns off or suppresses the eye with relatively weaker vision to prevent the child from having blurred or double vision. This suppression may occur when both eyes do not have the same visual acuity, both eyes do not focus together (strabismus), or one eye does not have a clear image because of cataracts or some other disorder. With time, the suppression may become irreversible; the brain can lose its ability to interpret visual information, leading to blindness in the weaker eye. Fortunately, if detected early, amblyopia can be effectively treated. Once the underlying problem—strabismus, impaired acuity, cataracts—is diagnosed, treatment of this problem can reverse the amblyopia.

Cataracts

Some babies with cerebral palsy are born with cataracts (clouding of the lens). Cataracts can block the visual images from entering the retina and cause visual impairments, including blurred vision and amblyopia. Cataracts can be due to genetic causes or to rubella, toxoplasmosis, CMV (cytomegalic virus), or other infections acquired while the baby is in the uterus. Children with cataracts usually have surgery in the early months of life to restore vision by removing the cataract on the lens. This surgery most often requires a hospital stay of only one to two days and is usually quite successful. If your child has a lens removed from her eye, she will need a contact lens to replace it.

Retinopathy of Prematurity

Retinopathy of prematurity (R.O.P.), also known as retrolental fibroplasia (R.L.F.), is common in babies born prematurely. In most cases, it is believed to result from the high concentrations of oxygen used when premature babies are on a respirator. R.O.P. affects the capillaries in the eye and can lead to myopia. It can also cause the retina to pull away from the back of the eye (detached retina), resulting in visual loss or blindness. Fortunately, treatment can prevent R.O.P. from progressing to retinal detachment. The retina can also be surgically reattached.

Cortical Blindness

Cortical blindness results from injury to the brain's visual centers in the cerebral cortex. A child with cortical blindness is able to pick up visual information with her eyes, but her brain cannot process and interpret the information correctly. The result is total or partial blindness. About 25 percent of children with hemiplegia have cortical visual impairments to parts of their visual field (*hemianopsia*). They are able to see objects in front of them, but can't see objects to one side. Total cortical blindness is rare and usually occurs when there is extensive brain injury—for example, in children with severe quadriplegia.

If your child has a visual impairment, you should seek both medical and educational treatment for her. Your child might benefit from an educational program that includes a specially trained vision therapist. This therapist can assess and enhance your child's useful vision and help your child learn to use information from other senses besides sight. The vision therapist, physical therapist, and occupational therapist can teach you special handling techniques to help your child learn where she is in space and to locate and place objects such as eating utensils. Visual aids such as bright lighting, bright colors, large print, and magnifying glasses may also help your child.

So, too, may tactile cues such as braille or raised markings on the wall near the stairs.

Orthopedic Problems Caused by High Tone

Cerebral palsy is not a progressive disorder. Once your child's brain injury has occurred, it will not get worse. Sometimes, though, abnormal muscle tone can lead to complications that make it *seem* as if a child's cerebral palsy is getting worse. Continuing tightness or spasticity of muscles can not only cause reduced function in the muscles themselves, but can also cause problems with the skeletal system—with the framework of bones, joints, ligaments, and tendons that support the muscles. These problems with bones, joints, or muscles are known as *orthopedic* problems. Common orthopedic complications that children with high tone may develop include contractures, dislocated hips, and scoliosis.

Dislocated Hips

Sometimes the strong pull of muscles around the hips can cause the femoral bone in the upper leg to partially slip out of joint where it joins at the hip. This tendency of the femoral bone to slip out of the hip joint is called *subluxation;* permanent displacement out of the joint is called *dislocation.* About one quarter of children with spasticity develop hip subluxation. Children with severe quadriplegia are especially prone to develop dislocated hips.

Hip subluxation and dislocation may be painful, and may cause significant problems with mobility, positioning, hygiene, and *scoliosis* (see below). Pain can be caused by degenerative arthritis (inflammation of the joint) as well as by chronic muscle spasticity. Anti-arthritis medications can help to control the pain.

An orthopedic surgeon will take hip X-rays to determine the extent of your child's hip joint displacement. To prevent dislocation, he can perform several surgical procedures, depending upon your child's muscular problem. Generally, if your child is three to eight years of age, the surgeon will begin by operating on the soft tissues (muscles, nerves, tendons). After your child is five, the orthopedic surgeon might consider an *osteotomy*—an operation to change the angle of the femoral bone and the hip joint. A total hip replacement might also be considered if the other procedures are unsuccessful. Surgery is very helpful in preventing hip dislocation in children with cerebral palsy.

Scoliosis

About 15 to 30 percent of children with cerebral palsy develop *scoliosis*, or an abnormal curvature of the spine. An unequal tension of the muscles along the spine can lead to this condition. Scoliosis can also develop as the result of faulty positioning or posture—for example, if a child habitually leans to one side in her wheelchair or has dislocated hips. Scoliosis can produce either an S-shaped or a C-shaped curve of the spine. C-shaped curves often result in unequal hips or shoulders.

If not treated properly, scoliosis can affect your child's posture, stature, sitting balance, walking ability, and heart and lung function. Scoliosis may also put additional pressure on the skin over the buttocks or back and cause pressure sores. Consequently, the orthopedic surgeon will carefully monitor the curvature of your child's spine over the years. He will also examine your child for any back or rib deformities.

Curvature of the spine can often be corrected or prevented from getting worse through proper positioning and physical therapy exercise programs. Molded seat inserts can improve sitting postures by providing support to the spine and can prevent pressure sores with padding to the pelvis. For early scoliosis, your child might also be prescribed a special plastic brace or orthosis worn around the trunk. If your child has a significant curvature of the spine, she might require surgery. The spinal vertebrae can be fixed in proper position with wire rods (segmental spinal instrumentation) or by fusing the vertebral bones together (spinal fusion). Unless respiratory complications make surgery necessary early in life, surgery is delayed until the major growth of the spine has occurred.

Contractures

Sometimes the constant pull of a child's tight muscles can lead to shortening of the muscles, tendons, and joint capsules (the cartilage that covers the end of a bone at the joint). If certain muscles around a joint pull harder than others, over time this muscle imbalance can lead to further shortening and to misalignment of the joints. This shortening of muscles and other tissues, with or without joint misalignment, is called a *contracture*. In children with cerebral palsy, contractures may develop because of limited active muscle movement or strong spasticity. Growth spurts can also contribute to contractures by putting additional stress on the muscle balance. Frequently children whose contractures get progressively worse over a short period of time are going through a rapid growth in height.

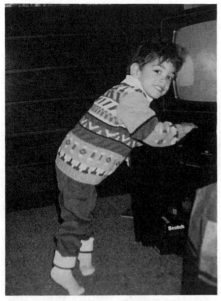

Generally, contractures further limit the movement of children with cerebral palsy. When they occur in the lower extremities, contractures can also affect your child's gait and posture. For example, children who develop shortening of the calf muscles and tendons tend to stand on their toes. This problem, termed *equinus,* is especially common in children with diplegia and hemiplegia. Children may also develop *flexion deformities*—abnormally flexed (bent) hips, knees, or ankles. This flexion can lead to a crouched or flexed posture in standing and walking and also affect balance. Occasionally, contractures of certain muscles around the knee may cause the knee joint to overextend backwards (*recurvatum)* and may lead to degenerative arthritis and pain. In addition, tightness of the adductor muscles in the inner thighs can cause a short stride, a narrow base of support, or—if severe—scissoring (crossing) of the legs. Contractures in the lower extremities are most common in children with spastic diplegia and quadriplegia, and may develop slowly over the years.

Contractures in the upper extremities affect a child's ability to reach for, grasp, release, and manipulate objects. Spasticity of the hand muscles frequently leads to a "thumb in palm" deformity. Not only does this position make it harder for children to handle objects, but it can also result in infections to the palm because of inadequate hygiene. A child's ability to grasp and release can also be affected by wrist flexion deformities. And flexion contractures of the elbow can interfere with reaching or with using a walker. Contractures in the upper extremities are especially common in children with spastic hemiplegia. In these children, muscles of the fingers, wrists, elbows, and shoulders may become progressively tighter.

Prevention and Treatment of Complications

Many of the complications of spasticity described above can be prevented or minimized with physical and occupational therapy. Therapists can use stretching exercises to improve joint movement and prevent contractures; handling and positioning techniques to improve tone; and strength-building exercises to improve movement. Chapter 7 provides more information on physical and occupational therapy exercise programs.

Besides the therapeutic methods that physical and occupational therapists use, there are several medical means of preventing or treating complications of muscle tone problems. For example, physicians may recommend a variety of special devices to minimize or prevent contractures. They may also perform surgery to correct deformities or to make a child's muscle tone more normal. This section describes the medical procedures most commonly used to treat the orthopedic complications of cerebral palsy.

Orthotics, Casts, and Splints

Orthotics. About 85 percent of children with cerebral palsy are prescribed an *orthotic* to supplement their therapeutic exercise program. Orthotics are plastic, leather, or lightweight metal devices

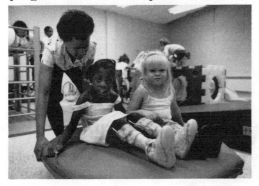

that provide stability to the joints or passively stretch the muscles. Orthotics may also help reduce tone, sometimes dramatically. Plastic is now the most commonly used material because it is light, easily cleaned, relatively attractive, and holds its shape under stress.

Orthotics most often used for children with cerebral palsy are ankle foot orthoses (AFOs) and knee ankle foot orthoses (KAFOs). These devices are worn inside the shoe and help to stabilize a child's foot, ankle, and lower leg, making it easier for her to make firm foot contact with the ground when walking or standing. When used in conjunction with physical therapy, AFOs can frequently help children who toe walk; the longer KAFOs can help children correct excessive knee flexion in standing and walking.

Orthotics are usually prescribed when a child is ready to stand upright. Sometimes, however, they are used earlier to maintain joint position. The use of an orthotic must be carefully coordinated with the physical therapist's exercise and stretching program and with other treatments such as casts and prone standers (equipment to enable a child to be upright at a table.)

Your child may wear orthotics for months or years as part of her therapy program. If your child needs an orthotic, your doctor should be able to recommend an *orthotist*—a professional skilled in custom making orthotics. These orthotics need to be made carefully and monitored by your physician and therapists so they can be periodically adjusted and refitted as your child grows and advances in skills.

When your child has new orthotics or adaptive equipment, it is critical to check her skin for red marks from pressure several times an hour. As they grow in size and weight, children with cerebral palsy run the risk of developing pressure injuries if they are unable to shift their weight every fifteen or twenty minutes to change the pressure on an area of skin. Children may also develop skin irritation, ulcers, and breakdowns if orthotics and other adaptive equipment do not fit properly. The weight-bearing areas of the spine, hips, buttocks, and feet are especially prone to pressure sores.

Prevention of skin ulcers is the goal, because once the sores develop, they are slow to heal. They are also painful, as is the treatment, which involves cutting away of the sores *(debridement)*, medications, and sometimes surgery. To prevent pressure sores, your therapists or orthotist can help adjust your child's equipment or provide padding over specific pressure areas.

Casts. Like orthotics, casts can help to maintain or improve a joint's movement, reduce tone, and prevent contractures. To further stretch the soft tissues, casts are sometimes made serially—that is, changed every few weeks as the contractures are stretched. Casts may be made in one piece, or they can be bivalved (cut into two pieces) so they can be taken off and put back on with straps. Bivalved casts are usually worn for longer periods of time than solid casts. Although plaster is sometimes used for casts, fiberglass is usually preferable because it is lighter, more durable, and easier to clean.

Casts are often used as part of a therapy program to improve toe walking, back kneeing gaits, and wrist or elbow flexion. In addition, a procedure known as inhibitive or dynamic casting is frequently (and successfully) used to reduce tone.

Casts may be worn for weeks or months. Usually they are used before orthotics are prescribed. They are also helpful for children who have trouble keeping orthotics on.

Splints. Splints molded of rigid plastic are sometimes prescribed to stretch the soft tissues in an upper extremity or to hold it in a position that makes movement easier. They can help prevent and treat wrist and elbow flexion deformities, as well as the "thumb in palm" deformity. They can be as tiny as an *opponens splint*, which holds the thumb in correct alignment, or as large as an entire resting hand splint, which supports a hand with very low tone. Splints are removable and may be worn for only part of the day or even at night.

Orthotics, casts, and splints are all expensive and custom made for your child, so you will want to learn the correct way to put them on and care for them. You may find it helpful to label them "Right" and "Left." If your child leaves the house with her devices, you will also want to make sure they are labeled with her name and phone number to guard against loss.

Medications

Although medications can sometimes reduce high tone, they are not routinely prescribed for children with cerebral palsy. This is because the medications are usually not effective and can have adverse effects on children's learning abilities and produce unwelcome side effects or chemical changes in the blood. They can cause sedation, dizziness, weakness, and fatigue.

Generally, drugs are reserved for children with painful spasms of severe spasticity and are used as only one small part of the treatment plan. Drugs most often prescribed for spasms include diazepam (Valium™), dantrolene sodium (Dantrium™), and baclofen (Lioresal™). Sometimes Valium may also help children with athetosis reduce their abnormal movements because of the relaxing effects of the drug.

Nerve Blocks

Spasticity in specific muscle groups can sometimes be significantly reduced through use of a nerve block. A nerve block is an injection of medication into nerves that go to the muscles. It impairs the conduction of impulses along the nerve, weakening or paralyzing the muscle, and sometimes causing numbness. Medications such as local anesthetics, phenol, or alcohol can block the nerve for several months or permanently, depending upon the dosage and type of medication.

For children with cerebral palsy, nerve blocks on the spastic muscles that pull the legs together (adducters) can reduce scissoring, and make crawling, sitting, standing, and walking easier. Nerve blocks are also occasionally used prior to surgery so that doctors can assess the desirability of doing a particular surgical procedure. This is because nerve blocks can sometimes temporarily produce the same results that a surgical procedure would produce permanently.

Although nerve blocks are often useful, there are several possible drawbacks to using them. First, the injection of a nerve block with a needle can be painful. Second, children sometimes lose—not gain—function from a nerve block. If a nerve block is suggested for your child, be sure to discuss all the pros and cons with the physician.

Surgery

There are several surgical procedures that can improve movement, correct deformities, or prevent further contractions in children with cerebral palsy. For the most part, these are orthopedic surgical procedures—surgery on the bones, joints, muscles, ligaments, and tendons. Children with cerebral palsy sometimes need surgery as early as their preschool years. Usually, however, surgery is not considered until after an attempt has been made to maintain and improve your child's mobility through physical therapy. Once surgery is approved, the orthopedic surgeon will coordinate with your child's physical therapist to make sure that pre- and post-operation therapy will maximize the benefits of surgery. Here are the types of surgical procedures sometimes used to help children with cerebral palsy:

Soft Tissue Procedures. Soft tissue procedures are operations on the muscles, tendons, or ligaments to correct deformities or improve movement. They are the type of surgery most often used with children under five. Examples of soft tissue procedures include:

- Tendon lengthening—an operation to correct contractures of the muscles or tendons. Lengthening the achilles tendon can improve the gait of a child who is toe walking; lengthening tight hamstrings at the back of the knee can correct a crouched walking position.
- Tendon transfers—procedures in which the tendons are moved to alternate places on the bones to provide better joint alignment and muscle control. Tendon transfers correct contractures and free up the joint, and can improve functional use of a limb. When a child has too much wrist flexion, a tendon transfer can strengthen her grasp and release by allowing better wrist extension. Transfers may also be used to correct contractures in the hand.
- Tenotomy—cutting the tendon to release muscle contractures and improve joint movement.
- Neurectomy—cutting the nerve to a muscle group to permanently reduce spasticity. Neurectomies are used in correcting or preventing hip dislocation.
- Muscle releases on recession (lengthening)—procedures that lengthen muscles and can correct problems such as thumb and hand contractures.
- Myotomy—cutting the muscle to release muscle contractures and to improve mobility.

Bony Procedures. Bony procedures are operations on the joints and bones to correct deformities. Because bony procedures can affect bone growth, they are not usually used until a child's major bone growth has finished. Normally, soft tissue surgery is considered first. Here are the two bony procedures most commonly used:

- Osteotomy—a procedure to realign the joints by removing part of a bone and repositioning it at a better angle. Osteotomies may be used to correct hip dislocation.
- Arthrodesis—an operation that fuses (joins) the bones to one another. Arthrodesis can stabilize the ankle and foot when there is severe foot deformity.

Selective Posterior (Dorsal) Rhizotomy. The traditional surgical procedures for children with cerebral palsy are all orthopedic surgical procedures. Recently, however, there has been much interest in a method of reducing increased muscle tone by using neurosurgical procedures—operations on the nerves and brain tissue. Selective dorsal rhizotomy, the new approach, involves selective cutting of the nerves of the spine to reduce the spasticity of muscle groups in the upper or lower extremities or trunk. By reducing spastic tone, the procedure can improve a child's control of voluntary movements and enable her to move more easily. Because the procedure is relatively new, neurosurgeons are still studying the long-term risks of the procedure. At present, the procedure does not seem to cause any significant loss of touch or position sensations. But some specialists believe the procedure may lead to spinal deformities in the future.

Since selective dorsal rhizotomy is still considered experimental, the surgery should be done only under well-controlled research procedures. Presently, it is recommended for only a limited number of children. Children with spasticity are considered for surgery, but children with low trunk tone or the involuntary, purposeless movements of extrapyramidal-type cerebral palsy are not considered good candidates. If this surgery is recommended for your child, discuss the procedure with a surgeon who can fill you in on the most recent research on the potential risks and benefits. Also make sure that the surgery will be closely coordinated with your child's therapy program for post-operative therapy.

Orthopedic Problems Caused by Low Tone

Children with low tone may have some of the same complications as children with high tone, but for different reasons. For example, their knees may bend backwards because their joints are hyperextensible (overly flexible), rather than because tight muscles force the knee back. Like children with high tone, children with low tone may also have subluxation or dislocation of the hips—but because the femoral bones in their legs are rotated out from their body.

Other common complications of low tone include a variety of spine deformities: *lordosis* (sway back), *kyphosis* (rounded back), and scoliosis. Since these conditions can lead to poor posture and serious deformity, an orthopedic surgeon should monitor them closely.

Finally, low tone in the foot and ankle can affect weight bearing and lead to flat feet (*pronation*). This condition can be painful and can impair walking because of poor foot and leg alignment. An orthotic device can help correct flat feet.

Most children with low tone do not need surgical procedures to treat complications. Complications of low tone can usually be effectively treated with orthotics and occupational and physical therapy.

Dental Problems

Common as they are in children, tooth decay and gum disease are not an inevitable part of growing up. As Chapter 4 explains, you can vastly reduce your child's likelihood of developing these problems by making preventive dental care a part of your daily routine. There are, however, several special dental problems that may arise as a result of your child's cerebral palsy. This section describes these problems as well as steps you can take to help minimize or prevent them.

Malocclusions

As they grow older, children with muscle imbalances in their faces tend to develop *malocclusions*—faulty bites such as overbites or underbites. Malocclusions significantly affect a child's chewing and speech, and in the long run can affect a child's appearance. In extreme cases, a child may not be able to bite because her teeth are so misaligned.

The speech-language pathologist, occupational therapist, and nutritionist can use oral-motor exercises to improve the tone around your child's face and prevent malocclusions. They can also work to reduce oral reflexes that cause faulty bites. Additionally, your child's dentist or orthodontist can use orthodontic devices to prevent and improve malocclusions.

Hyperplasia

Children with seizures who are treated with phenytoin (Dilantin™) may develop *hyperplasia*—excessive growth of the gums—as a side effect. This condition can lead to problems with oral hygiene and gum disease. If your child is taking Dilantin, she should have more frequent dental appointments so the dentist can treat any hyperplasia as early as possible.

Enamel Defects

Children with cerebral palsy are more likely than other children to have enamel defects—small areas in which the hard covering of their teeth is pitted or absent. Without proper treatment, enamel defects can lead to early tooth decay. If your child has enamel defects, the dentist can repair the enamel by applying sealants to the teeth.

Drooling

In children with cerebral palsy, constant moisture from drooling frequently irritates the skin around the mouth. To reduce drooling and the accompanying skin irritation, the occupational therapist and speech-language pathologist will work with your child to teach her to swallow her saliva and to improve muscle tone in and around the mouth. The ear, nose, and throat specialist can also do a surgical procedure to stop drooling.

Medical Insurance

Your child will probably require many doctor visits, medical procedures, and long-term therapies over the years. The medical costs are enormous and certainly can be a major financial burden on your family. Ideally, your family's medical insurance would cover all of these costs. Unfortunately, this is seldom, if ever, the case. Today, the tendency in the medical insurance industry is to try to keep costs down by limiting payments for long-term care of children with disabilities. Often insurance will cover medical visits, orthotics, surgery, and physical therapy services. Insurance is less likely to cover occupational therapy, speech and language therapy, and psychological services.

Because of federal and state legislation, insurance carriers feel that educational and health agencies should bear most of the costs. But even though the school system *does* pay for therapy to support your child's education, this therapy usually does not meet the true medical needs of your child. You may feel compelled to seek out private services for occupational, physical, or speech and language therapy.

Even when insurance theoretically covers services for children with cerebral palsy, the company usually requires more documentation of the medical need for services and equipment. It wants proof that your child's health will be worse if she does not receive the treatments. You may be asked to provide a letter from the doctor explaining the medical necessity of a procedure. You may also need to supply progress notes from therapists after the service is provided. To make filing claims easier, it is a good idea to keep a file with multiple copies of any documentation you may have gathered.

For help locating a standard insurance carrier with the best possible coverage for medical treatments and therapy, contact your local chapter of UCP or the ARC or other support groups. For information about "shared risk" insurance plans and your child's rights to insurance, see Chapter 9.

Selecting a Pediatrician

Finding a pediatrician who understands your child's special needs is crucial to your child's development and well-being. Even though your child will frequently see other medical and developmental specialists, the pediatrician will be your primary resource for help in dealing with medical concerns.

Your first priority is to find a pediatrician who is very knowledgeable about children with cerebral palsy. The doctor should know how your child's motor impairments may affect her health, behavior, and development—and he should share this information with you. For example, the pediatrician should tell you if your child's stiff legs will make diapering and dressing more difficult, or if tight abdominal muscles could lead to problems with having bowel movements. He also should listen to your questions and concerns and answer them in clear, nontechnical language.

Another factor to consider is the pediatrician's familiarity with community resources and specialists. He should be able to refer your child to the right person or place whenever medical, neurological, or developmental concerns arise. He should also be willing to coordinate your child's care. He should have regular contact with your child's medical specialists, therapists, and educational programs so he can tell them how your child's health will affect her education. Most importantly, the pediatrician needs to be a strong advocate for your child and take an active role in helping you find and secure appropriate treatment for your child.

Finding a pediatrician with all these qualities can be a tall order. By asking around, however, you can generally get the names of pediatricians in your area who specialize in treating children with developmental disorders. Good sources of names include other parents of children with cerebral palsy, members of your child's interdisciplinary evaluation team, teachers, or your local UCP or ARC chapter.

Conclusion

Despite the number of medical conditions described in this chapter, it is important to remember that most children with cerebral palsy enjoy good health. Although medical problems can arise, effective treatments are available for the majority of them.

As a parent, you are the one who is ultimately responsible for your child's medical well-being. But you can share this responsibility with many caring, competent professionals. If you select them well, together you can ensure that your son or daughter has the healthiest childhood possible.

Parent Statements

I feel extremely grateful that my child is healthy. One nice thing my pediatrician said early on is that he's an otherwise healthy child. People think, "ah, CP," but in fact it doesn't affect his health. He's not a chronically ill child, he's a disabled child.

❧❧❧

I used to hate to go grocery shopping. Everyone wanted to know why my seven-month-old wore glasses with bifocals. I got so tired of answering their questions. I began to feel like I had as much of a disability as he did.

❧❧❧

I think we were always a step ahead of our pediatrician. He never made suggestions unless we asked.

❧❧❧

It was really difficult to find a dentist who had the patience to work with my son. Most of them can't deal with it.

❧❧❧

You can't possibly rely just on your regular pediatrician. The best you can hope for is that you have a sensitive person, an upbeat person, and a person who will at least try to find answers to questions you have. And then you go to your specialists.

❧❧❧

We could accept the fact that he would never walk. My husband and I thought, "Thank God, he doesn't have seizures." Then at three and a half, our son had his first seizure.

❧❧❧

When our daughter had her first seizure and was in the ambulance, I wondered whether she was going to die or be brain dead. It was unbelievable. I thought, "I don't want her to die and I don't want her to be brain dead either."

❧❧❧

Right after Jason was born, we were told he had seizures in the hospital. When we took him home we were told to look for them but didn't know what they were. The hospital described what he had done there and we wondered and worried about almost every movement he made. I was terrified of him dying because I didn't know what to expect. I felt like we were handed a time bomb and told to go watch it. Because Jason is our only child, we didn't know what normal was. I hated him being on the medication but felt the seizures were worse.

❧❧❧

Sometimes when I saw seizures, I'd put off seeing the doctor because I didn't want Jason on more medicine.

❧❧❧

I've always assumed that my daughter's medical condition is so fragile that I will probably outlive her.

❧❧❧

When our son was first born, he had a shunt. I tried to think of somewhere we could go for a vacation. We had to go someplace where if he ever had shunt failure we could get to a hospital where they do pediatric neurosurgery.

❧❧❧

At eighteen months, Kelly started failing to thrive. The doctors wanted to give her a gastrostomy tube immediately. They said it was all due to the CP and that she would never eat correctly. I was convinced she was controlling the situation by refusing to eat, but nobody would believe me. We sought out alternative opinions. Both of the new doctors agreed with the first and explained everything very well. I fought getting the tube for about one year. We went through hell for about nine months while I force fed her, trying to avoid that tube. I finally had to give up when her health became too risky. By the time we got the tube, Kelly and I were the worst of enemies.

❧❧❧

After she got the tube, it was a tremendous relief to know she could be fed what she needed. I didn't try oral feedings for probably a couple of months after that. Then, when I started the feedings again, she continued to control the situation. About two to three months after the surgery, we moved and the new doctors said Kelly had a severe behavior problem with eating. I couldn't help but wonder, where was someone like that when I needed him? Finally someone agreed with me and it was too late. The tube was already there.

The hearing aids seem to bother her now, but I can tell they make a big difference in what she can hear. When she gets older, I'm sure she'll appreciate the difference herself.

Robby always seems to have the sniffles. Luckily, it's never developed into anything more serious.

Jennie's alcohol [nerve] block was more agonizing than her surgery.

I've never had a pediatrician I felt totally good about. I think most of them treat Linda as an object or disease.

They talk around her and just do things without telling her. I speak up now, but in the beginning I didn't. I make everyone aware that she's human, understands them, and has feelings. She deserves some respect.

I think that any time a child leaves the hospital with any kind of problem, the hospital should give the parents a file cabinet to keep track of all his records.

When I think of specific medical problems we have gone through with Keith, it brings back some painful memories. But when I think back on the whole five years, it's a blur.

✳✳✳

Devon went through years of discomfort due to constipation. I think it's because he doesn't get enough exercise to be regular. After years of mentioning this to my pediatrician, altering his diet, and trying various over-the-counter laxatives, we finally consulted a specialist and went on a mineral oil program. What a difference!

✳✳✳

Our doctor was great. He explained the hamstring release surgery not only to us but to Kevin as well. He explained that he would be making a little cut in the shape of a "Z" so Kevin could ZIP around. And sure enough, he's zipping right along.

✳✳✳

The hardest part of our daughter's soft tissue release was her first week home. Her legs were set in casts from her hips to her toes and she was very uncomfortable. Positioning her in these casts was very difficult—especially for toileting. After the first week she adjusted and began to feel better.

✳✳✳

Michael has gone through an assortment of orthotics. Too bad you can't recycle those things or pass them along. They are so expensive; it seems like such a waste.

✳✳✳

Katie's long leg braces are cumbersome. They have to be in a locked position when she walks or stands, which means that whatever she's doing—getting out of the car, going on the school bus, whatever—someone has to lay her down to lock or unlock her hinges.

✳✳✳

When our son had surgery, we were nervous wrecks. We tried to prepare our son by reading him all the kids' books about hospitals, assuring him that we would be there waiting, and visiting the hospital beforehand. Despite our worries, our son sailed through the whole experience.

❧❧❧

Getting my two-year-old to wear his inhibitive casts was really tricky. We tried stickers, happy faces on his toes, you name it. Eventually he got so used to them, he wore them all the time without complaining.

❧❧❧

My daughter slept in long, removable casts to stretch out her hamstrings and heelcords. It was hard for all of us. The stretching, of course, was uncomfortable which made it hard for her to relax and fall asleep. She would wake up several times during the night and I would have to talk her through her discomfort in order to keep the casts on.

❧❧❧

Patricia is so attached to her orthotist. She's been seeing her since she was about eighteen months old. She loves the whole process: the measuring, the casting, and even the sawing. I guess it's all in how it's presented and the parent's attitude. I know other kids who have a hard time dealing with it.

❧❧❧

FOUR

Daily Care

SHARON ANDERSON, O.T.R.*

If you have other children or are familiar with the day-to-day care of children, you already know that caring for babies and young children is both complex and time-consuming. When your child has cerebral palsy, daily care is often made even more complicated by medical concerns, movement problems, and developmental delays. For example, instead of simply needing to decide how and when to ease your child from bottle to cup drinking, you may need to find just the right nipple so that your child can drink out of a bottle at all. Instead of merely deciding whether or not to begin toilet training, you may need to track down the particular seat that will position your child so that he has the best shot at success.

To complicate matters further, there are hosts of medical and educational experts just waiting to advise you on selected aspects of your child's care. The physical therapist, for example, tells you to hold your baby like this and to be sure you do the range-of-motion exercises every day. The occupational therapist tells you how important it is to work on your child's hand control and provide varied sensory experiences. The speech-language pathologist suggests playing language games, making special tapes of your child's voice, and therapeutic toothbrushing. The special education teacher offers ideas to help your child master the concept of cause and effect and

---

* Sharon Anderson is an occupational therapist certified in neurodevelopmental treatment (NDT). She serves as the occupational therapist for the home-based program and the coordinator of occupational/physical therapy at the Ivymount School in Rockville, Maryland.

to learn social skills. The list of intervention strategies is endless, and each suggestion is a good one. Is it any wonder parents often feel overwhelmed by each new piece of information they are given about the care of their child?

This chapter will provide you with information to make the daily care of your child more manageable. Because each child with cerebral palsy is unique, it is beyond the scope of this chapter to give specific ideas for all areas of daily care. This chapter will, however, offer some suggestions for caring for most children with cerebral palsy, as well as some guidelines to help you assess your child's individual needs. (For more in-depth information on the day-to-day care and handling of your child, I recommend Nancie Finnie's classic book, *Handling the Young Cerebral Palsied Child at Home.)* The Reading List at the end of this book also includes other books on daily care.

As you read through this chapter, you should keep one thing in mind. Take only those suggestions that fit easily into your daily care routine and that can become virtually automatic. Do not take any suggestions that will only make more work for you. As the parent of a child with cerebral palsy, you probably already have a heavily burdened schedule. You want to avoid at all costs being caught up in the vicious cycle of "I'm not doing enough, often enough, for my child." Not only is this belief seldom true, but it can often be counterproductive.

It is human nature to shut down and become less efficient when you are overwhelmed, under stress, or feeling guilty. As a result, parents who can't do—or think they can't do—exactly as the experts suggest often do nothing. But in fact, the smallest suggestion or adaptation plugged into your daily routine may make a significant difference. I hope that among the suggestions that follow are some that will make a significant difference in your life—and the life of your child.

Holding and Carrying Your Child

Holding and carrying are crucial parts of the daily care of any baby. Before children walk or crawl efficiently, they rely on an adult to carry them to and from their crib and about the house. Throughout the day, any baby or young child is continually lifted, carried, and held so he can participate in activities such as feeding, bathing, playing, and exploring. Not only does carrying provide mobility for the child who has not yet learned to walk, but it also fosters social and emotional bonding between parent and child. In addition, carrying offers children important opportunities for sensory input. For example, when a mother walks, runs, rocks, or dances with her child in her arms, she gives her child input about movement, gravity, and position in space. And the close touch and warmth of a parent's arms and body give feedback to the child's *tactile* (touch) system.

When a child has cerebral palsy, how he is carried and held takes on even more importance. First of all, unless a child with cerebral palsy is carried properly, he will not be free to learn and interact with his environment. This means that he must be held in a way that 1) provides the support and control he lacks; and 2) controls any problems with muscle tone (tension) or abnormal movement patterns that he has. Secondly, in order to prevent later muscular or skeletal deformities, a child with cerebral palsy should be held with his body in correct alignment—that is, with his spine straight, his head centered and aligned with his spine, and his shoulders and hips level. In addition, because children with cerebral palsy usually need to be carried much longer than other children do, parents must learn to lift and carry their child in ways that minimize stress and strain to their back. They must also decide just how much carrying and holding is right for themselves and their child. A child who demands to be held all the time can be very trying to even the most patient parent. From the very beginning, it is important for your child to learn to entertain himself and to be content to be comfortably positioned where he can play, listen to music, or watch what is going on around him.

This section suggests a number of ways to hold and carry children with cerebral palsy. Some of them will be useful for your child, but others will not. To choose the best method of holding your child, you need to assess and understand your child's unique abilities and disabilities. You must also understand his basic problems with stability and mobility, since the first is the prerequisite to the second. For example, a child with athetoid cerebral palsy has mobility but no stability because his opposing muscle groups cannot contract simultaneously to hold a joint firmly in place.

As a result, his movements are poorly controlled and imprecise. The assessment and understanding needed to guide your selection of methods will come through your own observations, trial and error, and discussions with your child's physical and occupational therapists.

One of the keys to selecting an appropriate carrying method for your child is to understand his *muscle tone*. Muscle tone is the degree of tension in muscle fibers, and is discussed in Chapter One.

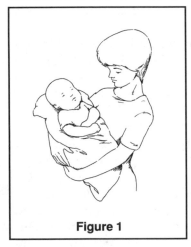

Figure 1

If your child has low tone, you have probably already noticed that he enjoys fast movements and being bounced around and responds with some desired increase in tone. Still, you may need to hold and carry your child in ways that support his body and keep joints and muscles in proper alignment. For the first six months, or until your child develops some head and trunk control, it is fine to carry your child as you would any baby. (See figure 1.) As your child gets a little older and larger, however, this type of carry will no longer be appropriate. First, your child would be unable to look out and see what is going on around him. Second, since he is fully supported in this position, he has no need to work on developing his posture control. Better carrying positions for children with low tone are shown in figure 2. Ask your physical therapist to help you choose the best carrying position for your child.

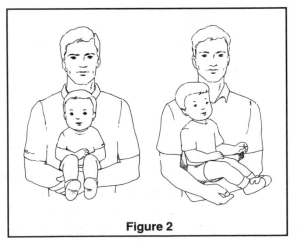

Figure 2

If your child has high tone, he probably responds best to slow movement and firm touch. Because your child's tone can easily increase with excitement and anticipation, it is best to keep interactions low-key. It also helps if you remember several basic principles to break up general high tone and *excessive tonal patterns* (abnormal distribution of muscle tone). These two techniques are *dissociation* and *rotation*.

Dissociation means position-ing the body so that it is impos-sible for the entire body to be in one rigid posture. This is ac-complished by "separating" one body part (such as a leg) from another, either by separating the upper half of a child's body from his lower half, or by separating one

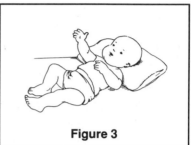

Figure 3

side of his body from the other. For example, if both of a child's legs are stiffly extended, the pattern can often be interrupted by flexing one leg. (See figure 3.)

The second technique for reducing tone, rotation, is actually a form of dissociation. Rotation means diagonal movement through the trunk. For example, a common position of rotation is to keep the child's hips stable and turn his shoulders in one direction, or vice versa. (See figure 4.) A common position of counter rotation is to turn the child's shoulders in one direction and his hips in the

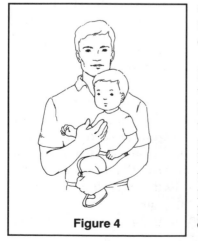

Figure 4

opposite direction. It may help you to think of your child's body as a corkscrew and turn it accordingly.

In holding children with low or high tone, how you position the pel-vis is of major importance. This is because the position of the pelvis is the key to the rest of your child's posture. If you hold your child so that his pelvic area is properly aligned, the rest of his body often responds positively, and you can hold and sup-port his upper body in a way that is comfortable for you and your child.

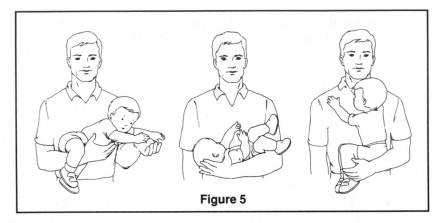

Figure 5

For instance, children with low tone often hold their legs far apart and bent at the knees in a "frog leg" posture. To position their pelvic area correctly, it is important to carry them with their legs together in good alignment, as shown in figure 2. Children with high tone, on the other hand, often extend and scissor their legs due to tight adductor muscles in the hips and inner upper thighs. This can be controlled by separating the legs and flexing the knees. So a good way to carry these children is straddled on your hip, or for a small baby, in a "football" hold with your arms separating the legs. (See figure 5.)

Sometimes in addition to problems in the pelvic area, tightness in the shoulders may make it difficult to hold a child with cerebral palsy. In this case, you may be able to carry your child more comfortably by bringing his arms up and forward over your shoulder,

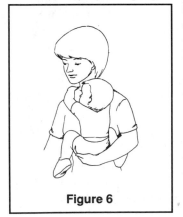

Figure 6

as illustrated in figure 6. Sometimes a child may be tight but with a predominance of *flexor tone*—that is, tone that brings the body forward or into a folded position. One of the more extended positions shown in figure 7 might be a good way to carry this child.

Don't be discouraged if it takes you a while to discover the best way to hold your child. Remember, too, that what works one day may not be as effective on another day; this is especially true

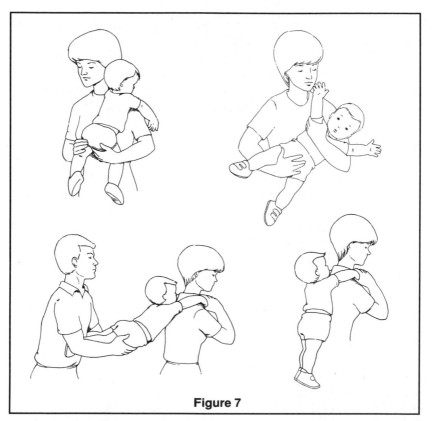

Figure 7

for children with fluctuating tone. If one position doesn't feel right, try another. When you finally find the right way to hold your child, you will be able to tell by the feedback you receive from his body. Your child's body will move easily with your movements and there will be no feeling of resistance or pushing or pulling away. If you have a good position, you'll know it and it won't make any difference if it defies all principles of handling.

One final note about holding and carrying your child: As important as good handling practices are in the daily care of your child, you must also have alternatives for proper positioning and mobility. It simply is not healthy for you or your child if you carry him with you everywhere you go, all day long. Every child needs time alone to entertain himself and to learn to interact with the sight, sound, touch, and play opportunities in his environment. This means that as your child gets older, you should gradually decrease the amount of time you spend holding and carrying him. Generally, once your child is about a year old, you should carry him only for the same reasons you would any other child his age—for long-distance mobility, for comfort when hurt, or for special times such as story time or bedtime snuggles. You may need to be actively involved in *positioning* your child most of the time, but not passive holding.

Positioning Your Child

No baby is able to control the position of his body when he is very young. If, for example, you place a newborn on his stomach with his head to one side, he may be able to turn his head from side to side, but will be unable to move from his tummy until you change his position for him. Babies who are developing normally do not remain physically helpless for long. Most babies instinctively learn to control first one group of muscles, then another. With little or no guidance, they learn to lift their heads, roll over, and sit up. Almost before you know it, these babies are able to position their bodies anyway they want in order to see, touch, or smell just about anything that catches their attention.

When you have a child with cerebral palsy, the story is somewhat different. Because of their neurological problems, children with cerebral palsy are unable to position their bodies as early or as competently as other children are. Not only is this highly frustrating for children with cerebral palsy, but it can also slow down their learning in many areas. For example, a child who does not crawl around on the floor and move his body over, under, through, and next to various pieces of furniture may have trouble learning spatial relationships. A child who cannot sit without using his hands for support will not be free to develop and practice fine motor skills because his hands are tied up in supporting his body. As Chapter 3 explains, children who cannot position their bodies properly may also develop complications such as scoliosis and contractures. For these reasons, you need to use positioning techniques to help keep your child's tone and posture as normal as possible.

Many of the principles involved in carrying your child correctly also apply to positioning him. The main difference is that when you hold your child, you use your own body to provide the support and control he needs. But when you position your child, you use an inanimate object such as a pillow, sandbag, or hammock to provide the support. Because inanimate objects cannot respond to your child's needs as you can, positioning often involves much trial and error and frequent adjustments.

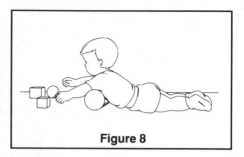

Figure 8

As you read through the positioning suggestions that follow, bear in mind that once again, your selection of strategies should be based on an understanding of your child's unique strengths and needs. Remember also that you should not place your child in positions he would not be developmentally ready for even if his tone and movement patterns were normal. For example, you should not try to prop a month-old baby in a sitting position. Motor milestones can occur only when muscles, bones, and reflexes are mature enough to support the next level of development. If you try to rush the process, you may slow or interfere with development or cause deformities. Your child's occupational and physical therapists will advise you which strategies are most appropriate for your child.

One of the first positions children use to play in once they have developed some head control is the *prone* (or tummy) position. Depending on your child's ability to support his head, you should begin placing your child in this position when he is about two to three months old. If your child has difficulty maintaining this position, you may want to place a rolled towel under his shoulder area to keep his arms forward. (See figure 8). If hip flexion (bending forward at the hips) makes it hard for your child to lie prone, you can help him with firm downward pressure on the buttocks from your hand or from a sandbag. (See figure 9.) As figure 9A

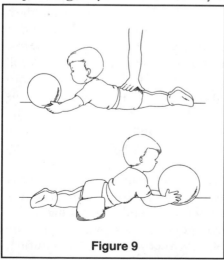

Figure 9

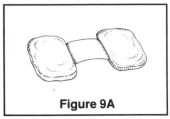

Figure 9A

illustrates, you can easily make sandbags using some sturdy, nonirritating fabric such as canvas or denim for the pouches and sand or rice for the filling. Sandbags can also be used to stabilize children who continually roll out of the prone position.

Yet another way to help children with cerebral palsy achieve a good prone position is to use a wedge. (See figure 10.) Wedges can be especially helpful for children who do not have adequate head control. Wedges can be purchased commercially, cut from foam, or constructed from wood and covered with foam and fabric.

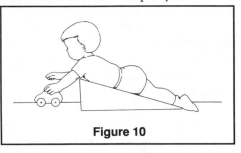

Figure 10

At the same time you are introducing your child to the prone position, you will likely also be working on the *supine* (back-lying) position. Playing while on their backs helps children to develop lower body control. It also gives them an opportunity to bring their hands together in the center of their body (midline)—a good position for manipulating and exploring objects. As in all positions, correct body alignment in supine is especially important for children with cerebral palsy because it is the key to efficient movement. It is necessary to take care not to exaggerate abnormal tonal patterns. If your child has mostly high tone, placing a small pillow or neck roll under his neck can help to reduce muscle tone. Flexing one or both knees while your child is lying on his back can also help to relax his body. (See figure 3.) Finally, for children with cerebral palsy who are totally extended and need more *flexion* in their muscles, a hammock is often helpful in encouraging a good supine position. (See figure 11.)

Besides front and back lying, another good position for many children with cerebral palsy is side lying. Like the supine position, it provides opportunities for developing hands-to-midline skills. Because your child's whole weight rests on an elongated area, he also receives good input from senses such as touch. In addition, children who cannot lift their heads to see what is going on around them while in a prone position have better opportunities to use their vision in a side-lying position. You can maintain your child in a side-lying position by placing sandbags on either side of him or by propping him with sandbags against a firm surface such as a wall or the back of a couch. Commercially built side lyers are also available. Whatever method you use, always be sure to alternate sides to give input to both sides of your child's body. (See figure 12.)

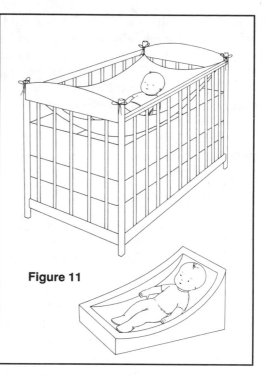

Figure 11

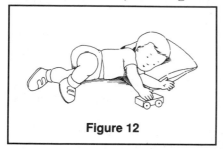

Figure 12

Once your child has some ability to keep his back extended and some head control (or a seating system that provides that control), you should begin working on sitting. It is from the seated position that children do most of their early play and exploration of objects, as well as learn self-help skills such as feeding, dressing, and bathing.

Although children who are developing normally usually learn to sit between seven and nine months of age, the age at which children with cerebral palsy are ready to sit varies widely. Children with cerebral palsy often have difficulty sitting because of their abnormal distribution of muscle tone, poor dissociation of body parts, and persistent primitive reflexes. If your child has trouble sitting, there are many commercially available infant seats and slings that can support him in a semi-reclined sitting position. Often, however, you will need to add rolled towels, foam pieces, or stuffed toys to correct your child's alignment. For more upright sitting on the floor or in a chair, a variety of specialized chairs can be purchased or constructed. The following section discusses these types of equipment, as well as equipment that can help support your child in a more upright or standing position.

Equipment

Many parents find their first purchase of a piece of "adaptive" or "special" equipment very difficult. It is a public statement that their child has a disability requiring specialized equipment. But special equipment can often help a child participate in life in some way that was not previously possible. Frequently a child has the ability to progress to a higher level of cognitive or social learning or play, but can be blocked from this progress by his movement problems. For example, a child may have the cognitive skills to use a communication board, but may be unable to sit in the upright position required for optimal hand use. This is when adaptive equipment can be just the catalyst needed to reach the next step of development.

Most parents are able to ease their way into the world of specialized equipment gradually. This is because much regular baby equipment can be adapted for the special needs of a child with cerebral palsy. For example, since even normally developing children are unable to sit independently much before nine months or walk before twelve to fourteen months, equipment that provides postural support or mobility for "normal" babies is readily available.

In fact, it is often the most practical and cost-effective strategy to use regular baby equipment as long as it fits your child properly and gives him the necessary support. The difficulty with equipment like this comes as your child grows and regular baby equipment is too small or does not offer the postural control your child needs. When this happens, you must ask yourself whether your child would benefit sufficiently by the addition of a piece of specialized equipment. A good guideline to follow is that if your child can achieve a position or skill with your help, it may be time to buy a piece of equipment that will allow him to expand on that skill independently. For example, if your child can sit with help, you might buy a corner chair equipped with a tray so that he can sit with total support and use his hands to play with blocks, draw, and eat. Several companies now make attractive, high-quality equipment for children with special needs. Most equipment can be used for several purposes—for example, a good floor sitter can also be used as a feeding chair and possibly also as an insert in a stroller.

In selecting or adapting both regular and special equipment for your child, keep several points in mind. First, *always choose equipment in consultation with your child's physical or occupational therapist.* Not only can therapists advise you what to consider when purchasing equipment, but they can also help you make minor adaptations to the equipment to give optimal positioning. For example, sometimes just a strategically placed, rolled towel alongside a child's trunk in an adapted chair can prevent an assymetrical position, or a non-skid surface on a chair can maintain the pelvis in a proper position, making the difference between useability and nonuseability. Secondly, always look for the simplest, least adapted piece of equipment that will benefit your child. For example, if your child has head control, he does not need a chair equipped with head support. Besides the obvious economic reason, there are several other reasons for this: 1) If something is over-adapted (provides too much assistance), your child will not have the opportunity to use the control he has or to learn more control. 2) There is no reason to make your child look more handicapped than necessary.

Before purchasing or securing any equipment, you may find it very helpful to talk with parents of children with similar needs. You can often benefit from their experiences. You should also consider these questions: How long will your child need the equipment? Will the piece of equipment need to be transported often? If so, is it lightweight and easy to handle? Consider looks, comfort, safety, and ease of care. Remember, too, that special equipment can be very expensive. Some equipment is covered by insurance, but you should always check on this before ordering. For equipment that your child may need for only a limited period of time, you may want to consider rental rather than purchase. In many areas of the country there are equipment exchanges that are often affiliated with schools or local United Cerebral Palsy or Easter Seal chapters. Remember, too, that you can sometimes make adaptations yourself at considerable savings. Foam, plywood, tri-wall cardboard, and non-skid materials are usually available locally at hardware or upholstery stores. You can also ask your child's therapists for sources.

The following are some of the more common types of equipment you may encounter. The list of Special Equipment Suppliers at the back of this book includes suppliers of these and other types of pediatric special-needs equipment.

Positioning Equipment

Adaptive Chair. (fig. 13) An adaptive chair positions the child optimally so that his feet, knees, and hips are correctly aligned at 90–degree angles. Adaptive chairs are provided with trays or fit up to a small table. Because these chairs are used for feeding and fine motor play, they should provide full support and control.

Corner Chair. (fig. 14) This chair provides back support in a sitting position. Its corner position keeps the child's shoulders forward and head optimally positioned, preventing the neck from over extending (hyperextending) and the shoulders from pulling too far back (retracting). Trays or tables are available to fit most corner chairs.

Floor Sitter. (fig. 15) A floor sitter provides the support a child needs to sit on the floor. The equipment can be as minimal as a back support or as complex as a complete semi-reclined sitting system.

Hammock. (fig. 11) A hammock consists of a length of fabric or netting suspended within a crib or a free-standing frame. Hammocks provide a more flexed resting position for children with high tone.

Prone Board. (fig. 16) These boards support a child in an upright position in which he needs very little control because his body weight is on a prone surface. Boards provide a good position to work on head control with the assistance of gravity. Because the child's leg bones bear some of his weight in this position, prone boards may also help minimize bone loss caused by disuse.

Side Lyer. (fig. 17) As explained earlier, side lyers provide weight bearing on one side of the body and place the child in an optimal position to bring his hands together in midline and watch what is going on around him.

Standing Frame or Box. (fig. 18) Standing frames or boxes support the child in a standing position or maintain a position without dependence on a child's balance.

Wedge. (fig. 10) Wedges are wedge-shaped platforms constructed of foam, wood, or other materials. When a child is placed prone on a wedge with his head uppermost, he is able to work on head control and also weight bearing on the hands and arms.

Movement (Mobility) Equipment

Crutches. (fig. 19) Crutches are used as aids to walking, sometimes in combination with leg braces. The type of crutch children with cerebral palsy most commonly use is the Loftstrand Crutch, which has an arm cuff, handle, and upright metal pole. Most frequently children with cerebral palsy begin to walk with the aid of a walker and then progress to crutches if feasible or necessary.

Strollers, Travel Chairs. (fig. 20) These can be any of a variety of wheeled chairs used to transport a child. Standard, "off-the-shelf" strollers or travel chairs are sometimes appropriate for children with cerebral palsy, but chairs built with special supports for children with motor problems are also available.

Tricycles. (fig. 21) Tricycles are three-wheeled, pedaled vehicles that can be adapted to accommodate motor problems. For example, tricycles can be fitted with pedal straps to help children keep their feet on the pedals, back supports to help them maintain their trunks upright, and adductor wedges to help them get their legs apart to relax tone and enable them to pedal.

Walker. (fig. 22) A walker is a light metal frame used for support in walking. Frames may be constructed either so they provide support in front of the child (forward push walker) or behind him (reverse or posterior walker).

Wheelchair. (fig. 23) A wheelchair is a chair mounted on large wheels. Wheelchairs come in a variety of styles and sizes and can be operated by hand or electronically. Often they must be used with seating inserts to ensure proper positioning.

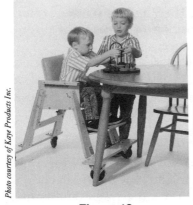

Photo courtesy of Kaye Products Inc.

Figure 13

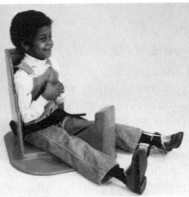

Corner Chair is provided exclusively by J.A. Preston © 1990 Bissell Healthcare Corporation and authorized Preston dealers.

Figure 14

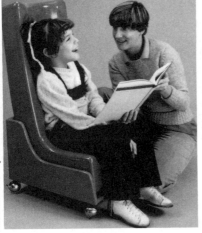

Mobile Floor Sitter is provided exclusively by J.A. Preston © 1990 Bissell Healthcare Corporation and authorized Preston dealers.

Figure 15

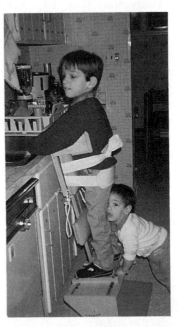

Figure 16

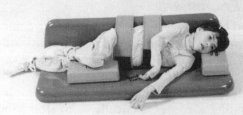

Side Lyer is provided exclusively by J.A. Preston © 1990 Bissell Healthcare Corporation and authorized Preston dealers.

Figure 17

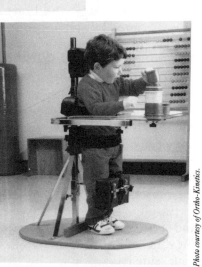

Photo courtesy of Ortho-Kinetics.

Figure 18

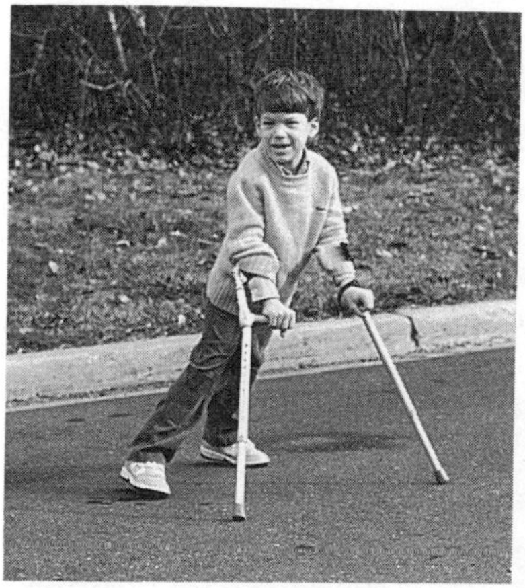

Figure 19

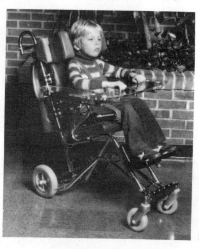

Photo courtesy of Ortho-Kinetics.

Figure 20

Communication Equipment

Communication Boards. The simplest form of a communication device is a communication board—a posterboard, plastic, or wooden board which has pictures or symbols arranged on it. A child can use the board by pointing with his hand or gazing with his eyes.

Electronic Communication Devices. More complex communication devices include electronically activated voice synthesizers which enable children to "talk" or print out what they want to say. Chapter 7 discusses communication devices in more detail.

Miscellaneous Equipment

Adaptive Switches. Adaptive switches enable children with limited movement ability to operate electric, electronic, and battery-operated toys or devices. Switches can be designed so that they require only a very imprecise pressing or swiping motion to activate a toy or to control a light, thermostat, TV, or other device. One of the major benefits of adaptive switches is that they allow even children with severe movement problems to experience cause-and-effect reactions.

Sandbags. (fig. 9A) Sandbags are fabric pouches filled with sand or rice and connected in saddlebag fashion by a length of fabric. They are often used to stabilize children with cerebral palsy in prone, side lying, or other difficult positions.

Helmets. (fig. 24) Helmets made of lightweight materials such as leather and plastic are sometimes used for head protection when a child has seizures or is first beginning to walk.

Vests. (fig. 25) Vests or straps are used to provide external support for trunk control and are often used in combination with seating systems or chairs.

Balls and Rolls. (fig. 26) Balls and rolls are therapy tools used in improving movement and balance reactions.

Benches. (fig. 27) Benches are therapy tools used for positioning and for improving movement.

Play Gym or Suspension System. (fig. 28) Play gyms are used to position toys within easy reach of a child and eliminate the frustration of dropping or losing the toy. They are available in most child furnishings or toy stores.

Feeding and Oral Motor Equipment

Cut-out Cup. (fig. 29) A cut-out cup is a soft plastic cup with a semi-circle cut out of one side. Cut-out cups make it easier for parents to monitor liquid intake and let children drink without overextending their necks. They are available commercially or can be made by cutting a soft Tupperware cup with scissors and then sealing the cut edge by quickly running it through a gas flame.

Adapted Silverware. Utensils with custom-made handles or bends to fit a child's unique hand use are available from baby stores or catalogs, or can be custom designed by your child's occupational therapist, physical therapist, or speech-language pathologist.

Oral Stimulators, Mouth Toys, and Toothbrushes. These objects provide sensory input inside and around a child's mouth and are used to help children who are over- or under-sensitive to touch. Believe it or not, pet stores are often an excellent source of soft, durable mouth toys. To clean mouth toys and toothbrushes, try washing them in the dishwasher with regular dishwashing detergent.

Exercise

If you watch a baby who is developing normally, you will see that he is seldom still; his arms and legs are in almost continuous motion. As he rolls, crawls, and gets into and out of sitting positions, he is exercising without making a conscious effort.

For babies with cerebral palsy, this kind of spontaneous exercise is usually limited. Because they may be capable of only a few movements, babies with cerebral palsy are often relatively inactive. But exercise is crucial for children with cerebral palsy. Movement through all ranges of motion can prevent contractures or joint limitations, thereby helping a child's body maintain its potential. Weight-bearing exercises can prevent bone loss. And the sensory and motor input that exercise provides is an essential building block for future development of cognitive skills.

As the parent of a child with cerebral palsy, it will be important for you to make sure your child gets all the exercise he needs. Consequently, if your child is passive and content to lie back and

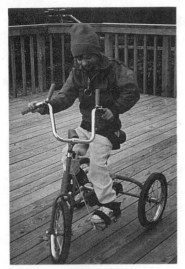

Figure 21

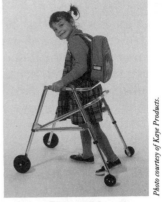

Figure 22

Photo courtesy of Kaye Products.

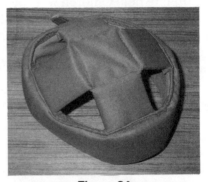

Figure 24

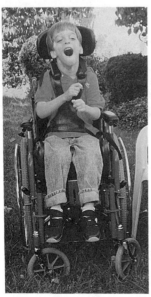

Figure 23

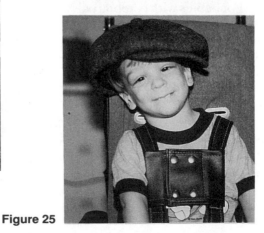

Figure 25

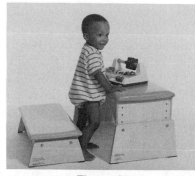

Photo courtesy of Kaye Products.

Figure 27

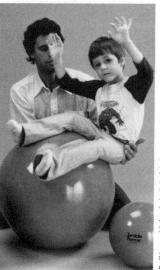

Ball is provided exclusively by J.A. Preston © 1990 Bissell Healthcare Corporation and authorized Preston dealers.

Figure 26

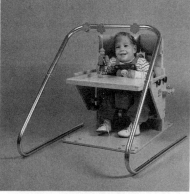

Photo courtesy of Kaye Products.

Figure 28

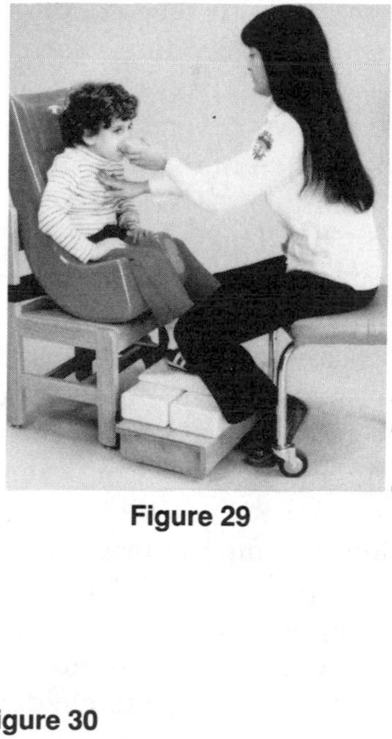

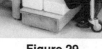

Cut-out Cup is provided exclusively by J.A. Preston © 1990 Bissell Healthcare Corporation and authorized Preston dealers.

Figure 29

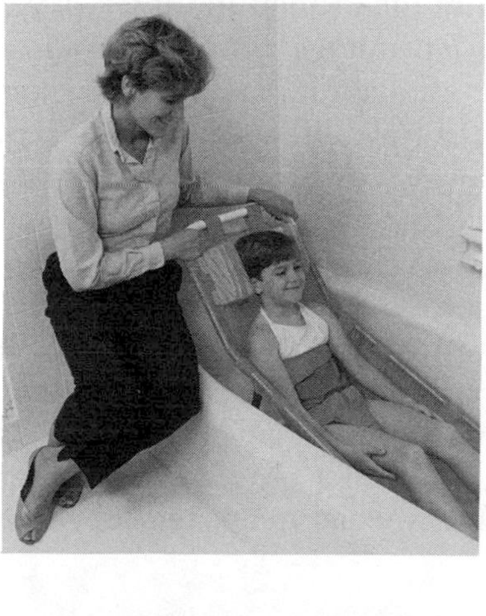

Photo courtesy of Ortho-Kinetics.

Figure 30

watch the world around him, you may need to impose movement upon him.

For young children with cerebral palsy, one of the best ways to encourage movement is through the roughhouse play that other children instinctively make a part of their regular exercise. The touch and movement input that is so much a part of this type of play is essential to the development of normal *tactile* (touch) and *vestibular* (response to movement) systems. Furthermore, your child will *enjoy* roughhousing, so long as you keep in mind the principles of good handling and pay attention to your child's body. For example, if throwing your child up in the air makes him stiff as a board, think of another, slower activity, involving some trunk rotation and leg dissociation (separation) to reduce your child's tone. A good alternative might be the human merry-go-round, in which you hold your child face-to-face with his legs straddling your waist and twirl around. Try to remember that children with low tone generally respond well to fast movements, while children with high tone respond better to a slower pace. Also remember that your child won't break, so don't be afraid to handle him.

Ideally, you will want to make your child's exercise a part of your daily routine by incorporating it into such activities as diapering, dressing, and feeding your child. Your child's occupational and physical therapists can give you specific tips on how to do this, but here are two general guidelines: 1) Place objects far enough away from your child that he needs to reach for them or crawl to them. For example, if you are working a puzzle with your child, don't simply hand him the pieces. Let him pick them up (or try to pick them up) from the table or tray. 2) Encourage your child to do all the physical activities he is capable of, even if it sometimes seems easier for you to do them. For example, if your child has the movement skills to put his blocks away in his toy chest but takes a very long time to do it, try not to get impatient and do it for him.

In addition to fitting exercise into their child's daily routine, some parents of children with cerebral palsy also enroll their children in formal physical fitness programs. Gym classes, movement experiences, and other programs for young children are blossoming, and many are quite receptive to children with special needs. It is not absolutely essential that you find a program with a staff trained in dealing with children with special needs, although you will want to have the help and cooperation of the instructor. Generally, it will be up to you to apply the correct principles of reducing or increasing muscle tone and encouraging normal movement as you assist your child. Your physical or occupational therapist can tell you whether your child might benefit from any program you are considering.

As your child grows older, it becomes increasingly important for his exercise routine to include outdoor activities. Walks in the stroller or in a backpack are good ways to provide opportunities for fresh air and learning about the world outside the house. Just spending time lying or sitting on the grass while parents do yard work can be a very special event. Birds, trees, flowers, and outdoor smells and sounds are all food for developing sensory systems. Your child may also enjoy rides on the back of your bicycle if you take the proper precautions. Because your child may make involuntary movements when riding on a bicycle or may shift his weight in ways that make it hard for you to keep your balance, always make sure that your child wears a helmet and that his seat provides him maximum support.

You may have to be a bit creative to think of outdoor play activities that are within your child's motor abilities. But since playing outdoors is the most enjoyable form of exercise for many children, the more activities you can come up with, the better. Often you can adapt indoor activities to the outdoors. For example, just crawling around outside can be exercise and especially fun if it is combined with a game of hide and seek. For children who are new walkers, pulling a wagon can be fun and can encourage walking backwards. Using a walker outside can be a new challenge; learning to maneuver a wheelchair outdoors enables a child to be at the same height as other children and to have the mobility to play with them.

Other new and pleasurable challenges for children of all levels abound in playgrounds. Riding a specially adapted tricycle can also be very exciting and provides excellent exercise. An outdoor activity that can benefit almost any child with cerebral palsy is swimming. Not only can swimming give children a freedom of movement they don't have on land, but it can also help improve respiratory ability. It is important to note that cold water can increase muscle tone, but warm water often has a relaxing effect and helps reduce muscle tone. This means you should look for a pool with a water temperature best suited to your child's tone. Other activities you may want to investigate once your child reaches school age include

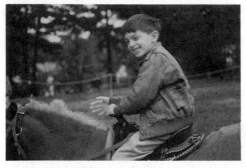

therapeutic horseback riding and Special Olympics.

As with many aspects of raising a child with cerebral palsy, much trial and error is involved in finding enjoyable exercises that are right for your child. Like any child, your child will have likes and dislikes when it comes to certain types of exercises. It is important to respect these feelings as much as possible so that your child comes to see exercise as a natural, enjoyable part of life, not a chore. Remember, fresh air and exercise are important for everyone, and if your child values them when he is young, he will likely value them for a lifetime.

Feeding and Nutrition

Feeding is a problem for many babies and children with cerebral palsy. For some children, the problem is a medical one. Some children, for example, are more likely to choke on food because they have no gag response. If your child has trouble feeding, you should naturally rule out all possible medical reasons before proceeding further.

If a medical examination fails to turn up any condition that would make feeding difficult for your child, the next step is to analyze your child's problems in the feeding process. In most instances, early difficulties with feeding will turn out to be related to problems with either movement or touch, or both.

Movement problems that can complicate feeding for children with cerebral palsy include problems with jaw control and with tongue, lip, and cheek mobility. These movement problems can usually be traced to problems with muscle tone—either too much or too little. To bring your child's feeding problems under control, you must therefore help him bring his muscle tone problems under control. Through your holding or positioning style, you should try to normalize your child's tone before beginning the feeding process, and to maintain it until you are through. If your child still has trouble controlling his jaw or closing his lips, you may have to provide some external support. For instance, you may need to use your hand to support your child's head or to help him close his jaws. As Chapter 7 discusses, a speech-language pathologist or an occupational therapist can help you customize these techniques for your child.

In addition to problems with movement, children with cerebral palsy sometimes have sensory problems that make feeding difficult. Some children, for instance, are overly sensitive to touch in and around the face and mouth. They find the touch of food, a nipple, a spoon, or even a hand unpleasant and may react to touch around the mouth by biting down, turning away, refusing to open their mouth, or even vomiting. This overreaction to touch around the mouth is referred to as *oral tactile defensiveness.* The condition may be so severe that it makes any attempts at feeding unpleasant and sometimes impossible, or it may be so mild that a child only rejects foods that combine more than one texture—for example, yogurt with chunks of fruit.

Some children with cerebral palsy have a feeding problem that is the opposite of oral tactile defensiveness. Instead of overreacting to touch around the face and mouth, they under react. Because they do not have adequate feeling in their mouth, it is hard for them to know how much food is in their mouth, where it is, or how to move it around their mouth and when to swallow. Children who have a mild form of this condition often do not know or feel when their chin is wet from drooling or that there is food in their mouth or on their chin.

A child who overreacts or under-reacts to touch can improve feeding skills through a careful program of *controlled oral motor input*—that is, through a program that gradually desensitizes or sensitizes him to touch in and around his mouth. If your child is oversensitive to touch, it is best to begin touching him (with your hand or a toy) outside the mouth and slowly work up to touching him inside the mouth. Remember that firm pressure is more acceptable to your child than light touch. If your child will not accept your hand, you may want to guide his hand to do the stimulation. If your child is under-responsive to touch, you will want to bombard him with input from different types of touch and texture. An occupa-

Age	Food	Feeding Style/Positioning
0–4 mo.	• Breast milk or formula	• Child held by parent or caretaker in semi-reclined position
4–6 mo.	• Breast milk or formula • Smooth solids (strained or pureed foods)	• Child held by parent or caretaker in more upright manner • Child fed with feeder spoon (small, narrow spoon with long handle)
8 mo.	• Breast milk or formula • Finger foods (baby cookies, crackers) • Lumpy solids (ground junior foods or mashed foods)	• Child seated in high chair or other feeder chair • Given choice of bottle so child can hold independently • Cup drinking introduced
12 mo.	• Milk • Meat sticks, fruit, vegetables • Coarsely chopped table food	• Child seated in high chair, or other feeder chair • Child is now active participant in feeding process • Uses fingers to feed and is introduced to spoon feeding (child-sized spoon) • Drinks mealtime liquid from cup
18 mo.	• Coarsely chopped table food • Most meats	• Child seated in high chair or youth chair at table • Independent spoon feeding (messy) • Drinks all liquid from cup

tional therapist or speech-language pathologist can show you how to use different food temperatures and textures to increase your child's awareness of what is in his mouth. You may also find that placing a mirror in front of your child during mealtimes helps his feeding skills.

Whether or not your child has the movement or sensory problems described above, he may have other problems that make independent feeding harder for him than for other children. For example, he may have trouble grasping a utensil or controlling his arm movements from the shoulder. If so, you may want to consider adaptive handles on his utensils. A nonslip placemat can help keep dishes in place, and special plates and bowls with suction cups are available through special equipment suppliers. For some children, drinking from a straw may be much easier than holding a cup or glass.

Your child's behavior at mealtimes can also complicate feeding problems. To keep behavior problems to a minimum, carefully analyze your child's strengths and weaknesses in feeding. Then provide the optimal in positioning and external support, feeding utensils, and choice of food. Try also to create a distraction-free, relaxing environment so that your child can focus his full attention on eating. For example, carefully chosen background music makes mealtime easier for many children. Remember, too, to let your child feel like an active participant in the feeding process. He needs to have some control even if he is unable to be physically independent in his feeding. You could, for example, let your child decide which food he wants when. You can offer him choices of two foods, or food and drink, and let him indicate his choice any way he can. Finally, don't forget that mealtime is an excellent time for socialization and communication. Perhaps your child's feeding needs are too complex to deal with when you are eating, but you can feed him before or after family mealtime and still let him join you when you eat.

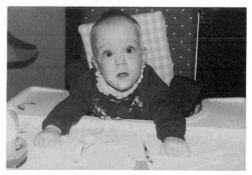

No matter what kind of feeding difficulties your child has, you will want to progress to new stages of food and feeding techniques as your child is ready for them. The chart on the previous page gives nutritional intake and stages of feeding development for children who are developing normally. Use these guidelines as a reference point, keeping your child's developmental age in mind.

The feeding chart specifies only types of foods, not amounts. But if amounts were specified, you would likely find that your child's caloric needs differ from other children's. Because of feeding problems, many children with cerebral palsy have problems gaining weight. In addition, children with high muscle tone burn calories at a higher rate than others do. As a result, you may need to find ways to supplement your child's diet and improve his growth rate. If your child has low tone, he may have a tendency to gain weight more easily. In this case, you will need to carefully monitor his caloric intake.

The goal in supplementing diets is to add calories without adding bulk (roughage) or empty calories to the diet. Supplemental calories should come from protein, fats, and unrefined carbohydrates. For example, you can add nutrients and calories to your child's diet with sprinklings of powdered milk, ground nuts, and cheese. There are also many infant formulas designed to give a high caloric, balanced diet, as well as supplements to increase calories. In addition, underweight children with cerebral palsy sometimes benefit from more frequent mini-meals rather than the usual three meals a day. Your child's pediatrician, speech-language pathologist, and nutritionist can advise you on these and other ways of increasing or enhancing your child's nutrition.

Dental Care

Growing up with healthy teeth and gums is just as important for your child as it is for any other child. It is also a goal that is just as attainable for your child, provided you make preventive dental care a part of his daily routine.

A good program of oral and dental care should begin early. Even before your child gets any teeth, you can use a child's toothbrush or your finger to massage and stimulate his gums. This will keep the gums healthy and prepare your child for later toothbrushing. Once teeth erupt—usually beginning around six months of age—you should clean them regularly. You can do this with a washcloth wrapped around your finger or with a small soft toothbrush and a small amount of toothpaste (not essential). In addition to cleaning the outer surfaces of your child's teeth by brushing, it is also important to clean the surfaces between the teeth with dental floss. Many parents find flossing easier if they use a floss holder. If your child has oral tactile defensiveness, see the previous section for tips on desensitizing his mouth.

When your child is young, you may find it simplest to clean his teeth while he is lying across your lap on his back. This not only makes it easier to keep him still, but also gives you a better view of his mouth. Usually it is enough to clean your child's teeth thoroughly once a day—preferably in the evening so your child does not go to bed with food particles on his teeth.

A hazard you should know about if your child is still nursing is the "nursing bottle syndrome." Nursing bottle syndrome refers to the very early rapid decay of teeth that sometimes occurs when children are given a bottle at bed- or nap-time. To avoid this problem, never let your child fall asleep with a bottle in his mouth.

Once your child has the motor skills to begin brushing his own teeth, you may need to get him a toothbrush with an adapted handle to help him maintain his grasp. Remember, too, that electric toothbrushes can provide some of the finer movements your child cannot do himself.

When your child is two or three, you should take him to the dentist for his first formal check-up and cleaning. Your dentist can suggest ways to improve your dental care program and also provide you with additional preventive strategies—for example, by applying plastic sealant to your child's teeth to make them more resistant to cavities. How you choose your dentist will likely depend on the severity of your child's handicap. A regular pediatric dentist who has the experience and equipment to work with young children might be right for your child. Or you may want to inquire around to find a dentist who has had special training in working with children with disabilities. Some major hospitals and medical centers maintain dental clinics for people with physical or mental handicaps. You can also contact the National Foundation of Dentistry for the Handicapped for names of qualified dentists in your area. See the Resource Guide for the Foundation's address.

Bathing

Bathing your child can and should be fun, a special time for both of you. Because bathtime is time-consuming, it is an ideal opportunity to do more than just get your child clean. It is a natural time to work on many of your child's self-help, motor, language, and cognitive goals in an interesting, different kind of setting.

Just as in bathing any child, the first item on the agenda is safety. For bathtime to be a success, you need to position your child in a way that normalizes his muscle tone as much as possible (see the previous discussion on positioning). You should also try to give your child a sense of security, rather than challenge his sense of balance. Many popularly marketed bath seats can provide your child the security he needs while giving you an extra pair of hands in the tub. You may also find a semi-inflated inner tube (from a compact car, or a swimming tube) helpful as a positioning device. If your child cannot maintain a sitting position, he may be more comfortable in a semi-reclined bath seat, which again is held in place with suction cups. Several such chairs are available through the special equipment suppliers listed in the back of the book. (See figure 30.) Finally, a bath sponge wedge can be used to bathe an infant in both sitting and lying positions. When using most of these positioning devices, you will need to keep the water level low and to pour or swish the water over your child to rinse him.

As your child gets bigger and heavier, you may need to rent or purchase one of the variety of bath chairs and hydraulic lifts available from special equipment suppliers. Some older children enjoy showering in a kneeling or sitting position. A shower sprayer on a long hose is handy for this purpose. Again, use the principles of good positioning for your child. You may also want to add grab bars or nonskid strips to the shower stall or tub to make it safer for your child. *Remember that no child, with or without disabilities, should ever be left unattended in a bathtub or shower.*

In devising ways to make bathtime a learning experience, think first about the process of undressing. If your child has the movement skills, bathtime is a natural time for him to begin independent undressing. It is also a great opportunity to quickly run through those range-of-motion exercises your physical or occupational therapist has suggested. As you do these routines, think about all the words and concepts it is natural to introduce to your child—for example, arm in, out, through; tub full, empty, slippery; water wet, warm, cold. If your child is around the developmental age of twelve to eighteen months, this would also be a wonderful time to work on the names of body parts.

In the bath, your child has many opportunities to learn cause-and-effect relationships, spatial relationships, wrist rotation, and tolerance of different sensations. And while your child is busy learning to float the duck, grab the soap, squirt the squeeze toy, dump and fill the cups, or paint the tiles with crazy foam, he may not even notice that he is also getting clean.

The time immediately following a bath can also be very productive. For example, a brisk rub with a terry towel can help your child learn to process sensations and can lead to better body awareness. And if your child is ready, pajamas are ideal for beginning to learn self-dressing skills. In any event, the period following bathtime is an excellent time to focus on calming activities such as a back rub, massage, or use of powder or lotion, and on using and understanding language.

For most children with cerebral palsy, bathing in a secure warm tub is calming, relaxing, and conducive to a successful bedtime. But for some children, bathtime has the opposite effect, and really stimulates and excites them. If your child reacts this way, you probably will not want to bathe him immediately before bed- or nap-time. Instead, you may want to schedule baths just before times when you want your child to be awake and alert.

Dressing

For most children, learning to dress and undress is a major step toward independence. Depending on the degree of your child's motor problems, independent dressing may or may not be a realistic goal. If your child has the motor skills, you will want to do everything possible to help him achieve the goal; if he has the desire and understanding without the skills, you will want to help him participate as fully as possible in the process.

Proper positioning is critical to success in the dressing process. Children with cerebral palsy usually find dressing easier when seated on a low bench or chair. If your child doesn't have the head and trunk control for this position, you may need to seat him on your lap.

Generally, you should work with your child on undressing first, as it is an easier skill than dressing. Many children find taking off socks the easiest skill of all. If you begin with socks, you may need to help your child by pulling the sock almost off and then let him have the final success of tugging it off. As soon as your child is able to accomplish one step in the dressing process, gradually reduce your help.

If your child cannot take off his clothes himself, encourage him to help any way that he can. For example, ask him to raise his arm as you pull off his shirt sleeve or to shift his weight so you can take his pants off more easily. If your child's movement skills are quite limited, you might ask him to look towards the appropriate clothing item when you ask, "What comes next?"

To make dressing as simple as possible for your child, you should put some thought into the clothing you buy. Some companies specialize in designing clothing for people with disabilities, and offer clothes that make dressing and undressing easier. The list of Special Equipment Suppliers at the back of the book includes names and addresses for several of these companies. You can also make dressing easier for your child if you buy clothes a little bit big and look for fabrics such as knits that have some flexibility. When shopping, bear in mind that zippers are easier than buttons, front openings are preferable to back openings, jackets with slippery linings slide on easier, and Velcro closures on shoes are more manageable than laces. Finally, always remember to let your child have some say in what he wears. Even if your child cannot dress himself, you should at least give him a choice of styles and colors.

It is so important to foster the desire for independence if it is realistic, and, if not, to make your child an active participant rather than a passive observer in his care. As your child strives for autonomy and independence in the "me do it" stage, you have a natural window of opportunity. If you miss this opportunity, your child may develop an attitude of learned helplessness, which hinders the development of self-esteem. So even when it seems like it would be easier and much more time efficient just to do something for your child, give him the encouragement and opportunity to try.

Toilet Training

When your child is ready to be toilet trained, you will know it. Like any child, he will give you certain unmistakable indications that he is physiologically mature enough to handle independent toileting. These indications include remaining dry for several hours at a time and being aware that his diaper is wet or soiled. No child who shows these signs of readiness for toilet training should be denied the chance to reach this milestone in independence.

To help your child achieve this goal, you will need to find a potty chair that offers support for your child's body and positions him in a way that minimizes abnormal muscle tone. It is critical that his feet touch the floor, not only for positioning reasons, but also to make it easier for your child to push with his abdominal muscles. Many of the chairs available for nonhandicapped children can be adapted to meet the needs of children with cerebral palsy. Special equipment suppliers also offer a variety of chairs for children of all ages and disabilities. Usually the insert seats that fit onto a regular toilet seat are not acceptable because they do not offer adequate support and stability. But depending on your child's disability, an insert may be effective if it has side supports and fits securely and tightly to the toilet seat.

If your first attempts at toilet training fail, wait several months and try again. Many children with cerebral palsy are toilet trained. But remember that developmental age is an important factor in learning this skill. Some children never achieve a developmental age where it is feasible. For them, diapers in larger sizes are available from medical supply stores.

A problem that complicates toilet training for many children with cerebral palsy is constipation. This is often a side-effect of medication, or the result of high or low muscle tone, a low-roughage diet, or a lack of exercise or movement. If dietary changes do not improve your child's constipation, your pediatrician can prescribe several types of medication. These include stool softeners, lubricants, bulk laxatives, and stimulants. For extreme cases of constipation, your child's doctor might recommend an enema. Before using over-the-counter remedies such as suppositories or mineral oil, always check with your pediatrician first. Overuse of laxatives can be dangerous.

Sleep

All parents long for children who are good sleepers. Unfortunately, children are just as likely to be poor sleepers as they are to be good sleepers. Babies with cerebral palsy, like all babies, are born with varying abilities to calm themselves in order to go from alert states to quiet states, and then to sleep. Some can go from state to state quite easily. Others need outside help to make these transitions. For example, a child may need the help of slow, rhythmic rocking, or the firm touch and warmth that comes from being swaddled or held. Music or slow, comforting talking can also be helpful, as can a ride in an automatic baby swing or a stroller.

When your child is very young, he may need these kinds of external assistance often—particularly after a period of hospitalization. The lights, noise, and pain from shots and IVs can all cause a child to be in a continual state of irritability or depression. Even just the lights, smells, and sounds in the home may be overstimulating. If these factors prevent your child's sleep habits from developing as expected, you will need to help him establish a regular sleep-awake cycle and ease his transition to and from sleep. Use the techniques described above to help him fall asleep, then gradually withdraw your assistance as your child learns to calm himself.

At first, your baby will need to sleep many times a day, usually once in every feeding cycle. As your child grows, he will spend more time in an alert-awake state. By about one year of age, your child should be sleeping about twelve hours at night and taking both a morning and afternoon nap. When he no longer needs these nap times, your child will give you clear indications—for instance, by remaining awake all through naptime. Once your child reaches this stage, it is a good idea to set aside some time for quiet play in his room. This gives you a much-needed break and time for some self-organization.

As children get a little older, sleep often becomes an issue of control. If you are sure your child is fed and comfortable, you need to be firm in sticking to bedtime routines. Habits that are hard to break and should therefore never be encouraged include: children sleeping in their parents' bed (you will never get them out!), falling asleep with a bottle (can lead to tooth decay), or falling asleep in front of the TV or in a place other than bed. Helpful bedtime routines include a warm bath, and a story or quiet play time with a parent. (If bathtime excites and arouses your child, you will, of course, not want to give a bath at bedtime.) Bedtime is not a good time for roughhouse play, because your child can quickly work himself up and then have trouble settling down and falling asleep.

Parents of children with cerebral palsy often wonder what kind of bed is best for their children. A crib is a safe place for a young child, and will probably be the best sleeping option for the first two or three years. After this age, you may want to think about a sleeping arrangement that will increase your child's self-esteem and help to foster bedtime independence. If you keep your child in a crib too long, you may be promoting the "baby" image, when your child may actually be at a much older developmental age in all areas but movement development.

When your child graduates from his crib, two issues become a concern: safety and independence. A child should be able to get into and out of his bed independently, if at all possible. Some of the options parents use are a youth bed with rails for safety, a regular bed with portable rails, or a mattress on the floor or in a box frame on the floor. This bed on the floor can actually be a good solution to both the safety and independence issues. As soon as your child can safely crawl into and out of his bed, you should consider a standard bed. Generally speaking, a firm mattress is the best, although some parents find that water beds are good because the warm temperature and gentle movement help their child to relax and reduces excessive muscle tone.

Play

Play is the work or occupation of babies and young children. It is through play that children develop motor coordination and an understanding of cognitive concepts. Play also gives children the chance to interact with others and to develop feelings of self-confidence and competence. But even though it *is* serious business, play should always be fun, spontaneous, voluntary, and done for the pleasure of the process rather than for the end product. In other words, the process of painting should be fun in itself, with the completed picture or adult praise only a byproduct, rather than the reason for painting.

There are three basic types of play: exploratory, manipulative, and imaginative. Exploratory play, the earliest form children engage in, helps children learn about themselves and their world. This play is based on *sensory motor awareness*—that is, on actions or movements made in response to sights, sounds, smells, or touch in the environment. For example, a baby exploring his own body by bringing his hand or foot to his mouth is engaging in exploratory play; so, too, is a child learning what a swing or see-saw does. The second type of play, manipulative play, begins as soon as a child can voluntarily hold an object. As children grasp, reach, and hold objects, they develop eye-hand coordination, visual perception, and hand dexterity. They also learn about size, weight, and spatial relationships. Toys that provide manipulative play include blocks, puzzles, play dough, and crayons. The final type of play, imaginative play, occurs when children use their imaginations to "make believe." Toys that encourage this kind of play include dress-up clothes, toy furniture, cars and trucks, dolls, work benches, and toy telephones.

Your child's readiness and interest level for these three types of play will depend on his cognitive (mental) development, social-emotional maturity, and, of course, his movement skills. If your child has the cognitive and social-emotional skills, he should have help bypassing or making adaptations for lagging motor skills. For example, if your child's problems with head or hand control prevent him from actually building a block tower, he may still enjoy watching you construct the tower—perhaps by choosing the color of each successive block verbally or by eye gaze. If possible, you should let

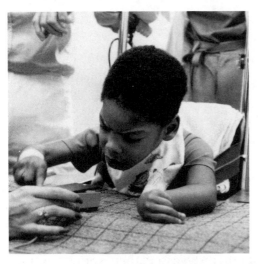

him experiment with making the blocks fall through some body movement. Let your child be the architect of the play situation, while you take the role of laborer.

When your child plays by himself, simple adaptations to toys can often help him overcome motor problems. For example, if your child has some hand control, he may enjoy constructing a tower using magnet blocks or large plastic snap blocks, or you can adapt some wooden blocks for him by gluing Velcro to them. Children with more limited movement can learn and play with the help of a computer. In this age of advanced technology, even children with serious motor problems can activate a switch to turn on a tape recorder or cause the toy piano to play or a mechanical dog to walk and bark.

Toys are the tools of play and they can be as elaborate and expensive as you desire, but often the best toys are simple household objects or throwaways. Pots and pans, measuring spoons and cups, cardboard paper rolls, and cardboard boxes are perennial favorites. When choosing these or any other toys for your child, you should first keep safety and ease of care in mind. Then think of the appeal of the toy, and how many different ways your child can use it. For example, a video game can only be used as a video game, but a truck or a doll can be used in many ways. Finally, it is important to remember your child's developmental age and choose toys for that age level.

Parents often buy toys that are too difficult for their child and beyond his developmental level. If you make this mistake, it may be a good idea to put the toy away until your child shows developmental readiness. For help in choosing toys that *are* appropriate for your child, you can consult your child's teacher or occupational or physical therapist. You may be able to get additional help if you live in one of the many communities that now have toy lending libraries for children with special needs. Usually these libraries not only have a tremendous selection of toys, but also a librarian equipped to guide you in choosing toys for your child. Also see the list of Special Equipment Suppliers at the back of this book for some mail-order sources of toys and adaptive devices.

Babysitters

If your child was hospitalized for an extended period following his birth, it is understandable that you may not feel ready to leave him alone again for some time. Sooner or later, however, all parents need time away from their children, whether their children have cerebral palsy or not. You and your spouse *need* some time together away from the continuous demands of child care. A trip to a movie, dinner with friends, or an outing to a local museum can seem like a mini vacation and offer a much-needed break. Other children in the family also need to have some time out with you and to have experiences that are not always influenced by having a brother or sister with special needs.

Time out means alternate care for your child or children. Some families are fortunate enough to have relatives close by who volunteer to take care of the children from time to time. But many other families must depend on babysitters. If this is the case with you, you need to take care in choosing and training your babysitter. You will want to find a sitter you have confidence in, and then have him or her spend some time getting to know your child while you are at home. This will give you ample opportunities to show the sitter how to handle your child and to familiarize him or her with your routines. Then, once you actually do go out, you should feel relatively comfortable with the sitter's ability to care for your child. For added peace of mind, always leave an emergency number where you can be reached, as well as general emergency information.

To locate babysitters, try getting recommendations from friends whose children also have special needs. Some families are very successful in working out cooperative arrangements in which they trade off babysitting duties with other parents of children with cerebral palsy. If you have met other parents, you may want to ask if they would be interested in such an arrangement. Who would have better skills in caring for a child with cerebral palsy than another set of parents whose child has similar needs? Other good resources include college students (especially nursing or special education students), high school child care programs, parent support groups, and local community organizations such as United Cerebral Palsy, the Association for Retarded Citizens, and Easter Seals.

In some communities, organizations not only maintain lists of qualified sitters, but also offer respite care arrangements. Through UCP, the ARC, and other agencies, you can qualify for several hours to several weeks of child care provided by someone with knowledge of disabilities. This care may be provided in your home, but more often in the respite worker's home. Pay is usually on a sliding scale and availability of care is based on need.

Remember, not only do you need time away from your child, but he needs time away from you. Learning to trust and to interact with other adults is a critical step in every child's development. It will be much easier for both you and your child if you make at least occasional alternative care arrangements when your child is young.

Conclusion

Caring for any young child can be a full-time job. But when you have a child with cerebral palsy, it sometimes seems as if you must work overtime every day just to keep him clean, clothed, and fed. Right now, when talk of high tone and low tone, oral tactile defensiveness, and adaptive equipment still makes your head spin, you may find it hard to believe that your day-to-day life will ever become manageable. But believe me, it will. Doctors, teachers, and therapists can show you efficient, effective ways to look after your child's special needs. More importantly, with time, patience, and persistence, you will master the child-care skills that will enable you once again to make your daily care routine just that—*routine.*

Parent Statements

Finding qualified in-home care for our child wasn't hard for us. It was always just an issue of money.

❧❧❧

Feeding was always a source of anxiety.

❧❧❧

Oddly enough, I've never worried much about her bath. What I did and still do is to lay her on a baby sponge in the tub. She's almost the length of the tub now and I'm considering a bath chair, but keep putting it off. She loves being in the water and I hate to take her out of it that much to be in a chair.

❧❧❧

When I became pregnant again, the doctors said no lifting. Who are they kidding? It's not even practical. I couldn't have done it if my husband didn't do the majority of the lifting.

❧❧❧

I didn't think he would ever be toilet trained. It was more my problem than his. It just took an incredible amount of time and discipline to get him to tell us when he had to go and then carry him down the hall. You can't just say, "Now go to the potty."

)<()(

Positioning wasn't a problem when he was small; now is the hard part.

)<()(

Sometimes I get mad at him. It may be wrong, but sometimes I just would like to say, "Why can't you just do it?" I don't do that, but sometimes I think it. I know he must think it too.

)<()(

Michael took pride in his eating abilities. Once he entered kindergarten, those abilities regressed. We think he's parked at the table and left unsupervised. It makes it hard for us.

)<()(

At first we didn't understand how important correct positioning is. The first stroller we had was the umbrella type. It had a semi-firm bottom and a padded and cardboard-reinforced back, which we thought was good for Caitlyn. She was a year old before she got therapy and that's when we started learning about positioning.

)<()(

The frustration with learning more about positioning is that you find out the market doesn't always have what is best for your child. We've always ended up adapting things even more for Caitlyn.

)<()(

Our therapists were a definite influence on our son's equipment. Initially, I trusted them fully. As I learned more, I began to question their advice or comments and gave some of my own. I researched the markets on equipment and tried to keep up on what was out there. I'd come up with things they had never seen which turned out to be pretty good.

❧❧❧

We never thought toilet training would happen. We tried for probably two to three years. It wasn't totally her fault. Sometimes the routine would be interrupted by an extended vacation and we'd lose the progress we had made.

❧❧❧

Stephen's always had a tremendous amount of patience with himself and others. As he's gotten older, it's gotten shorter, but professionals still tell me it's a lot considering what he goes through to do things.

❧❧❧

Initially, David definitely preferred me to a toy. It was like I was his body. He experienced things through me moving his body. It was almost like if you put the two of us together you had one person. He was totally dependent on me and it was extremely hard to break him from some of that. Teaching him to play by himself was a major job.

❧❧❧

It was very hard finding a sitter the first few years. I was overprotective early on and didn't feel anyone else could watch her. I've loosened up now and it's not as hard. When I find someone willing, I teach them what to do with her. If they feel okay with that, then we try it out. If the sitter, Annie, and I all feel okay with the arrangement, I can go out and not worry at all.

❧❧❧

FIVE

Family Life and Self-Esteem

NANCY S. COWAN, M.A., Ph.D., C.C.C.*

Being a parent is one of the most rewarding jobs around. But it is also one of the toughest, thanks to the unrelenting responsibilities that go along with raising a family. As a parent, you must not only look after your children's never-ending physical needs, but you must look after their emotional needs as well. In particular, it is up to you to foster the self-esteem that helps your children feel lovable and worthwhile.

For most parents, having a child with cerebral palsy makes an already complex job still more demanding. Because cerebral palsy is a *physical* disability, you may need to devote an enormous amount of time and energy to the *physical* aspects of your child's care—to the therapeutic exercises to improve movement, the special diets to enhance nutrition, the positioning of your child and her equipment. But at the same time, you must also try to keep your child's physical needs from becoming the focal point of family life. Remember, your child's emotional well-being is as important as her physical well-being, and the physical and emotional needs of other family members are as vital as your child's. *Everyone* needs to learn

* Nancy S. Cowan holds an M.A. in counseling from the West Virginia College of Graduate Studies and a Ph.D. in human development from the University of Maryland. As a parent educator, she has helped many families adapt to having a child with special needs. Currently, she teaches communication at the Model Secondary School for the Deaf, Gallaudet University, in Washington, D.C.

to see themselves as special, whether or not they have "special" needs.

Balancing everyone's needs can be a tall order, especially in the beginning. But as unbelievable as it may seem now, "normal" family life does not have to end because you have a child with cerebral palsy. By helping family members—and your child—to see cerebral palsy as just one acceptable part of their lives, you can do wonders to build normal family relationships. Your family can be just as well-balanced as any other family, as long as everybody feels good about themselves and each other.

Because accepting cerebral palsy and the difficulties it can bring usually poses different kinds of problems for children with cerebral palsy and their families, this chapter is divided into two parts. Part One discusses ways that having a child with cerebral palsy may complicate family life, and offers strategies to help you and your family adjust to your child over time. Part Two focuses on self-esteem and explains how it can help your child accept her strengths and limitations and achieve her potential in all areas. It then moves on to describe how your family's acceptance and actions can encourage your child to achieve high self-esteem.

PART I: FAMILY LIFE

Your Role as a Parent

How well your family adjusts to having a child with cerebral palsy depends on you, the parent. Children, other family members, and friends all follow the parents' cues. Because the way you view your child affects the way the whole family sees her right from the start, it is vital that you accept your child and her disability as early as possible.

What is acceptance? Marcia Lepler, the mother of a child with cerebral palsy, perhaps sums it up best:

> To me, acceptance means finding whatever
> pleasure I can in caring for [my child] day to day. It
> means looking at other children without always
> wishing that he were like them. It means looking at

the situation not in terms of what [my child] can do for me, but what I can do to enhance his potential. Acceptance means letting him progress at his own rate. It means being proud of him as my son and wanting others to know him. It means not deriving my own self-esteem from his developmental milestones. True acceptance means feeling that we can be a happy family as we once hoped.*

Unfortunately, learning to accept your child's cerebral palsy and to see her as a unique individual instead of someone with a handicap is often a difficult and lengthy process. The excitement parents usually feel at having a beautiful, perfect baby is dimmed. Instead, feelings of disbelief, shock, helplessness, and isolation may well up. These and other emotions can sometimes make it as hard to accept a child's disability as it is to accept a loved one's death. For many parents, paralyzing doubt about their own abilities to care for a special-needs child may complicate acceptance even more.

Emotions That Complicate Acceptance

Many parents react to the initial diagnosis of their child's cerebral palsy by denying there is a problem. They hope it is a bad dream, that it will go away, that it is not true. As Chapter 2 explains, intense anger at the unfairness of the situation may be overwhelming. Strong feelings of guilt, shame, and blame may also be present. Later, as the implications of having a child with a disability sink in, depression, sadness, and fatigue may follow.

The grief that most parents feel is no fleeting emotion, but a "chronic sorrow" that returns again and again as their child grows. Each time their child reaches a major milestone—for example, walking or talking, placement in special education, or the beginning of puberty—parents are reminded that their child is not developing normally and they are forced to work through some of the grief again.

Although grieving makes acceptance harder for most parents in the beginning, how long it continues to do so varies widely. I have

---

* Marcia Lepler, "Having a Handicapped Child," *The American Journal of Maternal Child Nursing*, January/February 1978, 32–33.

seen parents of high school students with cerebral palsy who also have hearing impairments or mental retardation still denying the existence of the disability, still making the rounds of doctors to find a different diagnosis for their child's difficulties, and still maintaining in parent support groups that their child will become "normal." On the other hand, I have seen parents of preschool children come to a clear understanding and acceptance of their child's disability and be able to help other parents through the grieving process. Why do some parents seem to have an easier time with acceptance than others?

Parents who come to terms with their child's disability relatively quickly can usually trace their success to three factors: communication, information, and support. They communicate as honestly and clearly as they can, and share their feelings with their spouse, family, and other parents. They seek information about cerebral palsy and disabilities in general by talking to medical professionals and by reading books and periodicals such as those listed in the Reading List at the back of this book. And they use whatever sources of strength and comfort they have available—support groups, church, meditation, exercise.

As you begin to be able to share your feelings, understand some of the implications of cerebral palsy, and put your role into perspective, your feelings of helplessness will start to give way to feelings of control. True, this may be a slow process with many setbacks. But every positive interaction with the unique and developing person who is your child will bring you closer to acceptance. Once you focus on what your child *can* do—return your smiles, make eye contact, make her needs to be fed or changed known—you will begin to see that your child has a very distinct personality and very definite potential. Even if your child has severe or profound mental retardation, acceptance will open your eyes to miraculous progress—you will see your child learn to respond to voices, to light, or to movement. You may come to appreciate your child's special abilities so well that you may disagree with how professionals rate her on developmental scales.

Chapter 2 discusses where to get the support and information that can help you accept your child when she is first diagnosed; the section on Marriage later in this chapter explores these issues *and* communication in more detail.

Feeling Good about Yourself as a Parent

Most new parents have little or no preparation for the major task of parenthood—guiding and supporting their baby's development. If their baby is healthy and develops normally, parents generally have time to pick up the parenting skills they need as they go along. But if you have a baby with cerebral palsy, you may think this trial-and-error method of parenting is not good enough for your child. You might occasionally doubt your ability to be a good parent, or even begin to question your own self-worth.

Worrisome as it can be, this sudden loss of self-confidence is completely understandable. It is hard *not* to question your abilities when you are being bombarded with child-raising advice from so many medical professionals, each of whom studied for years to learn how to treat one aspect of your child's disability. The very nature of cerebral palsy may sometimes also make you question your competence—no matter how good a parent you actually are. Because cerebral palsy often produces not 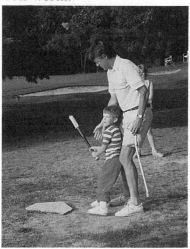 one, but multiple disabilities, each new disability you learn about can make your job seem more complex.

If this is not your first child, you will probably have an easier time adjusting to your role as parent of a child with cerebral palsy. You probably realize you don't have to be a superparent, and that your child is better off if she interacts with a variety of people instead of having Mom and Dad do everything.

If this *is* your first child, you will probably have to cope with the "superparent complex." When new parents bring a baby home from the hospital, most of them seem to think they are the only people in the world who can care for their child. This belief can lead to many problems, especially if you haven't been around other young parents much and don't recognize the normal feelings that come with caring for a child. You may become frustrated and depressed, and feel guilty when things don't always go perfectly—the baby isn't sleeping through the night at six weeks of age, she isn't drinking the amount of milk you heard was normal in your childbirth class, she isn't grasping a rattle and amusing herself at the right age. You may not be willing to leave your baby with a sitter and go out by yourself because something might happen if you aren't there.

Superparent feelings can be compounded if you and your spouse work outside the home. When a mother returns from work, she may feel she has to do everything when she gets home. She may try to give "quality time" to the baby, keep the house clean, cook meals for the family, do the laundry, maintain her relationships with her husband and other children, and get up in the morning to be a superperson at work, as well. Fathers may have many of the same feelings: they try to help out at home, share the care of the baby, and go to work and behave as if their family life has not changed.

Having a baby with cerebral palsy often magnifies feelings that you need to do everything yourself. For example, you may think you are the only one who can get your child to eat or who can position her so she can play comfortably. Fears about the safety and well-being of your child also increase. Even if child care is available, you may be more hesitant to go back to work when you planned, or to go out for an evening or weekend.

There are many ways you can help reduce the stress associated with an addition to the family and make your job as the parent of a special-needs child more manageable. To begin with, try to concentrate on one day at a time and plan for handling short-term situations only. Try to avoid being overwhelmed by vague, global fears about future issues such as independence, school, or your child's impact on your career. You might also try to simplify your lifestyle: for example, by modifying your home so that house cleaning and yard work is easier or by serving simple, potluck meals instead of formal, gourmet dinners when you entertain. Similarly, you can choose family activities that require less preparation time and energy—taking your children on an informal, come-as-you-are picnic instead of dressing everybody up to go to a fancy restaurant. To gain more time for essential child care activities, you might also reduce the frequency with which you eat out, wash the laundry, clean the house, mow the lawn, or do other chores.

If you suffer from the superparent complex, it is a good idea to carefully train someone else as a back-up care provider for your child. It may take some doing to find someone you trust who is willing to take on the responsibility, but it is an important step. You will be able to get your life back to a more normal state once you realize you do not have to do everything yourself. Chapter 4 offers suggestions for finding a reliable baby sitter who can help you make this adjustment.

Coping Together

The key to helping couples survive the diagnosis of cerebral palsy in their child *and* to helping them grow as a couple is, once again, open communication. Both of you must try to express your feelings without guilt and to accept your mate's feelings without judgement. It may help you to share openly if you remember that feelings are just feelings and are neither right nor wrong. It is perfectly normal for your emotions to run the gamut from guilt to anger, love to hate, helplessness to hopefulness. You should also remember that you and your partner will rarely have the same feelings at the same time. For example, one day you may be so discouraged that you find yourself wishing that your child had not survived, while your spouse may be especially hopeful and feel able to cope with whatever comes. Still, if you can recognize that you both have equally valid feelings, you can often give one another the emotional support you need.

Of course, if open communication has not already been a habit in your marriage, it is not automatically going to become one because you have a child with cerebral palsy. If you were lucky, the doctor and hospital social worker helped you to make connections with other parents who could provide initial support and strategies for developing communication skills. If you were not so lucky, you will need to request resources to help you develop those skills.

How easy it is to find the resources you need will vary greatly depending on where you live and what kind of help you are seeking. For years, I worked in metropolitan areas where parents could easily find resources. Generally, if parents contacted a doctor, therapist, school, social worker, county mental health service, or pastoral counseling service, they would eventually find the assistance they needed. Then I moved to a more remote area where very few children had the same disability. Imagine my shock and frustration when I realized how hard it was for parents to find help. In more rural areas, finding another parent of a child with cerebral palsy can be almost impossible, and even if you do find one, distance and transportation problems may prevent face-to-face meetings.

If you live in an isolated area, phone conversations, letters to and from other parents, or computer networks such as Specialnet may be the best support available to you. Rather than relying on local organizations, you may need to contact state or national organizations such as the National Information Center for Children and Youth with Handicaps (NICHCY), United Cerebral Palsy, State Department of Education, Crippled Children's Services, State Mental Retardation Agencies, and State Developmental Disabilities Agencies listed in the Resource Guide. Local universities with special education departments may also offer parent support programs.

Some parents find it easier to begin sharing feelings with support groups made up of members of their own sex before they are ready to share with their partners. Many times mothers discuss feelings with other mothers that they wish they could discuss with their husbands, but are not yet able to. This is a common concern I hear in support groups. It is always exciting when a mother makes a breakthrough and comes back to the group to share her delight in discovering that her husband not only accepts her feelings, but is anxious to share his own with her.

Until recently, it was harder for fathers to make the same kinds of communication breakthroughs because there weren't that many support groups just for men. Fortunately, more and more support programs are now being provided for fathers. You can contact any of the resources mentioned above for help finding the nearest father's group in your area. These organizations can also help you and other interested fathers start your own group. Your school district, too, may agree to provide the services of a social worker, psychologist, or parent liaison person as part of the Individualized Family Service Plan (IFSP) written for your child under P.L. 99–457. This professional could help organize a father support group.

Sometimes, even with the help of support groups, spouses have trouble expressing their feelings to one another. Some people are naturally more cognitive in their approach to problems and may find the idea of sharing their feelings difficult, frightening, or a silly, non-productive use of time. If you feel this way, "bibliotherapy"—

reading everything related to cerebral palsy you can lay your hands on—may help you accept your child and understand the implications for your marriage and family. Audiotapes for use in developing self-esteem, improving communication skills, and dealing with stress are also available. Keeping a journal about what happens and how you feel is also helpful to some parents, especially in the early stages of diagnosis. Sometimes parents say they feel so isolated at this time. But as they write, they can put things more into perspective, think of questions to ask the doctor, and go back and reread portions of their journal and see progress in their understanding, acceptance, and ability to discuss their feelings. Eventually, they can begin to share their feelings with their mate.

Take Positive Steps

Learning how to share your feelings is an important first step in opening up the lines of communication, but it is not the be-all and end-all of communication. Once you and your spouse communicate clearly and honestly about your deepest worries and fears, you can start working on resolving those feelings through positive action. For example, many parents of children with cerebral palsy have a long-term fear about what the future will hold for themselves and their child. They wonder whether their child will ever be able to hold a job or to live independently, or whether she will continue to depend on them for the rest of their lives. If you and your spouse discover you share this common concern, you can take steps now to quell some of your fears—for instance, you can find out what kinds of employment and independent housing options your community offers adults with disabilities like your child's, and then advocate for more and better services. You can begin financial planning for your child's future by using materials prepared by advocacy groups or by attending their workshops.

Most likely, many of your disagreements will center around day-to-day activities. For example, one partner may feel he or she is shouldering too many of the child care responsibilities. The ability to sit down together, calmly discuss feelings, and come up with a plan to more fairly divide home, work, and family responsibilities will help alleviate resentment before it festers. Afterwards, you will need to schedule a time one or two weeks down the road to evaluate whether your solution is working and to devise any further modifications necessary. Don't ignore this step. If your first plan still makes one spouse feel unfairly treated, he or she may hesitate to confront the problem again.

Take Time for Yourself

Parents expect to make sacrifices for their children. They expect to have to do without a new stereo system for the car in order to afford braces for their child, or to give up some evenings to help their child with her homework. They do not expect, however, to have to neglect all their own needs or to put all their dreams on hold until their children are grown. Nor should they have to. Unfortunately, parents of children with cerebral palsy sometimes have little or no time for themselves. As a result, they may feel as if they are stagnating. Their resentment and frustration may build as they watch opportunities for personal growth slip away. Their self-esteem may suffer and they won't feel as competent as they need to as a parent, a worker, or a spouse.

When you have a child who takes constant care and attention, you may need to ask yourself, "What am I doing for myself?" You may consciously have to analyze what people, places, and activities make you feel good about yourself and then schedule one of these activities with a person you enjoy in a place that makes you feel good. This may be as simple as getting up before the rest of your family for fifteen minutes of absolute "alone time" to drink a cup of coffee and think through your day. It may mean getting outside to take a brisk walk or pull some weeds in the flower bed to work off some nervous energy. It may take more planning—arranging to take a twice-weekly aerobics class, getting a sitter while you have lunch with a friend, or enrolling part-time at the local university to work on a long-deferred degree. Looking after your mental health in this manner can truly give you and your family a lift. Your refreshed outlook can only be a benefit to your family and yourself.

Not only do Mom and Dad need to do things for themselves, but they also need to do things together. Just to keep a marriage intact, you need some time together to discuss current issues in the home. To make a marriage thrive, you need time to enjoy each other's company without interruption, as well as time to communicate about your dreams, goals, and plans. You also need some time to just have fun, laugh, and enjoy yourselves. Becoming a parent is almost certain to change your social life, but you will need to continue doing some of the activities you enjoy most as a couple, with or without your friends. This makes it doubly important for you to find the reliable baby sitter mentioned earlier.

Your Marriage

There are no two ways about it: having a child with cerebral palsy puts a great deal of stress on a marriage. To begin with, the need to purchase special equipment or to pay for treatments and therapies not covered by insurance can produce tremendous *financial stress*—particularly if one spouse must quit his or her job to devote more time to caring for their child. Then there is the *physical stress* of constantly holding and positioning your child and her equipment; working with her on movement, feeding, and communication problems; chauffeuring her to and from doctors' and therapists' offices; overseeing her educational program; and advocating for services for her. These continual demands have a way of eating away at the time you have to spend with your spouse, and may also leave you feeling too exhausted to smooth out any rough spots in your marriage. On top of that, there is the sheer *emotional stress* that having a child with cerebral palsy places on a marriage. Not only must spouses come to terms with their own emotions about their child, but they must also cope with their spouse's feelings and their feelings about their spouse. For example, one spouse may resent the other for not shouldering his or her "share" of the child care responsibilities, or one spouse may secretly blame the other for having "caused" their child's cerebral palsy.

Some marriages grow stronger as a result of these shared stresses, while others break apart. It is almost impossible to predict how having a child with cerebral palsy will affect a particular marriage. But if your marriage does begin to buckle under the strain, do not hesitate to seek professional guidance. With counseling, even the most unbearable stresses can sometimes become bearable.

When parents of children with cerebral palsy do divorce, often the financial burden will fall on one spouse's shoulders, and the caretaking and medical burdens on the other's. This can lead to resentment on both sides. This is not to say that these problems are inevitable. Depending on your relationship with your spouse, your support system, and your financial situation, you may be able to work out a settlement that adequately serves everyone's interests. But couples who are seriously considering separation should fully discuss all child care, financial, employment, and medical insurance and treatment issues to ensure that their divorce does not compromise their child's future. A lawyer who is knowledgeable in advocacy and the rights of people with disabilities can help you resolve these issues, as well as advise you on the difficult legalities of divorce that involve extra financial needs.

Should you and your spouse opt for divorce, be sure to guard against scarring your child emotionally. So much of your child's reaction will depend on her age when you and your spouse separate. A very young child may not remember Mom and Dad ever living together, but may continue to fantasize about the "happy family life" until she is much older. You and your spouse have to be as consistent as possible in explaining to your child that you cannot live together, and must explain why in very simple terms. It is crucial not to make your child feel she is to blame. Try to avoid, at all costs, arguing over the responsibilities relating to your child (including money) in front of her. Explanations of what is happening and what to expect should be clear and simple and timely.

During the divorce process, counseling for spouses and children is often helpful. Local mental health agencies can provide assistance. Many schools and businesses now offer counseling related to family problems; you can contact your school counselor or social worker and your employee assistance program through your company's human resources department. If you are going to have custody of your children, you may also want to become involved in a single parent support group, subscribe to some of the materials and publications for single parents, and get acquainted with other resources in your community.

Siblings

The birth of a baby always changes the relationships in a family and presents fresh challenges for siblings. But when the baby has cerebral palsy, these new challenges can be especially stressful. Like their parents, brothers and sisters are usually flooded with strong, painful emotions that may get in the way of their acceptance of this new family member. They may worry, for instance, that cerebral palsy is "catching," or deeply resent the extra attention their special sibling gets.

If your child with cerebral palsy is the oldest sibling, the situation is a bit different. Small children usually look up to an older sibling and think they are pretty special. As younger children gradually begin to compare their brother or sister with others that age, parents need to give clear, honest explanations of what is different about the older child. For example, they can present differences in communication methods by showing the younger child how the augmentative communication device works, have them suggest words they want to use with their brother and add them to the communication board, or make a game out of using new adaptive sign language for communication.

It is vital that you be attuned to your other children's feelings and guide them to an acceptance of your child with cerebral palsy. Although this will not be easy for you, it will be well worth the effort. When helped to feel like equal, contributing parts of the family, children with cerebral palsy and their siblings can develop truly special, rewarding relation-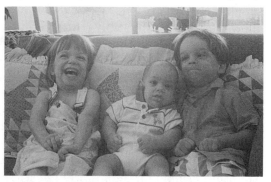ships. As you accept your children as unique, but equal parts of the family, they will accept each other and work together. Simple everyday tasks done together help develop strong relationships. Setting the table can be a family affair—one sibling can do the setting by asking her brother with cerebral palsy to choose the color of place mats or napkins, or which mug each person should use. Folding or sorting laundry, choosing food for the shopping list, and discussing places to go for family outings can also develop positive feelings among siblings.

Children's Feelings

Your other children's acceptance of your child with cerebral palsy is an on-going process, just as it is for you. How they view their brother or sister will change from day to day, depending on their emotional states and their developmental stages. To help your other children accept their special sibling, you need to be especially knowledgeable about the normal developmental stages and the emotional responses to expect in each stage. What follows is a summary of the thoughts and feelings siblings of children with cerebral palsy typically experience at different ages.

Preschool. At this age, a child's main fear is being separated from her parents. If a sibling seems to take all of Mom's and Dad's attention and concern, the toddler may feel unloved and displaced. She may throw tantrums, regress to wanting a bottle, withdraw, or even try to "super achieve" to win back your attention.

To help your child's pre-school brothers or sisters adjust, you should give them plenty of special time with Mom and Dad and allow them to feel like fully participating members in sharing their sibling. Bath and bedtimes are often good opportunities to share experiences. Choosing bathtub toys, and helping bathe, dry, and amuse the baby can be positive times. So can choosing the books to read or the story or music to listen to, or twisting the knob on the music box mobile to make the baby smile, relax, and fall asleep. Also remember that preschool children love to do "grown-up" things and to copy what their parents do. If their sibling with cerebral palsy is older than they are, they will naturally want to do some of the things Mom and Dad do for their brother or sister. As they fetch things for their sibling, fill in information about what's happening in another room or outside, or help with simple personal care, they will be rewarded by feelings of usefulness and appreciation. When pre-school children are involved in these ways, they usually fall in love with their brother or sister with cerebral palsy and want to help take care of her.

School-age. If siblings are about five to twelve years old, their responses to having a brother or sister with cerebral palsy will be different. Children of this age think it is important to be like peers and may worry about how to tell friends that their family is different because they have a sibling with a disability. They may also worry that if there is something "wrong" with their sibling, there may also be something "wrong" with them. They may feel they have to unfairly curtail their own activities to help care for their brother or sister, and as a consequence, may resent their sibling. On top of that, they may feel guilty about their resentment and any other negative thoughts they may have toward their sibling. Additionally, some school-aged brothers and sisters feel they are under increased pressure to perform for their parents to make up for the sibling who may not be able to achieve as much as they think parents expect.

Although this can be a difficult age, it helps if you can recognize that your children's feelings are normal. Try not to add to your children's guilt about their feelings; instead, encourage the positive interactions you see between your children. As long as you help your children handle their fears and guilt, they will be able to see and appreciate the unique qualities of your child with cerebral palsy on their own.

Adolescence. Teenagers often continue to have many of the same concerns of younger children, and develop other concerns as well. During this stage, they are working on their own identity, which is closely related to physical and sexual maturation. As a result, appearance and body image become increasingly important to them. Appearance of family members is also important, as any mother who has had a teenage daughter criticize her clothes, hair style, speech, and mannerisms knows. Having a sibling with an obvious physical impairment may be a source of great embarrassment to an adolescent. Adolescents may also worry that if they get married they will have a child with cerebral palsy of their own. Later in adolescence or early adulthood, they may worry about their role in caring for their sibling in the future—are they really capable of doing so, and will it mean changing their life?

As your teenaged children develop their own identity and strong self-esteem, they can move to a more adult relationship with their brother or sister. You can help to quiet some concerns by frankly discussing issues related to expectations for the future. If the siblings are fairly close in age and the future possibilities for your child with cerebral palsy are fairly clear—work, education, living arrangements—this is an opportune time for your whole family to honestly confront their concerns and plan for the future. If your child with cerebral palsy is very young and her potential is not known, you cannot help your teenagers overcome their fears quite so easily. You can, however, discuss possible ways your other children might be involved with their sibling with cerebral palsy in adulthood.

Dealing with Your Children's Emotions

If your child with cerebral palsy is your oldest child, you have already had some time to focus your attention on your own needs in coming to grips with the stress. If there are older children in the family, however, you will have to cope right away with both their emotional needs and your own emotional needs. It can be a difficult act, especially when you have a baby who needs so much attention, but you need to at least try to help your other children work through their emotions. Remember, your children will largely follow your lead in coming to accept your child with cerebral palsy. Here are some strategies to help you guide them to that acceptance.

Information. Every child fears the unknown—be it a spooky noise outside the bedroom window or a mysterious illness that makes her brother scissor his legs and drool. But no matter what the child's age, the best antidote to fear of the unknown is the same— clear, honest information. Even very small children can understand and accept a great deal about cerebral palsy if you explain it in terms appropriate to their age level. They definitely will understand your emotional tone when you discuss your child with cerebral palsy with your spouse, so honesty can help them to understand your feelings. On the other hand, if information is not shared with siblings, the emotional undertones may make them even more confused and frightened. The same holds true for the child with cerebral palsy, as the second half of this chapter discusses.

When a child is first diagnosed with cerebral palsy, there is usually a great deal of uncertainty about the extent of the disability and what the future holds. But if you tell your other children what is known *now* and what will be done *now*, they can begin to accept their brother or sister and feel less threatened by uncertainty. Small children are amazingly resilient and often come up with alternatives or solutions to the everyday care of their sibling that may surprise you. For example, children often interpret wants for other children. "He wants the cracker first and he'll stop crying." "She wants to play on the floor now." "He wants to sit where he can see you working." These suggestions frequently work.

Generally, the more information you give your children about this new situation, the better they will be able to accept some of the new demands that will be made on the family. You might say, for example, "Billy is going to start going to a special preschool. That means I have to get him ready for an early bus, pack his lunch and his bag, and write a note to the teacher about his sleep and breakfast. This will change how much time I have to help you get ready for school. Let's see if we can figure out how to make everything fit together."

Communication. As this chapter has emphasized, it is vital that all family members openly share their feelings about your child with cerebral palsy. But children may have just as much trouble expressing their emotions as adults do. Sometimes they simply cannot find the words to describe how they feel. Other times they may deliberately suppress their emotions because they feel guilty about having "bad" feelings such as anger, jealousy, and hatred toward their sibling. Parents, too, may inadvertently make siblings feel guilty about normal feelings. For example, it is normal for a sibling to resent the attention her parents give a new baby, but when her parents are so obviously concerned about the intruder, the sibling may be ashamed of her resentment.

If your other children cannot or will not voice their emotions, try to deduce their feelings from clues in their behavior. For example, if your nine-year-old son gives you a million and one reasons for not bringing his best friend home to play, you can probably assume that the real reason is because your son is reluctant for his friend to meet his sibling with cerebral palsy. Letting your son know you understand how hard it is to share your child with cerebral palsy with his friend can help him accept this "different" sibling.

Whether or not your children are able to share their feelings with you, they need the opportunity to share their feelings with others their own age. Your children need to know that they are not alone—that other children also have siblings with special needs. The Resource Guide at the back of this book describes several national networks for siblings of people with disabilities. Additionally, local school special education programs often provide sibling support groups. Pediatric hospitals or university special education programs also sometimes offer support groups for siblings. Check the

Resource Guide or contact United Cerebral Palsy for help in locating a group near you.

Balance. You should avoid at all costs making your child with cerebral palsy the center of the family. Difficult as it may be, you should never spend so much time looking after the needs of your child with cerebral palsy that you neglect your other children's needs. Your child with cerebral palsy does need encouragement when she takes her first steps with a walker, but her older sister also needs encouragement when she takes her first solo bicycle ride. You will be very excited when your child with cerebral palsy can make meaningful "yes-no" answers or type her schoolwork on a word processor, but also be sure to praise your seven-year-old's short story about the dog. If you don't balance all of your children's needs, you risk damaging the neglected children's self-esteem.

As part of your balancing act, try to give your children equal amounts of responsibility around the home. Although your child 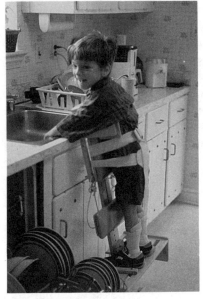 with cerebral palsy may be physically unable to master the variety of chores that your other children can, she should pull at least *some* weight. With help, even children with severe movement problems can handle jobs such as dusting, feeding pets, turning on the dishwasher, or putting away flatware. It would be unfair if everyone in the family except your child with cerebral palsy had household responsibilities, and the unfairness would definitely make it harder for your other children to accept their brother or sister.

While you are dividing up household responsibilities, keep a careful eye on how large a part your other children take in caring for their sibling. Children want to be helpful and are usually happy to be a part of family activities such as helping with their sibling's therapy. They may enjoy playing "teacher" and seeing small increments of improvement. These activities are more enjoyable if they seem to be the child's idea and do not limit their freedom and independence. Children do not like feeling forced to care for their sibling or to become the substitute "mother."

Especially as your other children enter adolescence, you should take care to allow them time to focus on developing their own identity. Rather than always asking them to babysit their brother or sister, you can ask them to help in more adult ways—for example, by asking them to suggest ways to improve your child's daily care or to suggest activities your family can enjoy together. It is important that you recognize the needs of all of your children and balance their demands.

Individuality. It is important that you give your other children the message that it's great to be the brother or sister of a child with cerebral palsy. But in delivering that message, take care that you don't unintentionally give your children the idea that their identities are limited to being siblings of a special-needs child. All children are unique individuals with kaleidoscopic assortments of interests and talents. To recognize their own individuality, your children need lives outside the family. You must encourage them to pursue their own interests and activities away from the home with their own friends. Success outside the family will help your children to be better adjusted within the family, and as a result, they will be more supportive of both you and their sibling.

Family Activities

In subtle and not-so-subtle ways, having a child with cerebral palsy complicates many family activities. Depending on your child's mobility and the special equipment she needs, certain activities may be difficult, if not impossible, to do together. And then there are the reactions of other people to deal with. There is no denying that whispers, stares, and rude questions can spoil even the most enjoyable outing. If you are proud of your child and her accomplishments, though, the whispers and stares become less important. Bear in mind, too, that many people ask questions not out of rudeness, but out of curiosity, ignorance, or even concern. Although it may sometimes seem simpler and less nerve-wracking not to do anything at all, remember: actions speak louder than words. If you truly want family members to believe that you are all one big happy family, then you must *act* like a family. That means doing things together—and not just going to medical appointments, therapy sessions, or evaluations—but doing things that are strictly fun.

Many of the activities your family enjoys doing together will be at home. For example, you may enjoy playing a game all the children can manage, having popcorn while you watch a favorite video tape, or reading or doing puzzles together. But it is also important to get out of the house and provide the kinds of activities that children need to help them learn to handle the outside world. All children—with and without disabilities—need opportunities to play in the park, select books at the library, choose food at the supermarket, eat out at restaurants, watch sporting events, attend religious activities, and go on picnics.

Outdoor activities such as canoeing, hiking, and camping may need to be reconsidered and modified to fit your new situation. For example, because portages with only Mom and Dad to carry the canoe would be difficult, family camping in more accessible areas may be a better alternative, at least for a while. If your child uses a wheelchair, renting a vacation cottage on a grassy lake shore may be

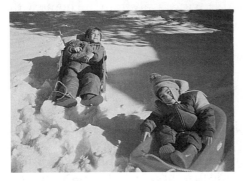

more practical than renting one on a sandy beach. Some amusement parks may not be as much fun if everyone can't go on the rides together. Unfortunately, although there is increasing awareness of the need to reduce physical barriers, provide sufficient handicapped parking spaces, and offer accessible transportation, many barriers still exist and may limit enjoyment of some activities. Still, you can often get ideas for fun, accessible outings from other parents, teachers, and therapists.

Of course, doing activities outside the home requires you to confront the issue of other people's reactions head-on. Since many parents of children with obvious disabilities say that socialization is one of their biggest concerns, this will probably not be easy for you. You may feel that your child's appearance or behavior will upset other people, or you may hesitate to expose yourself and your child to reactions you expect might occur. If family members or friends have been avoiding your family since learning of your child's disability, you may feel even more justified in your concerns. Once you actually take your child out in public, though, you may find that other people's reactions are related to your own attitude of acceptance toward your child. As you interact with your child in public, onlookers will take their cues from you. If you seem comfortable with your child, converse with her in whatever communication method you use, attend to her responses, and calmly go about whatever you are doing, onlookers will generally relax and be less obtrusive in their staring and curiosity. Besides, if you are genuinely involved with your child, you and your child will be less likely to notice what bystanders are doing.

One of your roles as a parent of a child with a disability is that of educator to the general public. This will also be a role for your child and her siblings. People will be curious, interested, fearful, and sometimes unintentionally rude, but generally, I believe, they want to understand and be helpful. How you deal with your child will help them learn how to behave with other people with similar disabilities. If people directly confront you with inappropriate or rude questions, you will need to respond as calmly and matter-of-factly as possible. If your child is old enough, questions should be directed to her to answer. "How old is she?" can be answered by saying gently, "Why don't you ask her yourself?" You might also face your child and say, "How old are you?" so as to model appropriate behavior for the person to pick up if the conversation continues.

Some parents find that sharing outings with other families of children with cerebral palsy is one way of making things a little easier. There *is* strength in numbers, and besides, it is refreshing to do things with others who understand the time it takes to get in and out of car seats, strollers, and wheelchairs, and how complicated it is to set up for eating in a restaurant. More importantly, having other adults and children along who accept everyone in your family as they are is great for everyone's self-esteem.

PART II: HELPING YOUR CHILD DEVELOP HIGH SELF-ESTEEM

Up to now, this chapter has focused on ways to help each member of your family adjust to your child with cerebral palsy. As mentioned earlier, your family's acceptance is the key to the development of normal relationships within the family. In turn, family relationships lay the foundation for the development of your child's sense of her own worth, or *self-esteem*. And self-esteem, as more and more research has shown, is essential to every child's success.

If your child has high self-esteem, she will not only be able to set high goals for herself, but also be able to take the risks needed to reach those goals. Additionally, she will have the basis for enjoying herself and others and for satisfaction with her life.

For children with cerebral palsy, the process of developing high self-esteem can sometimes be different or more difficult than it is for other children. For example, in her early school years, your child with cerebral palsy may dwell on her "difference" from peers and siblings when the need is to be "like" others. Each child's experience in the home, at school, and in the community will be different. There are, however, some typical stumbling blocks that children with cerebral palsy can run into on the road to self-esteem. This section discusses these obstacles, as well as ways you and other family members can help her around them.

How Self-Esteem Develops

Before a child can have a sense of self-esteem, she must first develop a sense of *self*. In other words, she must learn to distinguish her body from other people and things in her environment.

Most babies begin learning to see their bodies as physical objects quite early by experimenting with movement and touch—by discovering that playing with fingers and toes, for example, produces different sensations than does playing with a rattle or grasping a bottle. Gradually, as they interact with family members and other important people in their lives, babies also begin to see themselves as social objects. For instance, they learn to tell the difference between themselves and their mother or the person who feeds and cares for them.

By the time a typical baby has begun to move around a great deal (normally by the second year), she has usually developed a true sense of self. She imitates other people and can distinguish between them and inanimate objects. Her sense of *autonomy,* or independence, emerges, and she sees the world as "me," "you," and "mine." She begins to like herself as she plays and has a good time accomplishing physical feats. She also begins to react to other people's behavior—a smile or a frown, for instance—and social approval and blame become important to her.

Once an infant is capable of interpreting her experiences with things, people, and her own body, she is also capable of developing self-esteem. From now on, practically every experience she has will either boost her self-esteem or deflate it. The following section describes some typical experiences children have in their first few years of life and explains how these experiences can help or harm a child's self-esteem.

Different Feelings at Different Stages of Development

Age One. During the first year of life, a child usually learns to enjoy being with her mother and to trust that she will hold or feed her when she approaches. She also begins to feel some sense of accomplishment if she learns she can trust her body to do what she wants—to grasp a toy, reach something by crawling, or move something to her mouth. With proper care, even children with limited mobility can develop this basic trust in other people, the environment, and themselves. In fact, a baby whose cerebral palsy is identified early may have even more opportunities than usual to interact with people in ways that help nurture trust. For example, recently I was working with a baby with multiple physical and mental disabilities. He was being fed through a tube, but the occupational therapist encouraged his mother to hold and cuddle him so he could see her face, and to help him put his fist into his mouth to associate sucking and chewing with the sensation of having a full stomach. This baby received warm feelings from his mother and also became more aware of his body parts and sensations.

Ages Two to Three. Between the ages of two and three, children work on developing a sense of independence within the limits of their capabilities. Walking, talking, and bowel and bladder control are major goals of this period. Children are frequently frustrated by inability, but can accept the help and guidance of those they trust. With careful guidance, children can begin to make choices of activities within physical and social limitations. Choices should be limited and clear—for example, choices of two foods to eat or of two shirts to wear. As children choose activities and are successful in accomplishing them, their feelings of self-worth increase. But if children are not permitted to try to develop independence, they begin to doubt their self-worth. Because families of children with cerebral palsy often overprotect their children or limit their choices, both of these issues are discussed in detail later in this chapter.

Ages Four to Five. As the preschool years come to a close, learning through abstract thinking becomes more important than mastering physical tasks. Children can use symbols and language and can relate past and present experiences. Fantasy and imagination play increasingly larger roles in children's lives and children spend much time thinking about future possibilities—becoming firemen, astronauts, nurses, artists. Naturally, this cognitive development varies greatly with the extent of developmental disability.

During this period, children also develop consciences and begin to feel guilty for thoughts and actions. They see things as black or white, good or bad. They feel guilty when they think or do things people tell them are bad or they interpret as bad. Often they see a cause-and-effect relationship between their actions and a "bad" thing happening to someone else or to themselves. "Mother says I talk too much; that's why I have to get my tonsils out"; or "My baby sister is sick because I took her toy away and made her cry." Some guilt is actually important to development. Feeling guilty and coping with it leads to a sense of initiative and accomplishment. Overwhelming guilt, however, can lead to poor self-esteem.

If punishment and criticism of a child's behavior are handled judiciously, guilt can be kept to a minimum. Punishment needs to be consistent and understandable to the child. Parents sometimes need to try to understand their child's thinking process before labeling behavior "bad" and scolding or punishing. For example, why is coloring on paper okay, but coloring on a bedroom wall bad?

Why is giving the dog a biscuit fine, but giving one to the baby naughty?

Later in this stage, children with high self-esteem develop a clearer understanding of the consequences of their actions. They feel worthy, competent, and able to achieve through their own efforts. In contrast, children (and adults) with low self-esteem tend to feel they are not in control of situations and that things just happen to them. They attribute good results to luck and feel they don't deserve the results or praise. Small children will say, "He's lucky he got a smiling face on her paper." "I'm lucky I got a star on the chart." As children develop a good self-concept, though, they can relate the outcomes of their behavior to their own efforts.

Nurturing High Self-Esteem in Children with Cerebral Palsy

Don't Overprotect Your Child

A major part of the development process is coming to an understanding of our own strengths and limitations. Can you remember how you wanted to be graceful and athletic instead of klutzy and awkward? Were you the brain of the family when you would have preferred to be the beauty? Everyone must try out new things and experience both success and failure to arrive at a concept of self they are comfortable with. Ideally, everyone should learn to accept their strengths and limitations as part of their uniqueness.

Watching children try out their wings is often painful for parents. It is difficult to see your toddler sobbing in frustration because she cannot do something her older sister can do. When your child has cerebral palsy, it is even harder to watch her fail because you, too, feel her frustrations at her limitations. Frequently, parents of children with cerebral palsy try to shield their children from failure by overprotecting them. Parents may do everything for their child themselves and not even permit her to make choices or to have a baby sitter who does things differently than Mom and Dad.

This urge to overprotect, although understandable, can damage your child's self-esteem. To begin with, when you prevent your child from experiencing failure, you can set up artificial barriers to self-acceptance. For example, you may realize that your child will be very frustrated if she tries to use a spoon by herself. It may be better, however, to devise a plan to gradually encourage self-feeding than to not try it when your child seems to want to. In addition, your child may interpret your overprotection to mean that you think she is a failure and cannot do anything for herself. As a result, she may become shy, fearful, or withdrawn, and balk at trying anything new. Furthermore, children who are overprotected may seem immature, spoiled, or demanding. They may come to expect adults to do *everything* for them.

As hard as it may be for you, you must allow your child to test reality and experience limitations. Let her try progressively harder feeding skills, dressing herself, throwing a ball, communicating to express her needs and wants. Allow her to make choices—between banana or applesauce, the red or the blue pants. Remember, too, that not permitting your child to do things that other children with similar capabilities can do may be overprotection. Taking the bus to school with other children instead of being driven to school every day by Mom is an example. Riding the bus may take longer and may complicate your schedule, but if it is physically safe, it may give your child a sense of independence and of growing up and being more like her peers.

Like all children, your child must experience frustration and pain and decide what is important enough that she must find ways around the limitations that prevent her from reaching her goals. Your child needs the opportunity to accomplish what she is motivated to accomplish. She must come to accept her reality for herself.

Besides protecting their child from herself, parents may also try to protect their child from others. They may fear that strangers will react negatively to their child's disability, so may keep their child home as much as possible. But preventing your child from making social contacts and from learning how to get along in the outside world will do far more harm in the long run than any stares or insensitive comments will. Do not allow your own fears to limit your child's chances of independence and of having a normal social life. Instead, try to provide the encouragement and freedom that will allow your child to grow both inside your home and out. You can do this by demonstrating your enjoyment of your child as a unique person with characteristics that make her a valuable member of your family and of the world. Remember, other people's reactions are related to your own acceptance toward your child.

Talking about overprotection may seem very one-sided. Obviously you do not want to be an uncaring or neglectful parent. You want to permit your child with cerebral palsy to develop as normally as possible. To do so, you need to know about normal development at all stages and to help your child progress as well as she can. Each child is different and has different needs. If your child's disability has been identified early and a team of medical and educational specialists is working with your family, their opinions about when your child is ready for certain activities or skills will guide you. Be sure you voice your opinions and share your observations, as well as consider other ideas.

If you and your child are not a part of this kind of team and you feel that overprotection has already hindered the development of her independence, you will need to help her gradually begin to take some responsibility for herself. You certainly cannot suddenly stop doing things for your child until she has begun to acquire some of the self-help skills she needs. Professionals and other parents who have dealt with similar situations can suggest ways to help foster your child's independence.

It might be easier to keep your child with cerebral palsy in a protected environment at home with family members who love and understand her. But remember the words of the old saying: we must hold our children close and let them go. *Let* your child try her wings and learn to fly.

Be Honest with Your Child

Although your attitude and behavior toward your child will most strongly influence her understanding and acceptance of herself, what you tell your child is also important. As soon as your child is able to understand, you need to provide her with information about cerebral palsy and share your feelings and expectations.

In talking with your child, the cardinal rule is to be honest. Exactly what you say and how you explain it will depend on your child's cognitive and emotional development at the time. Gear the language you use to your child's development and avoid overwhelming her with very technical or extraneous information. A small child, for example, does not need to know what she will or will not be able to do in the future because she has little concept of time. Instead, she needs concrete examples and descriptive language— "this will feel like a pinch"; "this medicine will taste about like a cherry lifesaver." Later, clear discussion of school, work, and living options are appropriate and necessary, just as they are for any teenager.

Young children observe much more than we sometimes realize and draw conclusions that may be quite faulty. For example, a child may think that her 8:30 bedtime was set because of her cerebral palsy and not because the family decided that children in early elementary school should go to bed at that time. Her conclusion may be related to a casual comment or question about sleep asked by a doctor long before. It is important to help your child ask questions, express opinions, and share her observations. If your child has limited communication skills, you will have to try to interpret her thoughts and fears so you can give meaningful explanations. A knowledge of normal feelings of children at different stages of development can give you insight into what your child might be feeling. For example, when you leave your two-year-old at a center-based early intervention program, you can expect her to fear separation or abandonment. When your child is six or seven, you can anticipate that she will worry about being different from her peers. And once she reaches her teenage years, she will likely have concerns about physical attractiveness and sexual identity.

Besides helping your child understand and accept her disability and develop good self-esteem, open communication can also help her deal with her feelings about other family members. Naturally, we all compare ourselves to others and we need to recognize our comparative strengths as well as our comparative weaknesses. If a brother is a star Little League baseball player, the family will go to games, cheer, and take pride in him. But that brother may need assistance from his brother with cerebral palsy to do a computer problem for math class.

Your family's attitude in recognizing strengths and taking pride in each other will help your child with cerebral palsy resolve her comparisons with siblings. Recognizing accomplishments and strengths in all areas—social, emotional, spiritual, and intellectual, as well as physical—can help you identify ways to highlight the achievements of all your family members. Through open and frank discussion with your child, you can help her develop her own list of strengths to build on.

Set Realistic Goals with Your Child

Whether you realize it or not, you are constantly setting goals for yourself—whether it's to lose five pounds, to waste less electricity around the house, or just to make it to the end of the work week with your sanity intact. Goals give direction to our lives and help us to measure success. Setting and accomplishing goals is essential to self-esteem.

As the parent of a child with cerebral palsy, you will be called on many times to set goals for your child. Physical therapists, occupational therapists, speech/language pathologists, and special educators will all gear the services they provide your child to short- and long-term goals appropriate to her special needs. You will probably also set your own goals for your child within the family. To ensure that your child reaches her fullest potential, it is important to set the highest possible goals. To ensure that she achieves the success vital to her self-esteem, it is just as important to make sure that the goals are within her grasp.

The key to setting high but realistic goals for your child is that old standby, *communication*. Whether you are setting goals for feeding, physical therapy, speech activities, or social behavior, you need to involve your child in the goal-setting process as much as her developmental level allows. Your child will not feel motivated to achieve her goals unless she also feels encouraged, taken seriously, and carefully listened to.

Here is how you might involve a very young child in setting goals that would lead up to her learning to drink independently from a cup. You would begin by discussing with your child that you think she is both ready and able to master this skill. You would then set small, short-term goals—first for your child to learn to handle an empty cup, second for her to manage a very small amount of a favorite drink, and eventually for her to be able to drink a whole cup of milk or juice on her own. At every step of the way, you would encourage your child, watch for feedback that she is frustrated or fatigued, and modify your plan to fit the situation.

To set a goal for a school-aged child, you would again break it down into clear, manageable steps. Perhaps you and your six-year-old agree that she will learn to get your attention with a speech sound instead of a shriek. You might ask your child to approximate

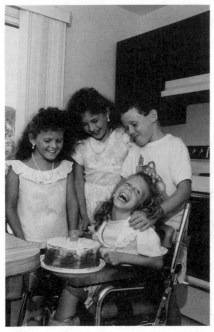

that sound twice each evening the first week, and then gradually increase the number of times your child makes the sound until she no longer shrieks for attention.

When your child reaches her later elementary school or teenage years, goal setting may become more difficult. For example, if your child drools, grunts, or has athetoid reflexes (uncontrollable movements), it may be especially hard to set goals that encourage social interaction. But if over the years you and your child have developed the habit of conferring about goals and ways to achieve them, you stand a better chance of setting goals with which you are both comfortable. For example, suppose your fourteen-year-old daughter refuses to wear her glasses because she thinks they make her ugly. If you can discuss her need for glasses during classes and also her need for peer approval, you and your daughter might compromise on the amount of time she needs to wear glasses in exchange for a promise of more attractive glasses.

Just as you should try to set realistic goals, you should also try to set realistic time frames for achieving those goals. Not all children with cerebral palsy learn at the same rate, and individual children may pick up new skills more easily at some times than at others. Try not to be impatient. Generally, if you can avoid feeling guilty that you aren't good at teaching and can avoid blaming your child for not cooperating, your child *will* achieve her goals. Remember, too, that being able to laugh together while working on goals will make life more enjoyable for the whole family. Laughing at your own mistakes will help your child put hers in perspective, too. For instance, think how much better you feel when a new recipe is a disaster and your family laughs with you instead of criticizing your cooking.

Let Your Child Make Choices

As mentioned earlier, permitting your child to make choices for herself is essential to the development of her self-esteem. Not only does making choices give children a sense of control, but it also gives them a sense of their own competence. Having this sense of control is especially important for children with cerebral palsy who may be unable to control their bodies or voices as they would like to. Making choices also plays a large part in the development of confidence and independence.

Perhaps you sometimes hesitate to let your child make choices for fear that she will make the wrong choices. But even children with moderate mental retardation can learn from the consequences of poor choices. They learn, for example, that snatching away someone else's toy leads to a slap from the other child or a "time-out." Nonverbal children, too, can make choices. You will know best how your child indicates her choices—through a smile or frown, eye gaze, a modified handshake for "yes" or "no," or other means.

Choices you offer your child should always be within her capabilities—not too easy, but challenging enough without being overly frustrating. For two- or three-year-olds, for example, permitting choices of food or clothing is usually appropriate. Even if the pants and shirt your child chooses do not fit your sense of color combinations, you can appreciate the delight she shows in her choices. The preschool teacher probably isn't going to think less of you because of your child's garish outfit, but if she does, so what?

In the beginning, limit choices to two things so as not to overwhelm your child. For example, if you are working a ten-piece puzzle with your three-year-old, she may feel overwhelmed and not be able to put in a piece. You can pick out two pieces and help her choose which one to put into a specific place. After she chooses the right piece, you can help narrow down subsequent choices until the puzzle is complete. As your child grows older, choices can be more complex and can involve more alternatives. For instance, your child can choose which friend to play with today, where to go on an outing, or which birthday toy to take to school to share with the class.

Children should also be involved in family choice-making to the extent of their capabilities. What to do for a special weekend family activity or where to go on vacation may be decisions your child can help to make. Even though your child's choice will not always be the one accepted, if you make sure that everyone's opinions are listened to and considered, your child's confidence and self-esteem will continue to grow.

Discipline and Self-Esteem

Parents of children with cerebral palsy may sometimes be reluctant to demand proper behavior from their child. They may think their child cannot understand rules and the need for good behavior, or may feel too guilty or too sorry for their child to discipline her. But if you allow your child to misbehave, she will undoubtedly continue to misbehave. Unless you use consistent, fair discipline to teach your child acceptable conduct, her safety, social relationships, and education will all be jeopardized.

Discipline is also important for another reason: it is vital to the development of your child's self-esteem. It can help to build your child's sense of being respected and cared about, as long as you dispense it with patience, kindness, and reason. Discipline should never be thought of as punishment for poor behavior, but rather as training to help your child make wise decisions. When your child experiences the logical consequences of poor behavior, she learns to behave more appropriately the next time.

For discipline to be effective, you need to set clear limits and think rules through carefully before making them. Remember, a rule is not a good one unless you can enforce it consistently. If rules change constantly, your child will be confused and not know when a behavior is right and when it is wrong. Try to keep rules to a minimum because children cannot work on everything at the same time. Families *need* rules that protect the safety, health, and rights of others: don't play with matches; don't open the door to strangers; ask before borrowing things. But many rules that families make are unnecessary or unenforceable: *everyone* does one hour of homework before dinner *every* night; your room must *always* be clean before you go to school. If you establish a few clear necessary rules, you can expect your children to respect them.

If possible, discuss rules in family meetings and involve all your children in making them. Discuss why certain rules seem to be necessary and what the consequences are if they are not followed. Listen to what your children have to say about the limits imposed by the rules. Your children will be more likely to respect and follow the rules if they have a part in making them.

All your children should follow the rules you decide are necessary. Naturally, the way rules are followed may differ according to your children's ages and intellectual abilities or the situation. A rule about respect for each other and your home may mean not throwing food on the floor during dinner time for a four-year-old child with cerebral palsy. For a teenager, it may mean cleaning up the dirty dishes after having snacks with a friend.

Generally, discipline should be timely and a logical, natural consequence of behavior. For example, cleaning up the kitchen is a consequence of making fudge and using every pan just before time for cooking dinner. A "time-out" is a logical consequence of behavior that is socially unacceptable or out of control—tantrums or aggressive behavior, for example. In a time-out, you remove your child to a quiet place where she can calm down and gain control. Always using the same place for time-outs helps small children understand why they are there. The time-out place should be non-distracting, quiet, soothing, and not frightening.

Just as there should be clear consequences for improper behavior, there should also be clear consequences—smiles, hugs, kisses, praise—for good behavior. Reward good behavior with praise immediately, and try to avoid criticizing when something is not done to your adult standards. For example, if putting away her toys is your child's responsibility, accept her work within her limitations. Don't say, "I'm pleased you picked up your toys this morning, but you didn't stack your blocks neatly." Instead, say something like this: "I'm pleased you picked up your toys this morning and you did it all yourself!" Keep it positive. If you give your child lots of love when she is on her good behavior, she will be secure enough to respond to discipline when it is necessary.

To further help your child accept the need for discipline, you should discuss your child's feelings about being disciplined and encourage her not to hide them. Let your child know that everyone feels angry, frustrated, or hurt sometimes. You should also share your feelings with your child. If you impulsively respond with anger and punishment to something your child does, share your feelings and understanding of what happened when you have calmed down. Then pay attention to your child's feelings when the same kind of situation happens with her.

Training any child to become responsible and self-reliant is a lifelong job. For parents of children with cerebral palsy, this process may be harder because of feelings of guilt, frustration, anger, and fatigue. There are many excellent publications that can guide you in encouraging positive behavior in your child or help you choose a procedure for establishing fair, consistent discipline within your family. Some of these are listed in the Reading List at the back of this book.

Cheering Your Child On!

Motivation. As your child matures, you will want her to develop an inner drive to go after the goals essential to her growth and happiness. You will want her to learn to decide for herself which goals are important and to pursue them without outside motivation. While your child is young, however, much of what she does will be to please the important people in her life, rather than herself—for example, earning stamps on her hand for meeting PT goals. Because your child will be more willing to tackle difficult tasks if she knows that everyone wants her to succeed, all family members should express their mutual respect by listening to and encouraging one another.

Your child's motivation will also be strengthened if she can see the positive aspects of trying to accomplish something new. For example, reaching a toy she wants makes the struggle to inch across the room worthwhile. As your child experiences success, she will begin to take pride in her accomplishments for themselves, as well as for the praise and attention the rest of the family gives her.

It is important not to undermine your child's pride in her accomplishments with criticism. Criticism makes children feel that their ways of doing things are not respected, and often leads to anger and resentment. To keep your child's motivation high, you should also try to avoid "taking over." When you take over, you are implicitly criticizing your child and showing you don't think she can do it right. If she is trying to get a shirt over her head and you take over and help, she may resent your interference before she is ready to ask for assistance.

Always stress the pride you feel in your child because she keeps on trying. "That was a great try; you almost did it." "You did that much by yourself. Soon you'll be able to do it all." "We all make mistakes. That's how we learn new things."

Praise. Praise is essential to developing good self-esteem. To believe in our own self-worth, we all need to be told we are successful and to feel love and appreciation from our families. I am always impressed when parents of very young children with cerebral palsy can recognize minute gains in movement, eating, speech, or social skills, and show their children such obvious excitement and pride in their accomplishments. Although the slow, painstaking training process can be very frustrating, the gains are worth it, and the spontaneous praise given by parents is so necessary to the child's feelings of self-worth.

Praise is a major part of the positive reinforcement needed to teach children with cerebral palsy. If you can remember that, you can create a positive learning environment in your home. Think of how a six-year-old feels after spending seven or eight hours in orthotics at school, followed by several more hours in physical therapy, and then homework, dinner, and a bath. Imagine how she would feel if you told her, "No bedtime story tonight—I've already spent my whole evening looking after you." Wouldn't she feel better if you said, "I'm really impressed with how well you're handling your new schedule. It must be rough to have to work so hard without any time out to play." A little listening, respect, and stressing of the positive can do wonders for the emotional tone in the family.

Praise can also be a secret weapon to use on your child's misbehavior. When your child is behaving badly, you may be able to improve her behavior by picking out a positive aspect of the situation, or by waiting for something positive to happen and them praising it. For example, if she is smearing her dinner all over her tray and making a real mess, when she suddenly takes a drink of milk through her straw you can comment on her good drinking skills and apparent enjoyment of her milk. This also may divert her attention away from food smearing. Of course, if a behavior is serious and dangerous, it must be dealt with directly. If your child is biting another child, you must tell her to stop at once. Many undesirable behaviors, however, can be ignored and will gradually diminish if you don't set up a power struggle by nagging excessively.

In praising your child, always be honest and don't go overboard. Many people have trouble receiving compliments because they do not feel they have earned the praise. Your child, too, will have difficulty accepting praise if she thinks it is excessive. Telling your child her drawing of you is the best picture you have ever seen may be too much for her to accept. If you express your delight at her choosing you as the subject for her drawing, the praise will be more honest. Try to keep praise genuine and related to the nature of your child's accomplishments.

Love from the Whole Family. After a child's basic needs for food, warmth, and clothing are met, the need for love is most important to emotional development. But when a child has a disability, parents may focus so much on differences in physical needs and demands they can forget that their child needs to be cuddled and loved like any other child. As your child grows, she wants to feel the same love she sees between other members of your family. This reinforces her feelings of worth and leads to high self-esteem.

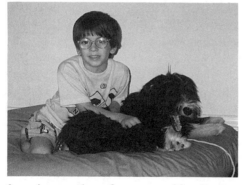 There are many ways of showing love that your child will understand. Some parents do a lot of hugging, kissing, and cuddling. Others verbalize love, tuck love notes into lunch boxes, or choose special cards for every possible occasion. Some show love by remembering little favorites and preferences of family members and by surprising them with tokens of love—a favorite food for dinner, a cartoon that reminds them of the loved one, a flower or sweet.

All of us want unconditional acceptance and love. So, too, does your child with cerebral palsy.

Your child with cerebral palsy needs to be accepted and loved by other relatives just as your other children or their cousins are. She doesn't want to be overprotected or doted upon any more than other children in the family do. She needs to be loved for her personal strengths and what she contributes to the family. And you need the support and acceptance this kind of love and caring can provide.

Fostering love from the whole family may be a slow, educational process, but can be well worth the effort. You must first explore and work through your grief, anger, and guilt so that you can openly communicate with the whole family. Then you need to judiciously share the things you are learning about your child with other family members as they are ready for information. Grandparents, aunts, uncles, and cousins all need to be given opportunities to accept this child for herself. Let them get to know your child—give them space together.

To help in the acceptance process, you may want to involve relatives with family support groups or with the professionals treating your child. A pediatrician I heard speak at a conference for parents of children with disabilities said he always tries to get to know the grandparents as soon as possible. That way he knows what kind of treatment to suggest to parents that will be acceptable to them and carried through successfully. Since parenthood is something we are generally not trained for, we tend to do things the way we saw them done in our own homes. This means your extended family can be very important in how you handle your parenting, even if relatives do not live close by.

I have found that acceptance and love from the extended family often makes a major difference in how children feel about themselves and how they see themselves in the world. An uncle who lets his teenage nephew help in his factory doing simple repetitive tasks during summer vacation makes him feel productive. A grandmother who invites her granddaughter with cerebral palsy and mental retardation to visit for a week makes her feel special. With your guidance, *every* member of your immediate and extended family can make valuable contributions to your child's self-esteem.

Conclusion

In my work and in this chapter, I emphasize the theme of acceptance. You and your family need to accept your child as she is so you can develop normal relationships and enjoy a normal family life. Your acceptance also equips you to help your child with cerebral palsy accept her disability and then go on to achieve high self-esteem. But remember: there are different shades of acceptance. There is the hangdog resignation that goes along with accepting defeat, and then there is the genuine joy that goes along with accepting the unexpected gift of something rare and priceless. Which type of acceptance your family will come to depends on many factors, but most of all on you. If you can see your child as a welcome, valued addition to your family, then no matter what problems you have integrating her into the family, you will be willing to work until you can find a solution.

As long as she has the acceptance of a caring family, any child with cerebral palsy can develop a positive view of herself. As she grows and experiences successes, praise and support from her family will encourage her to try for more difficult goals. Although the road to self-esteem is not easy, many children with cerebral palsy and their families have proven that it can be traveled successfully. No matter how cerebral palsy affects your child's abilities, your family's acceptance and support can help foster the self-esteem that will guarantee her a happier, more fulfilling life.

REFERENCES

Buscaglia, L. *The Disabled and Their Parents: A Counseling Challenge.* Thorofare, N.J.: Charles B. Slack, 1975.

"Children with Handicaps, Parent and Family Issues: A Guide to Readings." *News Digest,* National Information Center for Handicapped Children and Youth, November, 1985.

Cottrell, L.S., Jr. "Interpersonal Interaction and the Development of Self." In *Handbook of Socialization Theory and Research,* edited by D.A. Goslin. Chicago: Rand McNally College Publishing Company, 1969.

Dreikurs, R. *Children: The Challenge.* New York: Hawthorne Books, 1964.

Focus on Fathers (newsletter). Father's Program Outreach Project, Experimental Education Unit, WJ-10, University of Washington, Seattle, WA 98195.

Foley, G. Unpublished materials, Drake University.

Hermanson, E. "Securing the Future of a Disabled Child." Information from the National Information Center for Handicapped Children and Youth, October, 1984.

Kroth, R.L. Unpublished materials presented at Institute for Parent Involvement. Albuquerque, N.M.: The Parent Center, 1982.

Kroth, R.L. Unpublished materials. Albuquerque, N.M.: Manzanita Center, 1985 and 1986.

Lepler, M. "Having a Handicapped Child." *The American Journal of Maternal Child Nursing,* January/February 1978, 32–33.

Meyer, D. "Fathers of Children with Handicaps." In *Families of Handicapped Children: Needs and Supports across the Life Span,* edited by R.R. Fewell and P.F. Vadasy. Austin: Pro-Ed, 1986.

Richardson, S.A. "The Effect of Physical Disability on the Socialization of a Child. In *Handbook of Socialization Theory and Research,* edited by D.A. Goslin. Chicago: Rand McNally College Publishing Company, 1969.

Shafer, T. "Parents' Reactions to the Birth of a Severely Handicapped Child." *Division of the Physically Handicapped Journal*, 7 (1983), 34–39.

Smith, P.M. "You Are Not Alone: For Parents When They Learn That Their Child Has a Handicap." Washington, D.C.: National Information Center for Handicapped Children and Youth, March, 1984.

Terner, J., and W.L. Pew. *The Courage to Be Imperfect*. New York: Hawthorn, 1978.

Turnbull, A.P. and M.J. Brotherson. "Assisting Parents in Future Planning." Unpublished paper presented at CEC, May, 1984.

Parent Statements

I learned early on that when you have a child like this you don't take life day by day. It's more like hour by hour. Life moves in slow motion.

✺

I wasn't one of the lucky ones. My marriage didn't survive. My husband just couldn't handle it. He thought everything was my job, totally my responsibility. I would encourage anyone considering divorce to go through counseling first. You can't imagine how difficult a divorce is when your child's special needs are involved. Don't expect the lawyers and the courts to sympathize with you; it just doesn't work that way.

✺

Our daughter who doesn't walk asks us a lot if her baby brother will walk. We tell her yes. Right now she sees that the baby can't and pretends that she is the baby.

✺

Where we live and how we live—vacations, recreation, everything—have been affected by our child. All the heartache. . . we think of what might have been.

✺

Our lives have changed in every way imaginable. Economically, it's changed. Before our daughter's lawsuit came through, we scrimped by on one income with a lot of it going to pay for her needs. I haven't been back to work since she was born. There's a tremendous amount of physical and mental stress in dealing with all the different aspects of Annie and her needs.

✻❦✻

We've learned a lot. I sometimes feel like a doctor, therapist (physical, occupational, and speech), nurse, teacher, chauffeur, inventor, builder, computer expert, communication expert—so many things that I sometimes forget I'm still a Mom too.

✻❦✻

My son's handicap has opened my eyes to different things in the world. I'm more accepting of differences, especially if it's something that can't be helped. It's also made me irate at times with "normal" people. They take so much for granted and I can't stand to see them do something that hurts people with handicaps. It could be a stare, a comment, or even just taking a handicapped parking place wrongfully.

✻❦✻

I wish I could change the misconception of CP. Don't look at the shell; it's what's inside that is important.

✻❦✻

Sometimes I feel sorry for Zachary when his body won't do what he wants, but I won't cater to that. If it's been a particularly bad day, it's different—then he needs that extra hug or whatever. But for the most part I try to teach him to deal with it. I explain how his body doesn't always work like he wants but he just has to try. He now stops "to take a breath" before continuing. He's also learning how his body is sometimes separate from who he feels he is. I almost want to teach him that his body and mind are two separate individuals.

✻❦✻

I think I'm too soft on my son. My husband is very firm with him and Jared loves it. The firmness motivates him somehow.

❧

Lately my son's been saying that his legs are "stupid" because they won't do what he wants. The psychologist seems to think this is a healthy attitude, and it doesn't seem to hurt Brian's self-esteem any.

❧

Once I told my physical therapist that it bothers me when my daughter reaches out to regular people who don't know what her handicap is and they reject her. That breaks my heart. She said to me, "I don't think they are rejecting her. . . . I think you are too sensitive." So, ever since then, I've totally changed my attitude. I just let my daughter handle the situation. And she does great. It's phenomenal. She's really growing.

❧

When we discovered that Annie had problems, my mother became extremely depressed for a good two years. Now she has a very special grandchild in her life and says, "Just look how far she's come. I'm so proud of her—she's marvelous." She talks about Annie constantly. What a change we've seen in her.

❧

We look at Jared as if he has no handicap. I think that's how you have to be, because these kids will just walk all over you if you don't.

❧

When Jack was first born, our marriage was put in jeopardy. For some reason, I blamed myself; I felt guilty. I internalized my emotions. Once Jack started to show some progress, it became a joint goal to get him going. Now I realize that his disability has brought my husband and me closer together.

❧

We were hesitant to have another child after what we had been through with our first. Now to see them playing together is beautiful. The baby actually helps Sally and they each have a sibling to love.

❀

My two-year-old loves to help his sister. If her leg falls off the chair, he runs over to say, "Leg up, Nancy," and puts her leg back up on the chair.

❀

It was years before I trusted anyone other than family to care for my child. Then I got brave, went back to work, and made the separation. It was the best thing I could ever have done for my child or myself. My daughter became more independent than I ever knew she was capable of being. I suppose I was her crutch.

❀

There have been times over the years when friends, family, and even complete strangers have asked questions relating to CP in front of Melanie. I've tried to teach her to answer these questions with simple answers such as "my muscles work differently than yours." Of course, there are many times when she does not want to respond and I respect that as her choice. We just don't answer.

❀

SIX

Your Child's Development

JERRIE SCHMALZER BLACKLIN, M.S., C.C.C.*

Children are born magicians. They come into the world as tiny, helpless bundles who cannot do much besides eat, sleep, and cry. Then, right before your eyes, they turn into genuine human beings with personalities all their own. They learn to smile, babble, and laugh; to lift their heads, roll over, and crawl; to reach for their bottles, recognize mom and dad, and play peek-a-boo. Watching children go through this miraculous process of growth, change, and learning—or *development*—helps to form the infinite bond of love which binds parents to their children.

As the parent of a child with cerebral palsy, you undoubtedly find the developmental process just as fascinating as any other parent does. But you may also find it extremely frustrating because your child does not seem to be progressing as rapidly as other children his age. Perhaps he cannot sit on his own, feed himself with his fingers, or speak so that you can understand him. At times, the challenges these problems pose may even prevent you from developing the kind of relationship that supports your child's growth and development. And yet, even though cerebral palsy usually does cause delays in learning certain skills, this does not

* Jerrie Schmalzer Blacklin, M.S., C.C.C., is a speech and language pathologist. She is in private practice in Maryland and Virginia and is a consultant to the Reginald S. Lourie Center for Infants and Young Children in Rockville, Maryland.

mean that children with cerebral palsy do not develop. On the contrary, many of them make considerable progress when given the right kind of guidance. Parents play a critical and irreplacable role in helping their child grow both physically and emotionally.

This chapter provides an overview of the information you need to help your child maximize his potential. It discusses the basics of human development as well as some of the developmental needs children with cerebral palsy may have. More importantly, this chapter explains how you can work with teachers, therapists, and other professionals to make a tremendous difference in your child's development.

What Is Development?

Development is the lifelong process of wondrous change which occurs as children physically grow and intellectually and emotionally mature. The process is different for every child because it is based on individual genetic make-up and is influenced by cultural, emotional, physical, neurological, and environmental factors. The combination of these factors determines how and when each child acquires the skills he needs to mature.

Although each baby's development is unique, skills usually emerge in a predictable sequence. Each accomplishment lays the foundation for the next series of more sophisticated skills to emerge. For example, babies must learn to roll over before they can crawl; to babble and coo before they can say "mommy." Each of these skills which form the basis for future development is known as a *milestone*. Children may reach these milestones at different ages because so many different factors affect development. Often children reach a particular milestone such as walking or talking somewhat earlier or later than average, yet are still felt to be developing normally. For instance, although the average age to begin walking is twelve months, some toddlers who are developing normally do not begin walking until sixteen months of age. Figure 1 gives an idea of the wide range of ages at which a child can reach certain important milestones and still be within "normal" limits. Medical professionals look at a child's overall abilities and quality of growth to be sure that his development is progressing in a predictable and organized way.

Figure 1

AVERAGE MILESTONES

Milestone	Normal Range of Acquisition
Rolls from back to stomach	4 to 10 months
Walks alone	9 to 17 months
Babbles	5 to 14 months
First words	12 to 18 months
Plays pat-a-cake	7 to 15 months
Locates hidden object	9 to 17 months

Cerebral palsy has a definite effect on how well and how quickly children achieve milestones. Cerebral palsy, however, does not in itself predetermine the end result of development. Like all children, children with cerebral palsy have a variety of learning styles, strengths, and weaknesses. Through early intervention, you will be trained to identify your child's strengths and weaknesses, as

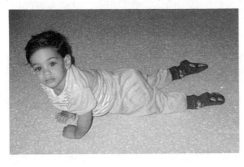

well as his readiness to develop new skills. With this knowledge you will be prepared to interact with your child in ways that will optimize his development. Your support of your child's growth will keep your youngster developing in a positive direction.

Developmental Areas

Development involves more than simply learning a series of isolated skills arranged in order from easy to more difficult. Rather, it involves mastering skills in several different, but interconnected categories. The developmental process is typically subdivided into six areas: 1) gross motor; 2) fine motor; 3) language; 4) cognition; 5) social; and 6) self-help. Because these areas are interrelated, progress in one area is often dependent on progress in others.

Gross Motor Abilities. Gross motor skills require the use of the large muscles of the body, such as those in the legs, arms, and abdomen. Examples of these skills include sitting up, walking, lifting, and climbing. By allowing your child to move around and explore his environment, these skills lay the groundwork for progress in other areas.

Fine Motor Abilities. Fine motor abilities enable children to control small and detailed movements. They include skills that involve muscles in the fingers, hands, eyes, face, and tongue. Skills such as picking up a small object, smiling, and following movements with the eyes are all important fine motor skills.

Speech and Language Abilities. Learning to communicate is probably one of the most important and remarkable accomplishments of childhood. Language development is usually divided into two stages: the development of *receptive language* and the development of *expressive language*. Receptive language is the ability to remember and comprehend words, gestures, and symbols. Expressive language is the ability to use gestures, words, and written symbols to communicate. Toddlers generally develop receptive language before expressive language, and the ability to communicate their thoughts with gestures before the ability to communicate with speech. Because speech calls for the ability to move lips, tongue, teeth, cheeks, and palate in a coordinated fashion, children often have a vast understanding of language before they are able to speak about what they know.

Cognitive Abilities. Cognition refers to the ability to think—to form mental images or ideas of objects and experiences—and to use this ability to reason and solve problems. Cognitive growth is thought to be influenced, in part, by the motivation to master more and more concepts. Typical cognitive concepts include cause-and-effect relationships, means-to-end concepts, and object permanence. Examples of these concepts include pushing a button to see a car move (cause-and-effect), climbing on a chair to get a toy (means-to-end), or searching for an object hidden from sight (object permanence).

Social Skills. Social skills enable children to establish relationships with adults and other children. How a baby bonds and interacts with his parents lays the foundation for feelings of belonging, trust, and love. Later, the toddler learns that he is a different person from his parents. He learns the right and wrong way to behave, but may start resisting his parents' guidelines just to show off his own independence.

Self-Help Skills. Self-help skills are those which allow children to care for their own needs of daily living. Feeding, dressing, bathing, and toileting are examples of basic self-help skills. When children master these skills, they become more independent and lighten their parents' child care burden.

In addition to the six distinct developmental areas described above, two other areas—sensory abilities and physical growth—affect readiness and skill acquisition. Sensory ability, or the ability to feel and comprehend sensations such as touch, sound, light, smell, and movement, is very important to a child's development. Looking at, listening to, and reaching out to touch the people and things close to them helps children understand the world around them. Unfortunately, some children with cerebral palsy have hearing and vision problems or sensory delays which make them over- or under-sensitive to touch, sound, light, or movement. Because these problems can make it harder for children to do the exploration essential to development, this chapter discusses sensory impairments in greater detail later on.

Physical maturation also plays a crucial role in a baby's development. Healthy bones and body tissue are essential to the development of motor, communication, and other skills. Children who do not get the proper nutrients in their early years often have delays in cognitive and language development later. By monitoring a baby's changes in height and weight and calculating his caloric needs, a pediatrician can determine whether physical maturation is proceeding as it should.

For children with cerebral palsy, feeding problems may initially make it harder to consume sufficient calories and may later restrict the variety of foods they are able to eat. Since young children need the right combination of nutrients in their systems for their bodies to mature properly, later sections review some reasons and treatments for these problems.

Although development is frequently broken down into the areas discussed above, you should try to view your child's development as a whole. All children have a unique set of strengths and weaknesses which contribute to their physical and intellectual growth. They may reach some developmental milestones right on schedule or fall behind in others, so that their learning profile crisscrosses the "normal developmental scale." Seeing the whole picture and getting to know your child's needs is a very real, but rewarding challenge.

The Sequence of Development

You have probably been asking questions about your child's development ever since he was born. "What can I expect from my baby?" "When will my baby walk or talk?" "How quickly can I expect my child to meet the goals his therapists set?" are typical questions posed by parents of children with cerebral palsy. In order to put your child's growth into perspective, you may find it helpful to learn about the sequence of human development—the order in which children normally acquire skills. Knowing what to expect can open new pathways to understanding and help you to aid your child's growth and learning.

Your Child's First Five Years

Studies have shown that the first few years of life are crucial to a child's future development. During this period, children make enormous strides in growth and learning, and progress from complete dependence on their parents to semi-independence. This section reviews ten developmental sequences or stages children typically pass through during their first sixty months. Bear in mind that the age ranges given for each stage are merely meant as guidelines and are not intended to imply fixed standards. Because your child has cerebral palsy, he will undoubtedly learn some skills later than most children do; he may also master other skills right on time or even early. What is important is the order in which skills are learned and their relationship to one another, not the ages they are acquired.

Figure 2 shows some of the skills that are usually achieved by most children during the first three years, and the ages at which they are achieved. Again, these charts are not meant to indicate exact times when children develop skills. Instead, you should view the skills as events which occur before a child reaches the next step on the developmental ladder. Refer to the charts and the information in this chapter for help in assessing your child's progress, but do not rely on them as a predictor of your child's future development.

Stage 1: Birth to Six Weeks. A baby's first few weeks of life are a time of wonder for parents. During this period, the baby becomes aware of the outside world, his own body, and his needs. He also begins to attach to his mother and form a mutual bond with her. At first, most of his actions, including sucking and eye, hand, and arm movements are *reflexive*—or not under his voluntary control. Typical skills a baby learns during this stage include turning his head from side to side while lying on his back or making throaty sounds associated with pleasure or discomfort.

Stage 2: Six Weeks to Four Months. Over the next few months of life, a baby's actions become more purposeful. As he gains better control of his muscles, he learns to keep his mother's attention by extending his neck from his shoulders, intently watching his mother, or even crying. As he begins to make sense of sights and sounds in his environment, he learns to look in the direction of noises and to focus on objects around him. At this stage, however, objects that are out of sight are still out of mind. Infants of this age begin to vocalize more than cry and can smile and squeal to show pleasure. Babies may also gaze at their own hands or reach for and grasp a rattle.

Stage 3: Four to Eight Months. During this stage, a baby gradually becomes more aware of his body. He recognizes that he can control his gross motor movements and may even be crawling or scooting about the house. He can shift toys from hand to hand and may be able to sit up without falling. The baby plays endlessly by experimenting with subtle variations of hand, arm, or leg gestures, and delights in keeping games going even when parents tire of the routine. He also plays early seek-and-search games if a toy is partially out of sight, and speech games involving babbling sounds with repeated consonants such as "mama" and "dada."

Stage 4: Eight to Twelve Months. Stage 4 marks the emergence of intentional behavior—behavior that enables the baby to achieve a desired purpose. For example, the baby can now use

Figure 2

	Phase I Birth to 6 Weeks	Phase II 6 Weeks to 4 Months
Gross Motor	• early reflexes present	• holds head erect • turns from back to side
Fine Motor	• grabs adults' fingers with tight-fisted hands	• holds a rattle • reaches for dangling objects with both hands
Language	• startles at sudden noises • makes gurgling sounds • breathing is regular	• coos and gurgles • turns head to mother's voice
Cognitive	• attempts to focus briefly on faces	• gazes at self in mirror • intently looks at people and objects • can wait for bottle when in sight
Self-Help	• completely dependent on parents	• can quiet self with sucking • recognizes bottle
Social	• begins to show preference for mother	• smiles, regards faces

Figure 2 (continued)

	Phase III 4 to 8 Months	Phase IV 8 to 12 Months
Gross Motor	• can hold head steady • sits alone • rolls from back to stomach	• stands alone • walks with help
Fine Motor	• picks up cube • bangs toys together • uses thumb and 　forefinger grasp	• stacks two cubes • releases hold on objects • uses pincer grasp • can hold a crayon
Language	• babbling begins • may say "mama" and 　"dada"	• responds to "no" • waves "bye-bye" • echoes words • may use one or two 　words • uses gestures to get 　things
Cognitive	• drops, looks, and follows 　fallen objects • bangs, hits toys together	• begins to look for 　hidden objects • puts toys in/takes 　them out of containers • nests three boxes
Self-Help	• lifts cup with handle • finger feeds self some foods	• takes off socks • attempts to use spoon
Social	• enjoys social games with 　gestures such as 　peek-a-boo	• wary of strangers • some parallel play 　(playing beside other 　children but not with 　them) • may be more negative

Figure 2 (continued)

	Phase V 12–18 Months	Phase VI 18–24 Months
Gross Motor	• throws ball • climbs upstairs • lowers self from standing	• stands up from stooping position • climbs onto chairs • stands on one foot • rides big toy cars • kicks ball
Fine Motor	• turns knobs • pushes, pulls, pokes toys • turns pages in hard-bound books	• scribbles with crayons • completes simple puzzles

Language	• many early words appear
	• jargoning or social babbling
	  occurs
	• may speak in sentences,
	  but often unintelligible
	• understands more than
	  can say
		• has 20–100 word
		  vocabulary
		• begins to have short
		  conversations
		• still echoes others' speech
		• begins to understand
		  questions

Cognitive	• uses objects as tools (bangs
	  toy hammer to hit
	  wooden pegs)
	• uses trial and error
	• knows functions of objects
		• can sort objects by
		  physical properties such
		  as color, shape, texture

Self-Help	• has more regular
	  bowel movements
	• can unzip clothing,
	  unwrap candy
	• feeds self with fingers
	  or spoon
		• shows interest in toilet
		  training
		• takes off clothes
		• can imitate mother
		  brushing hair

Social	• may have nightmares
	• makes intents known
	• may be attached to blanket
	  or pacifier
	• approaches new people
	  at own pace
		• pretend play with objects
		  (may feed doll with baby
		  bottle or use half-eaten
		  piece of bread as a gun)
		• plays near other children

Figure 2 (continued)

	Phase VII 24–29 Months	Phase VIII 29–36 Months
Gross Motor	• walks down steps with both feet • runs, jumps with two feet	• jumps in place • rides tricycle
Fine Motor	• strings beads • walks better • scribbles are more controlled	• works latches and hooks • uses scissors
Language	• listens to two-step directions ("Get your toothbrush and a comb") • rapid increase in comprehension • begins to make simple sentences with correct grammar • answers and asks questions	• follows directions • understands conversations and poses many questions • very intelligible
Cognitive	• begins to build block structures to house cars • knows attributes of objects—can group objects by color, identify big from little objects	• begins to classify objects by association and function (knows scissors and knives both cut) • has a sense of immediate time ("soon," "after lunch")
Self-Help	• participates in toilet training • puts toys away • helps dress and bathe self	• pours liquids • toilet trained • knows daily schedule
Social	• joins in nursery rhymes • frequently says "no" • likes to control own actions	• pretends to play with super heroes • belief in magic • egocentric

gestures to direct his parents to toys out of his reach. Greater control of gross motor movements allows the baby to actively explore his environment by crawling, pulling up to a standing position, walking with help, and reaching for objects. Greater control of fine motor movements permits the baby to grasp a crayon or begin to use a spoon. During this stage, the baby also becomes more aware of his environment and of others. He may try to communicate with gestures or short words, but may be shy with unfamiliar people. As cognitive skills increase, the baby begins to look for objects placed out of his immediate sight and learns that by searching, he can discover their hiding place. Additionally, he becomes more systematic in exploring sizes and shapes and learns to nest two smaller boxes inside a larger box.

Stage 5: Twelve to Eighteen Months. Between the ages of twelve and eighteen months, a baby begins to understand the power of language. His use of gestures declines and he learns to protest vocally when he does not enjoy an activity. He also begins to use words or short sentences to obtain toys, foods, or other objects, and he can follow simple directions. New avenues for physical exploration and game playing open up as the baby continues to expand his repertoire of motor skills. He can now pull up, stand, and walk on his own, and may even begin to run and flex his knees as though to jump. The baby enjoys the independence of playing with his food and feeding himself, yet is still very dependent on his parents and may be suspicious of strangers. At this age, babies often are interested in simple picture books. They can turn knobs, complete simple puzzles, place one block on top of another, and then smile at their achievements.

Stage 6: Eighteen to Twenty-four Months. This is an exciting stage for the toddler and his parents, marked by terrific progress in all areas. Communication skills become more sophisticated, and the child demonstrates that he can experiment with words and ideas and can hold onto thoughts. Rather than merely imitating others' speech, he now begins to create word combinations of his own. For example, he may pair the word "more" with "juice" instead of expressing his wishes by pointing. He can make known what he wants and does not want, and begins to use the word "no" at every opportunity to show his independence. Social skills also increase tremendously. The child seeks out other children and plays side by side with them. He is not yet ready to share, however, and may even take toys away from playmates. Physically, he can explore just about anything he wants, and can find his way around obstacles to reach a desired goal. He is beginning to run and to jump with both feet, although he still falls at times. He also delights in initiating hide-and-seek games, playing several rounds, and then changing the game at will. Fortunately, besides developing all these new skills, the child also develops the ability to wait for something, if only for a brief moment.

Stage 7: Twenty-four to Twenty-nine Months. In this stage, the toddler really begins to test his physical and mental abilities. It is no surprise that parents often spend a great deal of time developing regulations or rules for their toddler's sleeping and eating routines, as well as setting limits for their youngster's behavior. Children start to understand the concept of ownership, and "mine" becomes a favorite word. Play is more sophisticated and may include pretend play or trading toys with other toddlers. As the child continues to master communication skills, he becomes interested in carrying on short conversations and in asking and answering questions. In particular, toddlers like to question and explore the functions of objects as they work on understanding concepts related to texture, shape, and size.

Stage 8: Twenty-nine to Thirty-six Months. By their third birthdays, children begin to pick up social customs of their culture. Many children, for example, love to pretend to be adults. A child may wear his parents' shoes, or start to talk with his parents' own expressions. You may even recognize your own reprimands as your child scolds the dog! Children of this age may also begin to play games of make-believe with monsters and heroes. The world of monsters can become so real that children have more frequent nightmares. Do not be surprised if you find yourself searching the closets at bedtime to demonstrate that no monsters are hiding there.

During this stage, children become very social. They are now capable of initiating and maintaining intelligible conversations with strangers. And although they may not yet have a clear understanding of what is meant by "yesterday" or "tomorrow," they begin to express ideas using past and future tenses of verbs.

Stage 9: Thirty-six to Forty-eight Months. Between ages three and four, children become more active in the community. The neighborhood and preschool rank high in their social worlds. The world of the home blends into the world of the child's experience. Youngsters become curious about the world and ask many questions, usually preceded by the word "WHY." "Why does it rain?" or "Where do babies come from?" are common queries for them to pose, but they generally are content with a simple, direct answer to their questions. The three- and four-year-old can run, jump, kick, and climb, which opens up a new world of games with youngsters older and younger than himself. He may have a keen interest in pre-academic concepts involving numbers, colors, and letters and can classify objects and pictures according to similarities and differences in size, shape, and color.

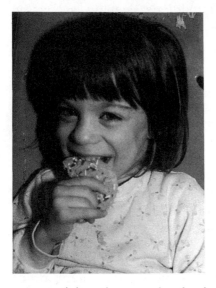

Stage 10: Forty-eight to Sixty Months. In this period, a child believes that he is the center of the universe. This self-centeredness is not the by-product of selfishness, but rather of the child's idea that the world is magic and he is in the center of it all. Consequently, he may feel that his own behavior influences all events around him. He may think, for example, that the moon follows him when he rides in a car. Or he may assume that his dog died because he wished earlier in the day that he did not have to care for it. Despite his egocentricity, the preschooler is very social. He still loves make-believe games, but now he may cast himself as the hero in a drama with many parts. Because of his school experience, activities such as cutting, pasting, and designing art projects become more important. He can now use his experiences and the order and predictability of his own routines to foresee future happenings and analyze past events. For instance, he now knows when it is Monday because his school week begins on that day.

The Development of Children with Cerebral Palsy

Perhaps you have just learned that your child has cerebral palsy. The diagnosis may have come as quite a shock since you may initially have heard from your doctors or therapists that your child had developmental disabilities, motor delays, or neurodevelopmental delays. Now the new label, cerebral palsy, adds a different dimension to what you may previously have considered to be a short-term problem.

You may wonder if your child's development will be normal. You may be searching the developmental charts to see where your child fits in. Remember that there is a wide range of what is considered to be "normal" development. Your child may have normal abilities in some areas, variable skills in other areas, or slower maturation in yet other abilities. Much will depend upon your child's particular strengths and weaknesses. For example, consider the baby who is not walking at 12 months. Perhaps the same youngster can use his eyes to direct you to obtain toys for him (a 9 to 12 month skill), can play peek-a-boo (also a 9 to 12 month skill), and can look for objects hidden out of sight (again in the 9 to 12 month range). Only the gross motor area lags behind the other areas of development. With time and motivation, walking may also be an achievable goal. Remember, how you adjust to your child's range of skills will help you to know your child's unique personality with all of its gifts. When you can see your child's whole developmental picture, it is easier to look beyond the immediate physical limitations.

For children with cerebral palsy, *quality* of development is just as important if not more so than *rate* of development. How rapidly your child acquires skills does not matter so much as how well he is eventually able to do them. Rather than push your child to achieve isolated milestones when it is "normal" to do so, it is far better to encourage skills that build upon those he already has. For example, if your child is at the age when children normally begin walking, but he has only just mastered rolling from his back to his tummy, you should help him work on crawling next instead of skipping right to standing.

Because every child's quality of development and rate of growth vary so remarkably, your child's therapists will *not* make predictions about your baby's future. Instead, the therapists will schedule regular re-evaluations of your child's growth and maturation. A skilled clinician can teach you how to recognize and appreciate your child's development in the various areas and help you plan for future progress. Do not be surprised if you come to rely upon the advice of a trusted therapist before scheduling a re-evaluation or planning an educational program.

Your child's therapists may also advocate for your child to get needed equipment that would support his growth and development. Therapists often act as the liaison with community agencies that provide wheelchairs, hearing aids, communication boards, or other needed equipment. In addition, your therapists should be able to guide you through the insurance and educational mazes that parents face when seeking treatment for their child.

Throughout the therapy process, the challenge is to learn how to observe your youngster so that you can motivate him when he is ready to be introduced to the next skill. As you recognize developmental shifts and spurts, you can open the door for each new achievement. Encouraging your baby to be curious without being critical of setbacks is the single most motivating guidance you can give your child. As Chapter 5 explains, this means it is important to cheer your child on by praising his attempts and by refraining from doing too much for him. If you help him capitalize on his strengths, he *can* learn to achieve on his own. And your reward will be discovery that growth and change *are* possible.

To plan for your child's future achievements, you need an overall impression of your child's strengths and weaknesses across all the developmental areas. As explained later in this chapter, you will probably not get this total picture all at once, but rather, in stages as your child's development is periodically evaluated and re-evaluated. Still, there are a number of conditions that affect the development of many children with cerebral palsy. To help you recognize and understand your child's developmental strengths and needs, the next sections review some of the more common conditions.

Persistent Primitive Reflexes

All children are born with a set of reflexes or involuntary responses which help them to survive until they develop voluntary control over their muscles. These reflexive movements usually disappear within a few months after birth as more sophisticated skills take their place. Because children with cerebral palsy often develop more slowly, reflexes may persist into childhood. When reflexes do not disappear on schedule, they are known as *persistent primitive reflexes*. Persistent primitive reflexes often interfere with development. For example, if the startle reflex persists longer than normal, a baby may have trouble learning to feed. This reflex, which usually disappears within the first six months of life, occurs in response to a sudden loud noise or a sudden shift in position of the baby's body. During a startle, a baby's arms and legs extend straight out away from his body and become momentarily stiff and inflexible. When a baby is slow to develop head control, it may be almost impossible for him to nurse if he is constantly being startled by slight changes in body position or noises in an adjacent room. With guidance, parents can learn techniques to help their baby relax so he can nurse more successfully. For example, it may help to swaddle the baby with his arms crossed over his abdomen or to nurse him in a warm, dark, quiet room.

Besides the startle reflex, there are a variety of other reflexes that may persist longer than usual in children with cerebral palsy. Figure 3 shows the more common reflexes that children have at birth and the relative rates at which they disappear. Knowing how the presence of these reflexes affects movement can influence the way you handle your baby. Your child's therapists can suggest handling techniques to help you optimize your child's development.

Muscle Tone

All children with cerebral palsy have problems with muscle tone; with the stretch and resistance, or give and take of their muscles. As Chapter 1 explains, some children have muscles that are floppy and relaxed, or *hypotonic*. Others have muscles that are abnormally tight, or *hypertonic*. In addition, some children have fluctuating muscle tone, which creates involuntary movements, tremors, or variation in the strength and weakness of the muscles

Figure 3

REFLEX MILESTONES

Common Reflexes	Developmental Influences	Reflex Appears	Reflex Disappears
Startle A sudden shift from sound sleep of the head in response to loud noise or sudden shifts in the baby's position result in startle. The baby's arms and legs come together, his legs shoot straight out, and his hips flex	• Baby can wake from sound sleep • Baby is fussy and irritable in response to speech and household noises • Baby has difficulty nursing because he is distracted by noises and movement	birth	4-5 mos.
Tonic Neck Reflex or "Fencing Pose" As the baby turns its head to one side, the arms and legs on the same side as the head straighten out	• helps the baby to breathe if his face is pressed downward • If identified when dressing the baby, the straightened arm can move easily into a sleeper before putting in the tight fisted arm	2–3 wks.	5–6 mos.
Neck Righting Reflex If the infant is on his back and the head is turned to one side, the shoulders and trunk turn to the same side	• This reflex is used when rolling from back to front. • If the muscles are weak in the trunk, shoulders, and neck, your therapist can demonstrate baby exercises which strengthen muscle tone and promote coordination	2–3 mos.	8–10 mos.

Adapted from: Rossetti, Louis. *High Risk Infants: Identification, Assessment, and Intervention.* Austin: Pro-Ed, Inc., 1986. p. 34.

during an intentional movement. Each of these types of muscle tone can have far-reaching effects on a child's development. The most obvious effects, of course, are on the development of gross and fine motor skills. For children with hypertonia, excessive muscle tension coupled with inflexible joints may make movement difficult. For children with hypotonia, overly flexible joints and weak and floppy muscles result in slower, imprecise movements. Fluctuating muscle tone can also make it harder for a child to control his movements. How your child's muscle tone affects his development of motor skills depends on how and where cerebral palsy affects his muscles, but you can expect at least some delays.

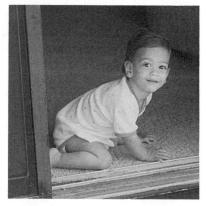

Besides delaying the development of movement skills, problems with muscle tone can also delay development in other areas. A child with hypertonia may have trouble taking part in activities which develop cognition. For example, he may have difficulty understanding the relationship between cause and effect if he cannot lift his hand to knock over a tower of blocks and watch them fall. If his gross motor system is greatly impaired, his handicap may even prevent him from watching someone else destroy the tower because turning his head and holding it up sets off a whole series of other movements in his body. In addition, hypertonia can interfere with a child's ability to acquire self-help skills such as dressing and feeding. For instance, he may not be able to grasp a spoon independently or to lift the spoon from his plate to his mouth.

Hypotonia can also delay skill acquisition in many areas, but for different reasons. For instance, a baby with hypotonia in the neck, shoulder, jaw, and speech muscles may have difficulty feeding because he is unable to keep his head up to drink from the nipple. Toileting is another self-help skill that may be harder to develop if muscles in the trunk are weak and floppy. Hypotonia may also affect a toddler's attention, and as a result, his cognitive development. For example, a child may exert so much energy maintaining an erect posture against gravity that he may not have any energy left over to pay attention to an exploratory game.

As Chapter 7 discusses, there are therapists who specialize in helping children with movement problems overcome their developmental delays. They are trained and skilled in identifying types of muscle tone and the changes in it, and in demonstrating techniques to improve your child's movement. They can show you ways to work with your child so that he can use his own muscles to achieve various goals. They may also devise special equipment to make movement easier. Your therapists will have many ideas to help your child move without undue physical and emotional stress.

Conditions Associated with Cerebral Palsy

As Chapter 1 explains, cerebral palsy is caused by damage to the part of the brain that controls movement. But when there is damage to a child's central nervous system, there is a chance that other areas of development besides motor development may also be affected. As a result, many children have conditions associated with their cerebral palsy that affect thinking, reasoning, communication, or sensation.

As you read through the following sections, keep in mind that these are conditions that children with cerebral palsy *may* have. Your child may have some, all, or none of them. If your child does have any of these conditions, understanding them and their effects on development will help you set realistic goals.

Mental Retardation

Mental retardation is a label loaded with fear for most parents. In the past the term usually implied mental incompetence and was often a ticket to institutionalization. But mental retardation does not mean incompetence, only slowed or delayed mental development. Children with mental retardation are not incapable of learning; they just do not learn as rapidly as other children do.

Until recently, about two-thirds of children with cerebral palsy were thought to have mental retardation. But now, thanks to early intervention and advanced technology, many children with serious movement and communication problems are better able to demonstrate their true potential. As a result, some experts believe the percentage of mental retardation may be as low as 25 percent.

Keep in mind that an IQ is based upon a standardized way of measuring cognition and achievement. Children with cerebral palsy often are penalized because their movement impairments can interfere with test-taking performance. A child who is in a wheelchair, for example, certainly cannot skip or walk on a line, two tasks required in certain tests of mental measurement. Similarly, a child with damage in the shoulders, arms, and fingers cannot perform the puzzle completion tasks on most IQ tests. Standardized tests may be viewed as a method of estimating where your child scores in comparison to other children his age. Intelligence testing, however, may very well not give an accurate indication of your child's potential.

If your child does score in the mentally retarded range, you can expect his development to be slower than that of others his age. But as in the "normal" population, children with retardation have a wide and varying range of abilities. As Chapter 1 discusses, the degree to which retardation affects the ability to think and reason is related to its severity. Your child may need more time to understand words and concepts, but if you filter information into simpler, more comprehensible units, your child, too, will learn new ideas.

Although your child's IQ may place some restrictions on what he learns and the rate at which he learns it, early intervention and special education programs can reduce the impact of mental retardation on your child's cognitive development. Sometimes the label "mental retardation" can even help your child obtain the most appropriate educational program. Programs for children with mental retardation tailor their curricula so that your child can learn at a rate which gives him confidence in his emerging new abilities. As Chapter 8 explains, this means it is important for you to recognize your child's developmental strengths and weaknesses so that you can help plan an educational program that will help him achieve his potential. When the curriculum is appropriate, a child is less likely to experience stress and more apt to appreciate his own achievements.

Remember, skill development, not high scores on an intelligence test should always be your goal. It is true that your child's pace of learning may be somewhat slower than other children's, but that does not make his achievements any the less meaningful. With your support and guidance, your child can continue to learn all his life.

Prematurity

Many premature babies develop more slowly than their peers because they need more time to adjust to life outside the womb. Within two years, however, premature babies usually recover from their rocky beginnings and catch up with other toddlers the same age. With the advances in medical technology, many "preemies" go on to have perfectly healthy childhoods. Most major cities have neonatal clinics which follow the "preemie's" development and offer support if a delay persists.

Premature babies most likely to have delays later in life often have very low birth weights in combination with other health problems such as breathing abnormalities or lung disease. And indeed, approximately 1 in 3 of the 300,000 children with cerebral palsy in the United States weighed less than 2,500 grams (about 5 pounds, 8 ounces) at birth. In the very early days of their lives, many of them needed a great deal of medical attention and specialized equipment such as incubators and monitors to help them survive. Often these youngsters also seem to be more susceptible to allergic reactions to medication and foods, or to other health problems.

Since chronic illness makes it difficult for a baby to focus on and explore people and things around him, his health needs to improve before he is ready to learn. Therapists can teach parents many different approaches to holding, stimulating, and feeding their baby that can help speed recovery. Babies who are healthy are more inclined to sleep, eat, and develop regular routines. . . then they can learn!

If your child with cerebral palsy was premature, frequent and regular developmental check-ups can keep you apprised of delays linked to his prematurity. The team of professionals working with your child can suggest intervention techniques when the need arises.

Seizures

As Chapter 3 discusses, seizures are frequently associated with cerebral palsy. According to some researchers, children with high tone may be especially prone to develop this condition.

The abnormal electrical activity in the brain that causes seizures can produce a variety of symptoms. The most common types of seizures include the grand mal, a massive convulsion with or without loss of consciousness, and the petit mal, more fleeting minor convulsions accompanied by temporarily diminished muscle tone and fading attention.

Because they disrupt a child's attention, seizures can interfere with information processing and make cognitive skills harder to learn. Children with seizures may also be unable to make eye contact with their parents at a young age, setting up further barriers to learning. Being able to observe a parent's facial expressions is crucial to the development of social skills such as smiling, as well as to the development of cognitive and communication skills.

If you think your child experiences seizures, discuss your concerns with your pediatrician. Your doctor can arrange for the tests necessary to diagnose seizure activity and, if indicated, can prescribe medication to reduce the frequency of seizures and increase your child's attention.

Vision Problems

Many children with cerebral palsy have some form of visual impairment. In addition to having nearsightedness or farsightedness, they may have several problems which interfere with development. Common problems include *strabismus*, a type of cross-eyedness in which one eye focuses on a target and the other eye drifts away; *diplopia* (double vision); and *nystagmus*, a jerky, involuntary movement of the eyes. These problems and their symptoms can be indicative of underlying disorders. Children with nystagmus, for example, may have underlying sensory delays that affect their balance and body awareness as they move from place to place. Consequently, they may have more difficulty achieving milestones such as walking or climbing. Children with double vision may have trouble discerning background from foreground and may trip over obstacles as a result.

If vision problems are detected early, their impact on development can be reduced through proper treatment. You, as the parent, can help in detection by monitoring your child for signs of potential problems. These signs include squinting, unusual or unexpected movements of the eyes at rest, or trouble focusing on people and objects. Once your child reaches three months of age, you can have his vision screened by a pediatric ophthalmologist.

Hearing Impairments

Children with cerebral palsy are more likely than other children to have hearing problems. The permanent nerve damage that affects their movement may also cause what is known as a *sensorineural* hearing loss. Sometimes mechanical problems in the middle ear may also cause hearing impairment. In *otitis media*, the most common type of middle ear problem, a vacuum or fluid in the middle ear impedes the transmission of sounds. Middle ear problems often are treated with medication, whereas sensorineural disorders require a hearing aid. Getting the appropriate treatment can make the difference between delayed acquisition of language and slower-paced, steady emergence of speech and language milestones.

Because hearing is vital to your child's development, you should monitor him carefully for signs of hearing loss. You should suspect hearing problems if your child seems oblivious to sound, does not respond to his name, or watches faces intently for meanings of words. Whether or not your child shows any of these symptoms, you should have his hearing checked regularly beginning at four months of age. An audiologist can test your child's hearing and diagnose problems affecting the transmission of sound. If necessary, your audiologist can help you choose the correct hearing aids and recommend programs that will help your child to learn language.

Speech and Language Disorders

In addition to having language problems associated with hearing loss, children with cerebral palsy may experience a variety of other speech and language disorders. For example, they may have difficulty understanding words and thoughts because they have trouble remembering what the words mean. Youngsters with cerebral palsy may also be slower to acquire language because they need more time to listen to words before they can comprehend the composition and order of spoken sounds. In addition, muscle tone problems in the face, neck, and shoulders may cause an *oral motor disorder*, an inability to coordinate the muscles to make sounds. Your speech/language pathologist can be very helpful in finding ways for your child to express himself. Gestures, picture boards, and computers can give your child the power to talk even when his muscles lag behind. Chapter 7 explains how you can work with your child's speech-language pathologist to optimize his development.

Sensory Impairments

Many children with cerebral palsy have sensory impairments, or trouble regulating the amount and quality of the many sensations they feel. They may have abnormal reactions to sounds, tastes, movement, sight, touch, or smell. For example, a child with cerebral palsy may have difficulty adjusting to the sensation of touch. Even the feeling of clothing against his skin could trigger tears because the feel of cotton is so uncomfortable. If a sensory impairment exists, any sensation can set off angry or fearful behaviors. As a result, children with sensory impairments are often fussy, cranky, or colicky.

If your child resists certain sensations, daily routines such as feeding, dressing, playing, or sleeping can be difficult and trying for you, and physically challenging for your child. In addition, your child may experience delays in cognitive, self-help, language, emotional, or motor skills. This is because a child's sensory abilities lay the foundation for exploring and learning about his world. If a child resists certain sensations, he may also withdraw from contact with the people and objects that can help him learn about his experiences. If a child is overly sensitive to the feeling of being wet or dirty, for example, he may be cranky whenever his diaper is wet. If the child is also hypertonic, he may not be able to control his voice to cry for his mother. The result can be a baby who is constantly moving and trying to avoid contact with his touching, caring mother. Similarly, a child whose gums are hypersensitive to touch might move his body away each time the nipple goes into his mouth. Feeding him could be a cumbersome, unending chore. The problem would be greatly magnified if, in addition, he overreacted to loud sounds and rocking while his mother tried to feed him.

Working with a therapist can make the difference in your baby's development and acceptance of various senstations and in your understanding of your child. An occupational therapist in particular can offer you invaluable support if your child has a sensory impairment. See Chapter 7 for further information on occupational therapy.

Feeding Disorders

Good nutrition is the key to physical and cognitive development. Children need an adequate supply of vitamins and minerals for their bones and tissues to develop normally. And research has shown that well-nourished children have fewer cognitive and language delays than malnourished children.

Unfortunately, malnourishment is frequently a problem for children with cerebral palsy. Not only are they more likely to have feeding disorders due to physical or emotional causes, but they may also burn more calories to make simple movements because of extraneous muscle movements caused by their condition. Consequently, their development is often delayed as they redirect their resources to survival, rather than development.

For children with cerebral palsy, feeding disorders are often the first sign that something is not right. The causes of feeding problems are as variable as the types of delays children can experience. Children with sensory problems, for example, may not like the feel of the nipple in their mouths or may avoid contact with their mother's milk, resulting in failure to eat, poor nutrition, and weight loss. An active baby who has trouble coordinating sucking and swallowing may choke on his milk or regurgitate it immediately after feeding. If the problem persists or is severe, your doctor may do some tests and prescribe tube feeding so your child receives the proper nourishment. He may also refer you to a therapist to help reduce feeding problems.

Besides physical problems related to cerebral palsy, some children develop emotional behaviors that get in the way of feeding. To compensate for the restricted mobility which limits their control over their environments, they may refuse to eat in order to have control of one routine in their lives. In these cases, establishing and maintaining a feeding routine early on is critical. Children must learn to see the feeding routine as an orderly and predictable time to receive nourishment, as well as the feelings of warmth and acceptance that help them feel loved and secure.

Feeding problems rarely have simple solutions. Usually a team of professionals must work together with parents to solve the problem. Teams may include a developmental pediatrician, nutritionist, developmental psychologist or psychiatrist, occupational or physical therapist, nurse practitioner, speech pathologist, or social worker. Chapters 3 and 4 provide more information about feeding disorders and their treatment.

Helping Your Child's Development

As this chapter has emphasized, it is impossible to predict how much a young child with cerebral palsy will be able to achieve. No one child with cerebral palsy is born with quite the same set of abilities and potentials as any other child with cerebral palsy. True, your child's development will be limited to some extent by his cerebral palsy and by conditions such as mental retardation associated with it. But there are ways you can reduce the impact of all these conditions. Chief among these is early intervention—a specialized way of interacting with infants and toddlers to minimize the effects of conditions that can delay development. Almost as important, however, are your expectations for your child and what you do to help make those expectations become a reality.

Getting Developmental Help for Your Child

The first step in getting your child the help that will minimize his developmental delays is to identify the problem. This means that if you have not already done so, you need to arrange for an *assessment* for your child—a complete evaluation of your child's strengths and needs in all developmental areas. The assessment will most likely be conducted by a team of professionals, including a physical therapist, occupational therapist, developmental pediatrician, social worker, and speech pathologist. Some teams also include nursing specialists, psychologists, nutritionists, and infant educators. For your first visits, you likely will work with a developmental pediatrician, infant educator, and physical therapist. By observing your child, these professionals will determine what skills your child already has and whether he is behind in achieving developmental milestones. At the conclusion of the assessment, the evaluation team should be able to present you with a picture of your child's development, pinpointing the needs he has and what specific therapies and educational interventions he should receive. Chapter 8 explains how to arrange for an assessment for your child.

Once your child's special needs have been identified, he will be eligible to receive developmental help from a variety of public and private sources. In some states, babies with cerebral palsy qualify for publicly funded early intervention education through local school districts or state-financed agencies. These programs—discussed in Chapter 8—provide services aimed at maximizing a baby's potential. As of 1991, all states will have designated agencies to identify and treat children at risk for developmental delays from birth onward.

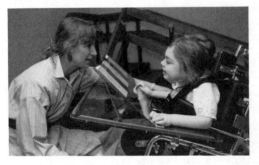

If public school services are not available, there are still many other sources of developmental help. Hospitals and health departments, for example, often provide assessment and treatment for children with cerebral palsy, as do special education and clinical programs in universities. Most communities also have physicians, therapists, psychologists, and educators in private practice who are trained to teach babies and young children with special needs. Their services are sometimes covered by medical insurance and group health plans. Particularly if you live in a rural or hard-to-reach area, you may want to locate and coordinate information from your own professional support team. See Figure 4 for a list of professionals and their areas of responsibility.

For information about services available in your area, contact your local chapter of United Cerebral Palsy or Association of Retarded Citizens, other support and advocacy groups, and, of course, other parents of children with special needs. The Resource Guide at the back of the book lists some associations that may be able to help you locate services or professionals qualified to provide them.

Your Expectations and Your Child's Development

When your child has cerebral palsy, it can be hard to "take it one day at a time." You want to know *now* whether your child will ever talk, or when he will learn to crawl. But concentrating on your child's day-to-day accomplishments—on his small victories—is one of the best ways you can support his development. As long as you and your child believe in his potential to make progress—however slight—he is much more likely to make that progress.

The reason your expectations can have such a profound effect on your child's development is not hard to understand. If you expect that your child will eventually be able to master a skill such as drinking from a cup, you will be more likely to allow him to try as many times as necessary before he succeeds. On the other hand, if you expect that your child will *not* master a skill, you will be more likely to give your child more help than he needs or to take over at the first sign of difficulties, thereby guaranteeing that he will never learn the skill.

For your child to succeed, you must set realistic, achievable goals. Observing what your child is doing and exploring is the first step. Your therapists will then help you decide what is possible based on your child's developmental stages. Your child can also give you important clues about the suitability of goals. Watch his face for signs of frustration. Look at his gestures and acting-out behavior if his speech is garbled. Talk to people working with your child and listen to your instincts.

Once your child's goals are set, your most important job is to motivate your child to develop his skills. To help your child accept his weaknesses and build on his strengths, be sure to notice and share in the joy of each achievement. Not only will your child's appreciation of his own accomplishments be heightened, but he will also be more encouraged to persevere in the face of frustration.

Of course, motivating your child to keep trying after repeated failures is often easier said than done. It can be very difficult to watch your child reach with awkward, clumsy movements, over-shoot his goal, and spill his milk. It is just as painful to encourage your child to walk when his balance is still insecure and his struggle may lead to a fall. But if the goal that you and your therapists set for

Figure 4—Areas of Development to be Assessed and the Professionals Responsible for Each

Area	Skills Assessed	Specialist
Speech/Language	Articulation, pronunciation, verbal abilities, vocabulary, understanding and following directions	Speech Pathologist
Gross Motor	Using large muscles—walking, skipping, running, throwing, balance & coordination	Physical therapist
Fine Motor	Using small muscles—handwriting, buttoning, puzzles, eye tracking, feeding, hand dominance	Occupational Therapist
Perceptual/Sensory Processing	Visual perception, design copying, planning of body movements, and such skills as toleration of touch and movement in space necessary for sensory motor development	Occupational Therapist
Cognitive/Learning	IQ, learning styles, achievement, thinking, reasoning, understanding	Special Educator/Psychologist/Educational Diagnostician
Hearing		Audiologist
Vision		Opthalmologist/Physician
Nutrition	Caloric intake, habits, variety of food, growth, nutritional status	Registered Dietician/Nutritionist
Medical	Brain maturation, related condition	Pediatrician/Developmental Pediatrician/Neurologist

Adapted from Reisner, Helen, ed. *Children with Epilepsy: A Parents' Guide.* Rockville, Md.: Woodbine House, 1988.

your child is achievable, allowing your youngster to take the risk and try to achieve his goal is the greatest gift you can give him. He will learn with time what is possible for him to achieve and what physical and other limitations he must accept. Children who develop an awareness of their talents and limitations are well suited to understanding the imperfections in themselves and the world around them. They can assess their possibilities realistically and go on to make the absolute most of their potentials.

Conclusion

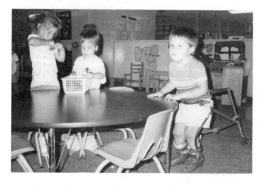

There is no denying that cerebral palsy will affect the way your child grows and learns. But there is also no denying that he *will* grow and learn. How well and how quickly he develops will depend to some extent on the type and severity of his cerebral palsy, and on the various conditions that may be associated with it. Fortunately, however, your child's developmental progress is also affected by factors that are under your control. If you and your child's teachers, doctors, and therapists provide a good educational program and a supportive home environment for your child, you can help offset delays in reaching achievable goals.

True, even with constant work and encouragement, your child may never be able to master some of the skills that other children learn automatically. He may or may not be able to play basketball, read fluently, or ride a bike. But even if your child is never able to shoot a basket, there is still no reason he shouldn't shoot for the stars.

Parent Statements

I don't wait around for him to reach milestones. He was never supposed to talk. There have been enough pleasant surprises that I feel there will continue to be more. That's what we have to continue to remember.

✽✽✽

It's really hard for me to watch my sister's baby crawling around and just naturally picking up all these skills Timmy has to slave over in therapy. I mean, I can't blame my sister for bragging, but I wish it weren't all so unfair.

✽✽✽

Initially, in the back of my mind I kept saying Ellen would show the doctors they were wrong. She would be okay. It's like finding the magic cure. I guess a lot of parents go through similar feelings. And not having an idea of what to expect didn't help at all. Always hearing "we don't know" was frustrating, to say the least.

✽✽✽

Frustration best sums up how I feel about her physical development. It's fantastic that she's come as far as she has. They said she wouldn't do this much. For the most part, though, her development is so extremely slow that you really get tired after a while. Mentally, I'm very pleased with her development.

✽✽✽

It was great when he could finally show professionals what I had believed all along, that there was a bright little boy in that body.

✽✽✽

Early on I looked forward to a developmental evaluation just to see where Jeffrey stood. After continually seeing how low he scored on their tests, it became depressing to have an evaluation. He's scored around the same level on his motor skills for several years, and you kind of get tired of seeing the negative side of things. You want a test that gives your child a fair chance.

❧❧❧

I take developmental tests with a grain of salt. I don't put a lot of value in them. There are too many variables that can influence a test score and the child isn't given a fair chance.

❧❧❧

It's sad that our society has to rely so heavily on tests to determine what services a child will receive and how a lot of them perceive the child differently depending on his scores.

❧❧❧

Every time Jeannie makes a speck of progress we fall all over ourselves congratulating her. Maybe as a result, her communication skills are really starting to blossom.

❧❧❧

I think his retardation is harder for me to accept than his cerebral palsy. I just think things would be so much easier if he had a better understanding about what is going on.

❧❧❧

People still ask me why I hold him so much. . . like I really have a choice.

❧❧❧

My biggest dream has been to take a walk down the street with my child. We do—we hold hands, he in his wheelchair and I along side. We may be slow, but these walks are very special to me.

❧❧❧

I recently gave my son a birthday party. Many of the parents were kind enough to call beforehand to ask what an appropriate gift would be for Scott. I thought that was just great. In the past, he has received countless inappropriate toys.

❧❦❧

The best thing you can do for your child is to accept him the way he is. Don't compare kids, even regular kids. All kids are just individuals.

❧❦❧

SEVEN

Physical Therapy, Occupational Therapy, and Speech and Language Therapy

LYNNE C. FOLTZ, M.A., P.T., GEORGIA DeGANGI, Ph.D., O.T.R., DIANE LEWIS, M.A., C.C.C.*

Cerebral palsy will present many challenges for you and your child. But you don't have to face these challenges alone. There are many professionals who have dedicated their lives to understanding the problems that cerebral palsy and other motor problems can pose for children and their families. They can help your child optimize her development; they can help her to live a life with as few limitations as possible.

Of the many types of professionals who *can* help your child, the three you are most likely to encounter are the physical therapist, the occupational therapist, and the speech-language pathologist.

* Lynne C. Foltz is the director of Footsteps Pediatric Physical Therapy in Silver Spring, Maryland, where she works with babies, children, and their families in a private practice setting. She received her physical therapy training at Stanford University and currently is on the faculty at Georgetown University. Georgia DeGangi is an occupational therapist and developmental psychologist at the Reginald S. Lourie Center for Infants and Children and also Director of the Cecil and Ida Green Research and Training Institute in Rockville, Maryland. Diane Lewis holds an M.A. in speech pathology from Michigan State University. She is currently working on a doctorate in Education of Severely, Profoundly, and Multiply Handicapped at Johns Hopkins University.

Depending on the nature and extent of your child's movement and communication needs, she will probably require the services of one or more of these therapists, for longer or shorter periods, sometime in her childhood.

To help you recognize your child's therapy needs, this chapter provides an overview of the ways that physical therapy, occupational therapy, and speech and language therapy can benefit children with cerebral palsy. It also discusses how to find the right therapists for your child and what to expect from therapy sessions. Finally, it offers some practical suggestions to help you and your child get the most out of all of her therapy services.

PHYSICAL THERAPY

What Is Physical Therapy?

The goal of physical therapy (PT) is to identify and treat problems with movement and *posture*, or body position. Originally, physical therapy was used to help World War I veterans reacquire skills they had lost due to nerve, muscle, or bone injuries. Today, physical therapy is used to help infants and children who are having

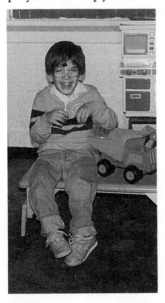

trouble acquiring movement skills because of injuries to their nervous systems. With special exercises, handling techniques, and constant encouragement, pediatric physical therapists can help children learn or become more proficient at a variety of movement skills, including rolling, sitting, crawling, and walking.

For children with cerebral palsy, whose movement problems are caused by brain injury, it is crucial that PT begin at an early age. This is because the central nervous system is most susceptible to change during the first five years of life. Specific problems that require PT vary from child to child, but here are some that children with cerebral palsy commonly have:

Posture. There are several important postures or positions that children need to master in order to acquire gross motor skills. These include: supine (on the back); prone (on the front); sitting; side-lying; kneeling; half-kneeling; and standing. Because of their brain injuries, children with cerebral palsy may be unable to hold their head, trunk, arms, or legs in proper alignment against gravity in one or many of these postures. In addition, children with cerebral palsy often cannot move one body part independently of another. For example, when a baby looks to the right, she may move her head and shoulders along with her eyes because she cannot keep her posture steady.

Transitional Movements. As Chapter 6 explains, the motor skills that enable children to move from one place to another usually develop in a specific sequence. For example, a baby normally learns to roll over, crawl, and walk, in that order. Before babies can master the more advanced movements, they must acquire the so-called *transitional movements* that enable them to connect one posture to another. For instance, one of the first transitional movements most babies learn is rolling from their fronts to their backs. Later, babies are able to get into a sitting position on their own by rolling from their backs to their fronts and then using their arms to push themselves into a sitting position. Once a baby can do this, she has mastered the "supine to sit" transition.

For babies with cerebral palsy, abnormal muscle tone makes many normal transitional movements difficult or impossible. Think, for example, about the way you would stand up from a sitting position on the floor. Usually you would kneel on both knees, put one leg up into a half-kneel position, and then push up with your legs into a standing position. A baby with high muscle tone, however, might have to use her arms to pull herself up on a chair because her legs are stiff and inactive. A baby with low tone might spread her legs far apart, place both arms in front of herself, push down on her arms, and stand up without distributing much weight to her legs. For both low-tone and high-tone babies, the half-kneel to stand transition is difficult or impossible.

Persistent Primitive Reflexes. Another factor which may affect a baby's posture and movement is the presence of primitive reflexes. These reflexes usually are present at birth and fade away before six months of age. Babies with cerebral palsy, however, may have what is called "persistent primitive reflexes," or reflexes that continue for longer than average. These reflexes tend to persist more frequently in children with high tone and often make it harder for babies with cerebral palsy to learn movement skills such as rolling and sitting.

One reflex that may persist is the *asymmetrical tonic neck reflex* (ATNR). ATNR occurs when a baby is lying on her back and turns her head to one side. As the baby looks and turns to the right side, her right arm involuntarily extends and straightens and her left arm bends and flexes. This response is often called "fencer's position" because it is similar to that used by someone who is fencing. Sometimes a baby's legs may also show this same involuntary response when she turns her head. ATNR can help a baby develop the eye-hand coordination needed to explore a toy or master other skills. However, when the reflex occurs every time a baby turns her head, it may prevent her from achieving milestones such as rolling or balancing herself while sitting. If a baby has a muscle tone problem, the influence of this reflex can be more pronounced on one side than on the other. See Chapter 6 for more information on persistent primitive reflexes.

Balance. Babies who are developing normally learn at an early age how to use movements to keep themselves upright. For example, if a ten-month-old baby loses her balance when she is sitting, she can use her head, trunk, and arms to prevent a fall. She can shift her body weight in the opposite direction from which she is falling and put out one hand to catch herself. In contrast, a baby with cerebral palsy may clench her fists tightly and bring her shoulders up toward her ears. When she loses her balance, she cannot free up a hand to catch herself, but falls over as one unit.

Sensory Impairments. If a child with cerebral palsy is over-responsive or under-responsive to sensations such as sight, sound, movement, and touch, the acquisition of movement skills becomes more difficult. Often what "feels good" to children with cerebral palsy is very different from the expectations of parents. Some children, for example, dislike being touched on certain body parts, especially the face, hands, and feet. This may discourage a child from exploring her own body. Other children do not enjoy being bounced on their parents' laps or being moved quickly from one position to another. When children have spastic muscle tone, this type of roughhouse play may cause their tone to increase, making controlled movement more difficult. Chapters 1 and 6 discuss sensory impairments in more detail.

Joint Mobility. Children with cerebral palsy frequently have abnormal joint mobility or flexibility. Depending on their muscle tone, they may have joints that are either more or less flexible than normal. Spastic muscle tone, for example, often makes joints such as the hips, knees, and ankles more difficult to move, and may result in limited range of motion. Limited range of motion occurs when muscles pull a joint more strongly on one side than on the other. If your child has hypertonia, you may hear about tight hamstrings (which can cause limitations in the mobility of the hips and/or knees) or tight heel cords (which make it difficult to place the heel on the floor and can cause "toe walking.") In severe cases, spasticity may even lead to joint *subluxation* or dislocation. The hips are the joints most frequently affected.

Children with low tone are less likely to have joint limitation, but may have excessive joint flexibility. This flexibility may hinder the development of efficient movement patterns. For example, children with extra joint mobility often lock their knees or elbows to help stabilize their feet and hands in space. Too much joint mobility may also stretch ligaments that support the joints, making injury more likely.

What Is a Physical Therapist?

The physical therapist is the professional who will evaluate and treat your child for the movement problems described above. She will probably be one of the most important people in your child's early life. She will help your child develop her motor skills to the maximum extent possible. She will also help you understand how to foster good self-esteem in your child, which is the critical element in how far and hard a child is willing to push to gain new skills. Most likely, the physical therapist will be your primary teacher about your child's disability and about her problems with specific movements. The physical therapist can also be an important link as an advocate for your child in the medical and special education mazes. She can advocate with you for needed services, serve as an intermediary, or give you the information you need to advocate on your own.

Physical therapists are required to complete a master's degree, which usually takes six years after high school graduation. They also must be licensed in the state in which they practice. Many therapists belong to the American Physical Therapy Association (APTA), which certifies specialists in the care of children (pediatrics). The physical therapist your child sees will probably specialize in pediatrics and may further limit his or her practice to infants and children with developmental disabilities. Your child's physical therapist may also have specialized training in neurodevelopmental treatment (NDT)—a therapeutic technique designed for infants and children with motor handicaps such as cerebral palsy.

Physical therapists may provide their services in children's homes, or in hospitals, early intervention centers, schools, or private offices. They may work alone or as part of a child's early intervention or special education team. And as Chapters 8 and 9 explain, babies and children with cerebral palsy are legally eligible to receive the services of a physical therapist free of charge as part of their special education programs.

How the Physical Therapist Evaluates Your Child

Before beginning to treat your child, the physical therapist must first develop a complete picture of your child's movement abilities and disabilities. Through tests and observations, she evaluates your child for each of the potential movement problems described earlier. To tailor a treatment program to your child's needs, the physical therapist also determines how your child will respond to therapeutic handling—to being held and moved in certain positions.

Standardized Tests. Standardized tests such as the Bayley Scales of Infant Development - Motor, the Peabody Developmental Motor Scales, or the Movement Assessment Inventory (MAI) may be used to measure your child's level of motor development. The therapist observes your child's movements to determine a motor age, which may be significantly different from her chronological age. The results of this testing help to determine whether or not your child has delayed motor development and if she can benefit from a physical therapy treatment program.

Observation. For additional insight into what is impeding your child's motor skill development, the physical therapist will observe your child's *movement patterns*—or how she moves. In particular, the therapist will try to identify postures your child likes to use which may delay or prevent acquisition of new skills. For example, if your child has low muscle tone, the physical therapist might observe that your child sits on the floor with her legs widely spread apart. She cries if toys are placed outside of her legs, but plays happily if the toys are moved inside her legs. The physical therapist might also observe that your child prefers to support herself with her arms placed on the floor between her legs and does not shift her weight from one side to the other while sitting. Because these preferred postures would prevent your child from reaching to the side or shifting from a sitting to a crawling position, the physical therapist would note the need to help her learn new, more efficient habits.

Besides observing your child's movement patterns, the physical therapist will also observe your child's ability to use both sides of her body in a coordinated manner. The physical therapist will observe, for example, whether your child leans to one side when sitting, can roll to the right but not to the left, or is able to use only one hand for reaching. Often these *asymmetries*—differing abilities to use either side of the body—are caused by *tone disturbances*, or any variation in tone from the normal (high tone, low tone, fluctuating tone).

After their child's initial evaluation, parents often expect that the physical therapist will be able to make specific predictions about how their child will progress. Unfortunately, predictions are usually impossible until after a child has been in active treatment for some time. Every child has her own style and rate of responding to treatment, determined in part by her motivation, ability, and degree of physical impairment. Your child's progress over time gives a much better indication of her potential than one isolated evaluation does.

To measure your child's progress, the physical therapist will periodically re-evaluate your child formally, usually every three to six months for a baby and every six to twelve months for an older child. The re-evaluation may be part of a developmental assessment performed to determine your child's progress in all areas. This time is often tense for hopeful parents who may have test anxiety watching their babies perform. You should try not to get caught up in the numbers, though. Bear in mind that the evaluation results are to help the physical therapist plan your child's treatment program, and are not a report card for your child.

How the Physical Therapist Treats Your Child

Once your child's evaluation is complete, the next step is to plan an individualized treatment program for your child. Planning usually begins when you and the physical therapist jointly decide on the movement goals that are most important to your child's future development. Goals might include standing up straighter, developing better balance reactions, using one body part independently of another, keeping hands or feet flat when supporting weight, spending more time in non-preferred positions, maintaining joint mobility, coordinating movements of different body parts, or increasing physical endurance. Also in the planning process, the physical therapist may suggest special equipment such as orthotics, special seating, and balls or other therapy equipment that will help your child reach her goals. In addition, the therapist will certainly discuss ways you and your family can work with your child at home.

Physical therapists may use one or more of a variety of treatment philosophies with your child. The Bobath approach, also known as neurodevelopmental treatment (NDT), is the one most commonly used for infants and children with cerebral palsy in the United States. It was introduced in the 1950s by Karl and Berta Bobath, a husband and wife team working in London, England. The goal of the Bobath approach is to prepare the child's posture and movement to permit the development of "functional skills"—that is, skills such as feeding, dressing, and bathing that a child needs to live as independently as possible. Treatment focuses on encouraging the child to use normal, rather than abnormal movement patterns, and on preventing deformities or muscle contractures that would make developing movement skills more difficult.

In addition to using Bobath techniques, a therapist may integrate some concepts from other approaches into your child's PT program. For example, if your child has sensory integration problems, the physical therapist may incorporate the treatment techniques of Jean Ayres into the session. Brunnstrom techniques are often used with children who have hemiplegia, whereas Rood techniques are helpful in treating oral-motor problems.

Whatever approach your child's physical therapist uses, she will probably schedule your child for at least one or two therapy sessions each week. During periods of rapid change or surges in your child's motor development, the physical therapist may want to see your child more often to capitalize on her readiness to learn new skills. Most likely, you will bring your child to the office, school, center, or hospital where the physical therapist works, but the physical therapist may also provide treatment in your home. This is called *home-based* treatment and is often used for babies who cannot travel to a school or office because they have medical problems. Chapter 8 provides more detail about the therapeutic and educational settings you may encounter in more detail.

Your Child's Therapy Sessions

In initial therapy sessions, the physical therapist will likely concentrate on gaining your child's trust and on building a good relationship with her. This is because children between the ages of eight months and two years are frequently anxious about being separated from parents and can be afraid of strangers. To get some idea of how well your child separates from you, the physical therapist will probably ask you to place her on an exercise mat by herself. Later, the physical therapist may use a large doll to demonstrate treatment techniques while you try them with your child. Sometimes just seeing the same doll at each therapy session helps a child feel more at ease with the therapist. Eventually, the physical therapist will hold your child herself and move her around to observe her response to being held and moved in certain positions. If your child adapts easily and seems to enjoy the new movement sensations, the physical therapist will begin therapeutic handling.

The goal of therapeutic handling is to make new movements possible for your child. For example, in treating a child with high muscle tone, the physical therapist uses specific positions and handling to reduce the child's tone. These positions may include side-lying on your lap, supported sitting on a ball, or prone lying on your legs. To a child who is used to having a stiff body, these new positions may feel strange at first. As the child's body becomes more relaxed, however, she will find many movements easier. For example, it will be easier to hold her head up against gravity when support is provided at the shoulders or trunk. The child may be very pleased and stimulated by this new ease of movement.

In handling your child, the physical therapist will look for positions your child especially likes and will use these frequently. She will also investigate the positions your child dislikes and introduce activities in these very gradually. For example, your baby may prefer to lie on her back and avoid rolling over to her tummy. This may be due to your baby's awareness that it is difficult to hold her head up against gravity. But without the ability to hold her head up, your child's visual stimulation is limited. The physical therapist may try to introduce prone positioning with your baby placed on her lap. By providing support at key points, especially the head, shoulders, and pelvis, she will make active movement easier for your baby.

Besides therapeutic handling, there are other methods the physical therapist will use to stimulate your child's movement. For example, she may use equipment such as balls and bolsters to provide a mobile surface. A mobile surface can help to alter your

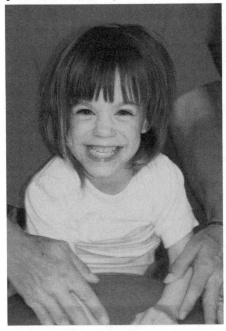

child's tone to make movement easier for her. She may also encourage your child to experience a variety of sensory stimuli—objects or activities that appeal to your child's senses of hearing, sight, touch, smell, or taste, or to her *vestibular* (movement) awareness. For example, the physical therapist may sing or play a tape to help your child pay attention, or may use a cue such as placing her hand on your child's chest to remind her to position her head a certain way.

The physical therapist will probably also use all sorts of toys in different shapes, sizes, and textures to help your child reach her movement goals. For example, the physical therapist may introduce a toy bar with interesting toys hanging at midline to encourage your child to use her arms and shoulders to reach and grasp. Or she may use blocks, finger foods, small magnetic balls, or bean bags to help your child work on voluntary release of objects. To help your child feel more at ease in standing, she may encourage your child to stand or walk with a vacuum cleaner, doll stroller, or other push toy which offers support at shoulder level. As an added bonus, these toys will also teach your child about object permanence, cause-and-effect relationships, and other important cognitive concepts discussed in Chapter 6. Your physical therapist will help you to select the toys most appropriate to your child's developmental level—that is, toys suitable for your child based on the skills she has mastered, not her chronological age.

After you have been working with the physical therapist for a while, you will notice that she uses a great deal of repetition. Practice and repetition help children to become familiar with and to refine skills. Sometimes, though, if a child practices a skill in only one setting, she will only learn to do that skill in that particular setting. For example, a baby might begin crawling on a specific mat in the therapy room. When she goes home, however, she may continue to roll, rather than crawl, across the kitchen floor. To help your child transfer the skills she learns in therapy to a variety of "real-life" settings, the physical therapist may visit her at home, at school, or on the playground.

Special Equipment

For use at home, your physical therapist may suggest that you buy or make some of the same equipment she uses in therapy sessions—for instance, a small bench, therapy ball, or mat. As Chapter 4 explains, your child may also need more specialized positioning or mobility equipment. For example, your child might benefit from a prone stander for table top work; special seating for feeding, bathing, or transportation; or a walker or crutches for support while walking. Your child's physical therapist will help you to select any potentially helpful equipment, then work with you and your child to learn how to use it. She may also discourage you from buying certain popular baby products that could interfere with your child's therapy goals. Suspended jumpers and walkers with a sling seat and four wheels, for example, may significantly increase your child's tone and make controlled movements more difficult. These "baby walkers" may also threaten your baby's safety.

Sometimes your child's doctor and the PT may jointly decide to try an *orthotic.* An orthotic is a custom-made device used to support the foot and/or leg in proper alignment for weight bearing—in what therapists refer to as a "neutral" position. A neutral position is the most efficient for standing and walking. Orthotics include:

1. shoe inserts, which help position the foot only;
2. supra malleolar orthoses (SMOs), which support the ankle joint and foot and extend just above the ankle joint;
3. ankle foot orthoses (AFOs), which hold the ankle and foot in a neutral position (a ninety-degree angle to the floor), and extend high up on the calf;
4. inhibitive fiberglass casts, which also hold the ankle and foot in a neutral position, but are more supportive than AFOs; and
5. knee ankle foot orthoses (KAFOs), which hold the knee, ankle, and foot in a neutral, functional position, and extend up on the thigh.

Orthotics are made by specially trained orthotists. Your orthotist will consult with the doctor and physical therapist to make adjustments needed because of your child's growth and change. Orthotics can be used on a short-term or long-term basis, according to a child's specific needs.

Physical Therapy after Surgery

As Chapter 3 explains, surgery to improve function by heel cord or hamstring lengthening or to prevent or correct deformities such as scoliosis or hip dislocation is sometimes recommended for children with cerebral palsy. After surgery, your child's movement abilities can temporarily deteriorate due to immobilization, weakness from disuse, and lack of practice. Following the initial period of healing, however, surgery may enable your child to learn many new skills. For example, if tight muscles are released in the legs, tone in the trunk or arms is often reduced. This can improve hand function tremendously and bring skills such as handwriting, eating, using a touch talker, or propelling a wheelchair within your child's grasp.

Physical therapy may begin within 24 to 48 hours following surgery, and is a critical force in maximizing your child's progress. Children need to learn new movement patterns immediately while motivation is high and fear and anxiety are low. Because your child will make her greatest improvements in the first six to twelve months after surgery, your physical therapist may ask to see your child for more frequent treatment during this period. Working with your child at home is also crucial.

Although movement gains may be very dramatic just a few weeks after surgery, it is important not to push your child too hard. She may feel some pain or discomfort and movement may be slow and labored. Casts may be used for optimal positioning for several weeks after surgery or may not be used at all. This decision will be made by the orthopedic surgeon. If your child must wear a cast, you may have to do much more lifting, carrying, and other hands-on care than you did prior to surgery. The physical therapist is therefore concerned about *your* body during this recovery period and will provide suggestions and demonstrations to reduce the likelihood of injury. You may need a wheelchair or special stroller for a short period of time until she becomes more mobile.

Getting Involved in Your Child's PT Program

When your child is very young, you will play an active part in her physical therapy sessions. In addition to helping your baby adjust to her therapist, you will learn new ways to carry her, feed her, and play with her to encourage new movement patterns. Once your child is two or three years old, however, the therapist may request that you leave the room during treatment for a while. This not only helps your child develop some independence, but also gives her the chance to show off new skills when you return.

Whether or not you are actually present during therapy sessions, your role in your child's physical therapy program is vital. To begin with, you can give the physical therapist invaluable input about the movement goals most important for your child and your family. For example, when your child starts preschool, she may need to be toilet-trained. The therapist can offer ideas for achieving success with independent or assisted use of the toilet. Likewise, your insight into your child's problems with day-to-day activities such as eating can help the physical therapist choose the special equipment that your child needs. In addition, it is up to you to make sure that your child practices the new movement skills she learns in therapy when she is home. Your therapist will teach you how to move, handle, and position your child to make it easier for her to use these new movement patterns.

Sometimes children with cerebral palsy learn that they can get their parents' attention by rebelling against their therapy program. They may sit in a "w" position, climb out of a prone stander, or refuse to wear orthotics. The therapist will help you to identify these attention-getting behaviors and to deal with them in a positive way. For example, the child who refuses to wear orthotics may need a specific time of the day (after school, perhaps) when she can "relax" and move freely without wearing the orthotics. The therapist and parents can work together to set up an orthotics-wearing schedule that is acceptable to the child.

It is important not to let your child control her home follow-up program. This is often an area of struggle for families. Even though parents really want their child to cooperate with all therapy goals, their child may learn to manipulate them to avoid meeting their expectations. Your physical therapist is familiar with these conflicts and can help to negotiate a compromise, perhaps first with your child in therapy sessions, and then at home with you.

Because your support and encouragement are crucial to your child's progress, the therapist will probably also show you how to praise your child at each small step along the way. Major milestones such as walking *are* important, but you won't want to miss your child's excitement at being able to hold her head up straight, play with a challenging toy, keep herself from falling, or stand with support.

The specific techniques your physical therapist will teach you depend on your child's needs, but instruction often involves learning about:

1. feeding;
2. carrying;

3. dressing;
4. seating;
5. locomotion (independent or assisted);
6. providing sensory experiences;
7. reading your baby's cues;
8. combining motor goals with language, cognitive, and educational goals; and
9. fostering your child's independence and self-esteem.

Although the physical therapist may give you specific therapeutic suggestions at each session, how you integrate them into your life is up to you. If you can adapt techniques to your family's lifestyle, you are more likely to succeed at helping your child reach her goals.

Often the physical therapist will use a notebook to record her therapeutic suggestions and to keep track of your child's progress through notes and photographs. This is an excellent way to help you and everyone involved in your child's physical therapy program coordinate their efforts to help your child.

How to Find a Physical Therapist for Your Child

Many early intervention centers provide physical therapy treatment for children with motor disabilities such as cerebral palsy. Other centers offer only generalized infant stimulation without the expertise of a physical therapist. In this case, you may need to seek private services for your child. This expense may be covered through your family medical insurance policy.

The Neurodevelopmental Treatment Association (NDTA) directory listed in the Resource Guide at the back of this book lists physical therapists, occupational therapists, and speech-language pathologists who are certified in NDT. These specialists work in all kinds of facilities—Easter Seals, UCP, and Kiwanis clinics; private offices; schools; hospitals—but tend to be concentrated in the larger cities. If you live in a small town or rural area, it may be harder to find a physical therapist with the pediatric expertise your child needs. You and your child may have to see a physical therapist who works primarily with adults and make periodic visits to a consultant pediatric physical therapist in another city. Visits with the pediatric specialist can reassure both you and your therapist about your child's progress and can give you the chance to develop new treatment ideas together.

Aside from educational qualifications, there are other considerations to take into account when choosing a physical therapist. Some of these include professional expertise, experience in dealing with babies and children with cerebral palsy, the use of toys and equipment that can motivate your child, and the ability to establish good rapport with your child. For your child's sake, you will want to find someone with enthusiasm, as well as someone who can set limits. For your own sake, you will want to find a therapist with whom you feel comfortable discussing your thoughts, feelings, and concerns. Your child's pediatrician may be able to recommend a physical therapist with these qualities, as may United Cerebral Palsy, Easter Seals, and the NDTA. Local hospitals with developmental centers and other parents of children with cerebral palsy can also be excellent sources of names.

OCCUPATIONAL THERAPY

What Is Occupational Therapy?

When advised to seek occupational therapy for their child, parents typically react by saying, "My child doesn't need to learn an occupation!" Actually, the name "occupational therapy" is misleading. Occupational therapy, called "OT" for short, got its name in World War I when therapeutic activities were used to help soldiers regain function in their arms and hands. At that time, treatment centered mainly around arts and crafts activities.

With the development of new theories and treatment methods, occupational therapy has changed dramatically. It now includes specialties in physical disabilities, mental health, and pediatrics. In each of these special areas, the purpose of OT is the same: to help people function as effectively as possible in their environments. By "occupying" adults or children with meaningful therapeutic activities or exercises, occupational therapists help them to overcome sensory, motor, and perceptual problems affecting learning and daily living skills. Treatment programs are highly individualized and are geared to individual intellectual, language, and social-emotional abilities. For children with cerebral palsy, receiving OT in the first few years of life is often critical and may determine whether they are ever able to use their hands for dressing, feeding, grooming, handwriting, and other skills.

Often parents are confused about the differences between OT and PT. This is understandable, since there is some overlap between the areas that occupational and physical therapists treat. For example, both may work on motor skills such as sitting up, crawling, and walking, as well as on problems with balance and reflex development. In general, however, PT focuses more on the development of gross motor skills—on movements involving large muscles such as those in the legs and trunk. OT, on the other hand, focuses on the development of fine motor skills—on movements involving smaller muscles in the arms, hands, and face—and on processing and using input from senses such as sight, hearing, touch, and movement. Here are some of the areas an OT might work on with a baby or child with cerebral palsy:

1. problems with muscle tone or movement quality (stiffness of movement) that prevent a child from using her hands and arms efficiently—for example, problems keeping head, trunk, and shoulders positioned correctly to allow independent movement.
2. basic hand skills such as holding, manipulating, and releasing objects. Also accuracy of aim in activities such as stacking objects or placing pegs in a board, and grasps such as the pincer and palmer grasps described in Chapter 6.
3. more complex hand skills such as cutting with scissors and writing.
4. skills that require eye-hand coordination—for example, throwing and catching a ball.
5. use of the arms for weight bearing—when crawling, for example—and for reaching in different directions for objects.
6. dressing, grooming, and other self-care skills.

7. feeding skills and *oral-motor* skills such as chewing and swallowing that involve the use of muscles in and around the mouth and face.
8. perceptual skills that require an understanding of spatial concepts—for example, puzzle completion, depth perception, constructing structures such as block bridges, and pre-reading readiness (letter and shape recognition).
9. *sensory processing* functions—that is, receiving and interpreting information from the senses. For example, awareness that a body part has been touched or moved in space involves sensory processing.
10. *sensory integration*, or using information from the senses to learn and develop skills. For example, infants typically rely on their touch, movement, and position senses to develop balance, to coordinate the two sides of their bodies, and to learn how to plan and sequence movements. The senses of touch, movement, and position are linked together with hearing and sight during play and daily activities. For instance, a child first looks at her hands while she manipulates a toy in a new shape. Later, she can recognize the shape just by feel.
11. basic nonverbal communication (making and understanding gestures) and functional play skills (learning to play with a toy in a variety of ways).

What Is an Occupational Therapist?

There are different types of occupational therapists. Some work in rehabilitation facilities with adults who have physical disabilities, some work in mental health settings with people who have psychiatric disorders, and still others work exclusively with children. This third type of occupational therapist—the *pediatric occupational therapist*—is the specialist you will want to find for your child.

Pediatric occupational therapists are specially trained in the diagnosis and treatment of infants and children with a variety of developmental disabilities. They may have either a bachelor of science or a master's degree in occupational therapy and must complete a six to nine month internship to become certified and licensed. Like physical therapists, occupational therapists may also have training in neurodevelopmental treatment (NDT), the form of therapy especially for people who have abnormal movement due to central nervous system disorders. In addition, pediatric occupational therapists may have training in sensory integration (S.I.)—a therapeutic technique designed to help children who have trouble with fine motor coordination or perceptual skills such as reading due to problems sorting out and organizing sensations.

Occupational therapists work in a variety of settings, including hospitals, schools, and families' homes. They are often members of early intervention or special education teams, but may also work alone, in private practice.

How the Occupational Therapist Evaluates Your Child

Whether your child should have both OT and PT will depend on her needs. Sometimes children under the age of eighteen months have difficulties only in areas which either an occupational or a physical therapist can treat—for example, head control or sitting up. In this case, it may be appropriate for the child to see only a physical therapist or an occupational therapist until it becomes clear that either one or both is needed. Other children with cerebral palsy have multiple needs or could benefit from different therapeutic approaches to the same problem. These children might benefit most from a combination of physical, occupational, and speech and language therapy.

To find out what, if any, occupational therapy services would help your child, she should have a complete occupational therapy diagnostic work-up. If your child has not already had a complete developmental evaluation, you will want to arrange one so that the occupational therapist can make the most appropriate recommendations for your child. Chapter 8 discusses developmental evaluations in detail.

To evaluate your child, the occupational therapist will give your child tests in fine motor, perceptual, and oral-motor development. The therapist will observe how your child responds to touch and movement in a variety of activities such as handling a textured toy or balancing on a therapy ball. The therapist will also interview you to find out more about how your child can dress and feed herself and to find out your concerns.

The precise elements of your child's evaluation will depend on her age and the degree of her disability, but will probably include assessments in most of the potential problem areas described earlier. Most young children with cerebral palsy need to be re-evaluated every six to nine months to determine progress and further therapy needs.

How the Occupational Therapist Treats Your Child

After the occupational therapist has finished evaluating your child, she will plan a treatment program geared to your child's individual needs. Once again, your role in the planning process will be to help pinpoint the goals most important for your child to achieve. For example, you might like your child to learn to spoon feed or to fasten zippers and buttons on her clothing. Or you might like your child to be able to draw with a pencil or to use both hands to take off a jar lid or to do other tasks.

To help your child reach her goals, the occupational therapist may use a number of therapeutic techniques. The techniques most commonly used for infants and young children with cerebral palsy are neurodevelopmental treatment (NDT) and sensory integration (S.I.). Because an important goal of occupational therapy is to help children become as independent as possible, occupational therapists also train children to use special equipment that encourages the development of self-care skills and to use computer techniques that promote fine motor control and perceptual development. This section describes how occupational therapists typically use NDT, S.I., and special equipment in treatment programs for children with cerebral palsy.

Neurodevelopmental Treatment

Before your child can develop fine motor skills, she needs good upper body control—that is, she must be able to position her trunk, shoulders, and pelvis properly and to rotate her trunk so she can reach freely with her arms. As discussed in the physical therapy section of this chapter, improving children's posture and movement so they can better use their hands is a major goal of NDT.

To prepare your child for functional skills, the occupational therapist will first use a variety of physical handling techniques to 1) relax your child's spastic muscles or increase the tone in her floppy muscles; 2) obtain good alignment of your child's spine, pelvis, and shoulders; and 3) help her use her arms and legs more effectively for weight bearing. To accomplish these goals, the therapist may hold your child in her lap and move parts of her body in many different patterns or use special equipment such as therapy benches or inflated bolsters or balls.

Once your child has achieved good alignment, the therapist will use a combination of physical handling techniques and therapeutic activities to work on your child's reaching, grasping, and releasing skills. For example, if your baby has tightly clenched hands and cannot reach for objects, the therapist will first position her carefully. She might place your baby so that her body is completely relaxed, with her neck, spine, and pelvis in good alignment and her arms and shoulders optimally positioned to bring both hands together to hold an object. The therapist might then loosen the muscles in your baby's shoulders and hands with rhythmic alternating shoulder movements. Next, the therapist may work with your baby on reaching for and holding her own feet, a position that requires her to use her whole arm to reach and grasp. The therapist might follow this activity by having your baby hold an appealing ball toy in wide open hands and bring it up to her mouth. This type of activity would not only motivate your baby to develop reaching and grasping skills, but also prepare her for the hand-to-mouth skills she needs to feed herself.

When your child is preschool-aged, the occupational therapist will use NDT treatment techniques to help her learn more complex hand skills such as feeding herself, working zippers and buttons, cutting with scissors, or drawing. For instance, a two-year-old with spastic diplegia may have difficulty scooping with a spoon because she cannot turn her wrist into a palm-up position while holding onto an object. In the effort of trying to feed herself, the toddler may raise her shoulder up high and bend her elbow toward her body. To treat this problem, the therapist may first work with the child on keeping her shoulder down and elbow extended, perhaps by placing the child in a side-sitting position on the floor with both knees to one side of her body so she must use her arms to support herself. Next, the therapist may use various handling techniques to free up the movement of the child's forearm and wrist.

Finally, to motivate the child to work on the troublesome movements herself, the occupational therapist will select an activity that not only addresses her fine motor and feeding needs but also involves enjoyable play and language skills. For example, the therapist might give the child a magnetized stick to hold and have her make a pretend ice cream cone by rotating her wrist in a scooping motion to pick up magnetized balls. Later on, the therapist might help the child carry over this skill for feeding by having her scoop foods such as peanut butter or pudding that stick to the spoon. Eventually, by isolating and working on the separate movement problems that prevent the child from scooping with a spoon, the therapist will improve the child's feeding skills.

Often parents are confused about how OT and PT differ because both occupational and physical therapists may use NDT techniques. Although both receive identical training in basic neurodevelopmental treatment techniques, how they use their training is somewhat different. Whereas the physical therapist trained in NDT concentrates on improving gross motor skills such as crawling and walking, the occupational therapist with similar training concentrates mainly on the upper body control needed for fine motor, feeding, and self-care skill development. For example, both might work with your child on standing and walking, but for different reasons—the physical therapist, to help your child become more mobile; the occupational therapist, to help your child keep her arms at her sides or to carry an object or hold onto a table without her arms becoming stiff.

This overlap of physical and occupational therapy goals can be very beneficial to children with cerebral palsy. For instance, your child might find it easier to reach her PT goal of standing with good alignment after her occupational therapist has worked with her on reaching upward to place magnets on a refrigerator or on carrying a large ball with both hands. As the speech and language therapy section of this chapter explains, OT goals may also overlap with speech and language goals.

Sensory Integration (S.I.) Therapy

Sensory integration refers to the ability of the central nervous system to take in, sort out, and inter-relate sensations received from the environment. These sensations include what we see, hear, taste, and smell, as well as what we feel from our senses of touch, from the pull of gravity, and from moving around.

Most children begin learning how to detect and interpret information from their senses during infancy. Learning to process touch, movement, and position sensations is particularly important at this stage because of the impact of these sensations on motor development. Infants use information from these three basic senses to learn to plan and sequence movements, to coordinate the two body sides, to develop balance and stability in their movements, to coordinate eye and hand movements, and to develop a sense of their own body. Later on, these skills lead to refinements in perceptual-motor development, or the ability to discriminate shapes and positions of objects. This is needed for skills such as reading, writing, and math.

Unfortunately, many infants and young children with cerebral palsy have *sensory integrative deficits*, or problems receiving and processing sensations. These problems may include *hypo-* (under) or *hyper-* (over) sensitivities to touch and movement, and difficulties planning and sequencing movements. S.I. therapy—an approach developed by the occupational therapist A. Jean Ayres—can help children with problems in these areas. The following sections discuss sensory integrative deficits children with cerebral palsy often have, as well as how occupational therapists usually treat them.

Tactile Hyper- and Hypo-Sensitivities. Children with high muscle tone frequently have a condition known as *tactile defensiveness* or *tactile hypersensitivity*. They have a severe sensitivity to being touched and may react adversely to types of touch that other children would tolerate or enjoy. For example, children with spasticity often have difficulty placing weight on their hands and feet, and as a result, do not experience normal touch-pressure to these body parts. A child may bear weight on her fists instead of her palms, and when her hand is opened, she may withdraw her hand and resist touching objects because her palm is very sensitive to touch. Typical postures of children with high tone—extending the neck backwards, raising the shoulders up, and flexing the arms—may compound hypersensitivities to touch. If children with these movement problems also dislike being touched around the face, neck, and shoulders, dressing and bathing become two-fold problems involving both touch and movement difficulties.

Children with low muscle tone sometimes have a combination of hyper- and hypo-sensitivities to touch. They usually develop strong preferences for certain body positions, and when positioned differently resist not only the new position, but also the contact of different parts of their bodies with the floor. For example, a child might habitually sit with her legs drawn up on the floor beside her in a "w" position, but become upset if placed on her side or stomach. A child with low tone may also place weight on the backs of her hands to avoid contact on her palms, or she may walk on her toes to avoid contact on her heels or soles. Along with these signs of *hyper*-sensitivity, the low-tone child may also have signs of *hypo-* sensitivity. For example, she may laugh when she falls off furniture, sit half on and half off a chair without seeming to notice, catch her arm beneath herself without flinching, or even bite herself without seeming to feel pain.

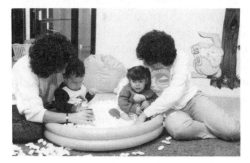

To treat *hyper*sensitivities to touch, the occupational therapist tries to give the child tactile (touch) experiences that will desensitize sensitive body parts such as palms and soles while stimulating touch pressure all over the body. For example, the therapist may have the child work on weight bearing on her hands and feet in bins of styrofoam chips or dried beans, may roll the child up like a "hot dog" in a cotton blanket or rub her palms and soles with a plastic hair brush, or may have the child play with bristle blocks, which give more tactile input to the hands.

For the *hypo*sensitive child, treatment focuses on providing firm, deep pressure to stimulate the sense of touch. The activities are similar in many ways to those described for the hypersensitive child.

Movement Insecurities and Cravings. Another area of sensory integration that sometimes poses problems for children with cerebral palsy is their sense of movement and position. For example, many children with spasticity do not shift their weight from side to side or forward and back when lying, sitting, or standing, and as a result, do not stimulate their own movement sense as other children do. (The movement sense, also known as the *vestibular system*, helps control posture and balance and is also important for movement security and normal muscle tone.) When they do move, children with high tone often do so in abnormal ways. For instance, they may arch on their backs to get across a room, or hold their necks tipped backwards most of the time. Usually children with high tone are very fearful when therapists introduce new movement patterns, especially those involving changes in neck position. They may also dislike being moved on therapy balls and the amount of movement that occurs in therapy.

Unlike children with high tone, children with low tone are more apt to enjoy movement. Much to their parents' dismay, they love to bounce on furniture or rock forwards and back very vigorously. They, too, have their favorite ways to move, however, and may be quite reluctant to move in new ways. For instance, they may cry if placed on their stomach and may resist rolling or other movements that involve body rotation. Characteristically, low tone children are slow to start movement and may be content to lie or sit still for long periods of time. Thus, children with low tone often paradoxically crave certain movement activities while fearing new and different movements.

To treat children with cerebral palsy who have movement insecurities or cravings, occupational therapists must often use a combination of S.I. and NDT treatment approaches. For instance, a child with spasticity may love roughhousing with her father, but when they play together this way, the jostling in mid-air makes the child's legs stiffer. The therapist may suggest that the father continue to roughhouse, but with his daughter's legs straddling his waist to keep them from stiffening.

Motor Planning Problems. Many children with cerebral palsy have motor planning problems or *dyspraxia*—trouble planning their movements and putting them into sequence. For example, they may be unable to figure out how to get themselves into a new body position or how to put separate movements together to produce a more complex movement such as skipping or drumming a rhythm. In some children, motor planning problems affect their ability to get from one place to another. For example, a child might go around in circles and make all kinds of movements before she can figure out how to get onto her therapy bench herself. In other children, motor planning problems affect more sophisticated perceptual skills such as constructing a design out of blocks or creating a drawing. Usually children with motor planning problems have difficulty playing with their peers, mainly because they tend to rely too much on their parents to get themselves organized. Generally, they also have trouble learning the movement sequences needed to manipulate zippers, buttons, shoelaces, and other fasteners.

The occupational therapist works extensively on helping children with cerebral palsy overcome their motor planning problems. A major part of the therapist's work lies in carefully diagnosing the problem, then determining how to unlock the block that prevents the child from learning new movement skills. The therapist must also consider factors that may contribute to the problem: frustrations, resistance to new and different tasks, and manipulative behaviors such as throwing a tantrum if the smallest thing is changed. Next, the therapist must work on ways to motivate the child to try new ways to learn skills and to help reduce frustrations. For instance, suppose a child cannot hold paper and snip with scissors because she cannot put the movements into sequence. To reduce frustrations, the therapist may give the child a play dough snake, which is easier to hold than paper is. To motivate the child, the therapist might then ask her to snip the snake into little pieces to feed a favorite stuffed animal.

Often the therapist needs to backtrack and lay the sensory basis for motor planning—that is, to give the "feel" of moving in new ways. To learn this "feel" of movement, many children need to work on touch and movement activities in combination with sequenced motor activities. For example, the child may practice crawling on sticky contact paper or walking with shoe boxes on her feet to give extra tactile feedback.

Functional Activities

As mentioned earlier, one of the major aims of OT is to help children master the functional skills they need to live as independently as possible. Often occupational therapists must invent new ways to allow children to learn these skills. Frequently the new ways they come up with involve the use of customized adaptive tools, positioning devices, and computer technology.

Adaptive tools help children with cerebral palsy learn skills such as feeding, dressing, and writing that they might not otherwise be able to acquire. The tools are specifically developed with an eye to the children's individual developmental needs. For instance, suppose a three-year-old boy with floppy muscle tone cannot pull up his pants himself, but this is a major priority for his family, since they are working on toilet training. The occupational therapist may adapt a pair of loose sweat pants by sewing loops on each side of the waistband so that the child only needs to slip his hands through the loops and flex his arms to pull the pants up. At the same time, the therapist would work with the child on his hand grip, which may be what is preventing him from dressing the traditional way. Then, after the child masters the skill using the adapted method, the therapist can help him practice grasping his pants by the waistband.

Besides designing adaptive tools specifically for one child's needs, occupational therapists may suggest special equipment that is commercially available. For example, adaptive devices can often help children with cerebral palsy gain independence in feeding. There are spoons with built-up handles to promote grasping, specially designed cut-out cups to encourage a better neck position while drinking, and a variety of other adapted utensils. In addition, there are many positioning devices that make it easier for children with cerebral palsy to achieve the upper body control they need for fine motor skills when lying down, sitting, or standing. Chapter 4 discusses these kinds of special equipment in more detail.

Recently, occupational therapists have embraced computer technology as a means of helping children with cerebral palsy master new skills. On the simplest level, this means that many occupational therapists now use electronic toys to help stimulate skill development. They can adapt battery-operated toys with special switches so that even children who cannot manipulate toys with their hands can play with them. By enabling children to turn toys off and on at will, the therapists help them learn about cause-and-effect relationships first hand. By giving children the ability to act on their environments, the therapists help unlock communication and cognitive potential that may not otherwise have been tapped. For example, a little girl who cannot speak may be able to press one of several switches to make the computer say "pop." Her mother then blows a soap bubble for her daughter to pop after the computer's voice gives the signal.

On a more sophisticated level, occupational therapists may use a variety of computer programs to promote perceptual, coordination, and writing skill development. Many computer programs have been developed for infants through school-aged children. They range from fantastic color and action displays that a child can start and stop, to coordination and learning games that require making choices and timing responses. These programs can be operated by simple switch pads or keyboard adaptations that just require a child to press a picture on a board to activate her choice. Occupational therapists who specialize in this aspect of pediatrics usually work to develop the switch or keyboard adaptations that will help a particular child make the best use of this technology.

Getting Involved in Your Child's OT Program

Every family has different expectations for what they hope to get out of therapy. Some families want to learn everything the therapist does so that they can do the exercises and activities at home with their child several times a week. This is an excellent way to optimize therapy and helps children make good progress. This is also a good option for families who have limited financial resources and cannot schedule therapy sessions as frequently as they would like.

Not every parent wants to or is able to learn an extensive home program, particularly if the family is going through stressful times. Other parents start out wanting to learn all they can and may work very hard, but then reach a "burn-out" point and want to reduce their involvement. A good OT will be sensitive to your needs and will not pressure you to do more than you can cope with.

Since your role in your child's OT program is largely up to you, it is a good idea to let the therapist know how you want to be involved. You must decide what you need to learn from the therapist to allow you to enjoy your child in play, to make daily care manageable, and to help your child be part of everyday family experiences. For example, would you like the therapist to help you identify good toys for play and learning or to find a toy-lending library for special-needs children? Would you like the therapist to teach you good positions for play and everyday care activities? Or, more important-ly, would you like the therapist to help you integrate the therapy goals with your own personal goals for your child and family? For example, you might want to learn some simple water play activities for your child so that your whole family can enjoy playing in the pool together. By deciding exactly what you want your child and your family to get out of OT, you can help shape the course the therapy will take.

Finding an Occupational Therapist for Your Child

Many excellent occupational therapists work in the public school systems. Unfortunately, these therapists often have enor-mous caseloads and cannot dedicate as much time to an individual child as might be needed. If your child is seeing a school-based therapist and you feel frustrated because you would like to learn more about how to help your child or because you think she should have more individualized attention, you may want to seek the services of a private occupational therapist. If your financial resour-ces are limited, you can arrange for services on a more advisory basis (e.g., once a month to plan home programming) rather than on a once- or twice-weekly basis.

To find the right occupational therapist to treat your child, you must match your child's needs with the therapist's skills. Even within the field of pediatric OT, there is considerable specialty. Some therapists work only with children with learning disabilities, while others work primarily with children with severe disabilities. Some therapists use neurodevelopmental treatment exclusively, and others use only sensory integration. More and more occupation-al therapists are becoming trained in both NDT and S.I., however, and can provide a more comprehensive treatment approach for children with cerebral palsy.

It is a good idea to find out what the therapist's skills are before making your first appointment. If the therapist is not the same one who evaluated your child, you may even want to meet the therapist and have a few trial sessions to see how things go. To guide you in selecting the right therapist, here are some questions you should ask:

1. Is the therapist trained and certified in NDT? If not, does she have experience in using this approach and has she participated in NDT workshops or worked under an NDT-certified therapist?
2. Is the therapist experienced in sensory integration techniques in addition to NDT? This is important if your child has a combination of sensory integrative and movement problems. Generally, it is more important for the therapist to have experience in S.I. and in applying its techniques to children with cerebral palsy than it is for her to be certified. Certification in S.I. is required only to administer a battery of tests to children with learning disabilities.
3. Does the therapist have a primary age specialty? Some therapists are most experienced with infants and young children, whereas others prefer to treat older, school-aged children.
4. If you already know what your child's primary occupational therapy needs are, you may want to ask the therapist about her experience in those areas. For instance, if your child needs work on handwriting or feeding skills, does the therapist have experience in these areas?

Besides choosing an occupational therapist with the skills your child needs, you may also be able to pick one who offers services in the type of setting that most appeals to you. Some therapists will come to your home. This is especially good for young infants who may tire quickly on a long drive to a therapy session. Other children, particularly toddlers and preschoolers, learn better in a center-based program that has interesting toys and a variety of equipment. Even for young infants, a center-based program may be the best option. This is because some centers not only offer excellent therapy services for children, but also family services ranging from advocacy to supportive counseling.

Good sources for names of occupational therapists are the Neurodevelopmental Treatment Association and the American Occupational Therapy Association, both of which are listed in the Resource Guide at the back of this book. Your child's pediatrician and other parents of children with cerebral palsy may also be able to recommend a therapist with the qualities you are seeking.

SPEECH AND LANGUAGE THERAPY

What Is Speech and Language Therapy?

In everyday conversation, we often use the words "speech" and "language" interchangeably. For example, when we say, "Watch your language," we are really asking somebody to be careful about what he says. But there *is* a distinction—a distinction it is important to grasp in order to understand what speech and language therapy is all about.

Technically, speech is the process of producing sounds and combining them into words to communicate. Language, on the other hand, means any set of spoken words, written symbols, or gestures one person uses to communicate with another. In other words, speech is only one type of language. Besides spoken languages such as English, Spanish, and Chinese, there are also languages such as American Sign Language made up entirely of gestures, and languages such as braille made up entirely of symbols.

As Chapter 6 explains, to communicate in any language we must have both the ability to get our message across to others (*expressive language)* and the ability to understand other people's messages (*receptive language)*. Since the goal of speech and language therapy is to evaluate and treat any problems with expressive language, receptive language, or speech, this means that speech and language therapy is concerned with any difficulty with communication.

The part of the communication process that children with cerebral palsy usually have the most trouble with is speech. This is because speech depends on the coordination of the muscles involved in *respiration* (breathing), *phonation* (voice production), and *articulation* (sound production). Any abnormality of muscle tone anywhere in the body will affect speech production. For example, low muscle tone in the trunk makes it difficult to control the respiratory muscles needed for speech. As a result, some children with low muscle tone may have very breathy speech and may run out of air before they reach the ends of words or sentences. The same low tone is often mirrored in the lips and tongue and may make it difficult for children with cerebral palsy to produce a variety of speech sounds. Low tone in the lip area, for example, often makes it difficult for a child to produce [m], [b], [p], and [w] sounds. And the [t], [d], [n], [l], [s], [sh], and [z] sounds are more difficult to pronounce if the front of the tongue is affected. The term *dysarthria* is used to describe the slow, sluggish, monotone quality of speech in children with cerebral palsy who have these types of muscle tone problems.

Speech and language therapy can help children improve muscle tone and other problems such as motor planning difficulties that impede clear, fluent speech. It can also help children who are permanently or temporarily unable to master the physical aspects of speaking learn to communicate in other ways—for example, through sign language, photographs, picture symbols, or Morse Code. In addition, speech and language therapy can help in the treatment of problems with feeding, drooling, or other *oral-motor* functions—that is, movements involving the muscles in and around the face and mouth.

Usually, children with cerebral palsy can start speech and language therapy as infants, provided their medical condition is stable. Because communication problems often translate into delays in social, emotional, and cognitive development, it is vital for children to begin speech and language therapy at an early age. By beginning therapy as soon as possible, a child can be encouraged to develop normal patterns of movement, and discouraged from developing abnormal patterns which would have to be corrected later. Problems connected with tube feeding can also be minimized. Finally, young children with cerebral palsy can learn alternative communication strategies before they become frustrated at their inability to communicate intelligibly.

What Is a Speech-Language Pathologist?

Professionals trained to provide speech and language therapy go by a variety of names—speech-language pathologist (SLP), speech therapist, speech teacher, and speech clinician. These different titles reflect varying amounts and types of education. It is usually best to seek the services of someone who uses the title speech-language pathologist and holds the Certificate of Clinical Competence (C.C.C.) issued by the American Speech-Language-Hearing Association (ASHA). This will assure you that the specialist has made a substantial commitment in undergraduate- and graduate-level university training and supervised internships. To receive the C.C.C., a therapist must complete a master's degree and clinical fellowship program and pass a national exam. To use the title speech-language pathologist, a therapist should have completed a master's degree and received the C.C.C. from ASHA.

Like occupational and physical therapists, speech-language pathologists may specialize in pediatrics and developmental delays. They may also have special training in a number of techniques helpful in treating children with cerebral palsy. For example, they may have certification or training in neurodevelopmental treatment or in *augmentative communication*—the use of nonspeech techniques such as signs, gestures, or pictures to supplement a child's speech abilities.

How the Speech-Language Therapist Evaluates Your Child

Just as occupational and physical therapists do, SLPs must first evaluate your child's abilities and disabilities before planning a treatment program. Before you schedule an evaluation, however, it is important that an audiologist see your child to rule out a hearing problem that could affect communication development. A list of certified audiologists may be obtained by contacting ASHA, as listed in the Resource Guide at the back of this book.

Most often, the therapist begins the evaluation process by reviewing reports of anyone who has previously worked with your child, including PTs, OTs, audiologists, psychologists, special educators, and teachers. To obtain a clearer picture of your child's background, she will also ask you for information about the pregnancy, and about your child's medical and developmental history. After briefly considering this information and observing your child interact with you, the therapist will plan the order of evaluation procedures. Depending on your child's age, skill level, and ease with the therapist, the SLP will either start the evaluation by sitting back to observe how your child moves, plays, and interacts with you, or by giving your child a variety of standardized tests.

At least once a year, the SLP should thoroughly evaluate your child's abilities in two areas: oral-motor skills such as feeding and speech, and language skills. The therapist should also assess your child's need for augmentative communication to supplement her speaking abilities. The following sections explain how the therapist will assess your child's needs in each of these areas.

Oral-Motor Skills

At the outset of the evaluation, the SLP needs to get a good idea of your child's sensory motor skills—that is, how she responds to input from senses such as touch, smell, sight, hearing, and how she moves her body. This is because your child's muscle tone and any sensory integration problems she has will definitely affect her *oral-motor* functioning—or how she uses her tongue, lips, jaw, and facial muscles. For example, an oversensitivity to touch might make it difficult for your child to eat foods with different textures and at different temperatures. And low muscle tone, as mentioned earlier, can pose problems in the production of certain sounds. Depending on how much training the therapist has had in working with children with these types of problems, she may ask an occupational or physical therapist to help with this part of the evaluation.

While assessing your child's sensory motor skills, the SLP will probably evaluate how your child breathes, since adequate respiratory support is critical to both feeding and speech. The SLP will determine whether your child primarily uses her abdominal (belly) area to breathe or whether she uses her thoracic (upper chest) area, too. Normally, infants six months and younger breathe mainly with their abdominal muscles. As they develop, they are able to breathe more efficiently by using both their abdominal and thoracic muscles. Children who do not have this ability have trouble taking in enough air and controlling it to produce multisyllabic words and longer sentences. The SLP will also measure your child's rate of respiration since this, too, affects a child's ability to pronounce the final syllables of words. In addition, the SLP will check whether your child can breathe with her mouth closed when she is at rest. Many children with cerebral palsy have difficulty keeping their mouths closed due to frequent head colds or muscle control problems in the trunk, head, and neck areas. As a result, they cannot use their nose to filter and warm the air before it enters the lungs.

Next the SLP will probably evaluate your child's feeding skills. Because your child will actually be eating during this part of the evaluation, try to bring her to the appointment slightly hungry. Also bring along any special chair, cup, utensil, or other equipment your child uses at home for feeding. If your child is still an infant, the SLP will probably ask you to demonstrate how you feed her. If your child is older, the SLP will want to see how she feeds herself. But whatever your child's age and abilities,

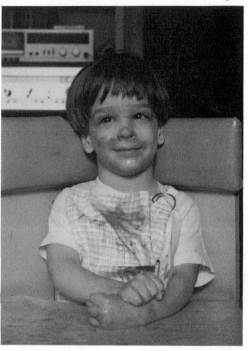

the SLP will investigate the following areas: 1) how much your child eats; 2) the variety of food textures and temperatures your child tolerates; 3) the positions in which your child is able to eat; and 4) how your child uses her lips and tongue to suck and swallow and her jaw to bite.

If your child has certain feeding problems, various other members of a "feeding team" may assist the SLP during the feeding evaluation. For example, if there is a possibility that food is leaking into your child's lungs, a specialist in digestive disorders known as a *gastroenterologist* might prescribe a type of X-ray test called a modified barium swallow study. A nutritionist would evaluate and monitor your child's caloric needs. And a psychologist might observe how you and your child interact at mealtimes to suggest ways to encourage your child to eat.

An evaluation of drooling should follow the feeding evaluation, since your child's feeding skills determine how efficiently she can swallow and how well she can feel saliva pooling in the front of her mouth. The SLP will begin by deciding whether your child's drooling is due to sensory problems, motor problems, or a combination of the two. For example, if your child drools all the time, a sensory problem in her mouth and face could be decreasing her awareness of the wetness. If she only drools when she is sick or tired or when she is kneeling, walking, or in some other position difficult for her to maintain, then the drooling is probably due more to a motor problem. It will also be important for the SLP to determine how your child reacts to others' feedback about her wet chin. For example, if your child feels badly when another child complains that her drooling has ruined a toy, this reaction could be channeled to motivate your child to control her drooling.

Other skills the SLP may assess during the oral-motor portion of the evaluation include "nonspeech movement support" and articulation (speech sound production). In the area of nonspeech support, the therapist will examine how well your child is able to imitate lip and tongue movements essential to speech—for example, kissing, blowing whistles and bubbles, and sticking out and wiggling the tongue. She will also determine whether your child can imitate a series of nonsense syllables such as "pu-tu-ku." To evaluate your child's ability to articulate various speech sounds, the SLP will administer a standardized test. She will also gauge whether your child can be stimulated to produce these sounds correctly when given a model to imitate or other assistance. Finally, the therapist will note how your child produces speech sounds in conversation.

Language Skills

After completing her evaluation of your child's oral-motor skills, the SLP will assess your child's language skills. Most likely she will use a variety of standardized tests to evaluate your child's abilities in these areas:

1. receptive and expressive language.
2. *vocabulary*—the words your child recognizes and understands—and *concepts*—generalizations made about a class of things (for example, recognizing the difference between things that are edible and things that are not).

3. *auditory processing*—how your child's brain uses information arriving through the sense of hearing. For example, how does your child's brain process *sequencing* information, or information that requires understanding the order in which actions must be performed (before you pour soda out of a can, you must pull up the pop top). What are your child's *word retrieval* skills—or ability to say a word she knows after seeing a picture or other cue? What is her short-term memory for words and other sounds?

4. *pragmatics*—understanding how and why language is used. For example, you say "no" when you'd like someone to stop offering you spinach.

To evaluate your child's language skills, the SLP has a wide range of tests to choose from. The choice depends on your child's age, ability, and extent of physical limitations. Even if your child has no intelligible speech, her receptive knowledge of grammar, vocabulary, concepts, and pragmatics can still be tested if she can indicate her response by pointing or eye gazing. The SLP can modify the test presentation depending on your child's physical abilities. For example, if your child cannot control her hand movements well enough to point to one picture from an array of four, the SLP could enlarge the pictures on a photocopy machine and cut them out to space them further apart. She could then arrange the pictures so your child could indicate her response by eye gaze or with a less precise hand movement.

Besides giving your child standardized tests, the SLP will also observe how your child communicates. Does she use words? phrases? sentences? vocal approximations such as "bu" for "bubbles"? an augmentative communication system? Does she initiate communication or wait for someone to prod her? That is, if your child wants a snack, does she make a gesture or sound to indicate her wishes, or does she just look longingly at the cookie jar until someone prompts her to say "cookie"? Does she appear frustrated with communication? The SLP will probably make a tape recording of your child's vocal communication and analyze the kinds of consonants and vowels she uses, her sentence structure, and how and why she uses speech sounds (for example, using "hi" to greet someone).

Augmentative Communication

In the final portion of the evaluation, the SLP will look at your child's need for augmentative communication—for supplemental communication devices and techniques to help her compensate for difficulties with speech. It is important to identify a child's need for augmentative communication as soon as possible, because waiting too long for speech to develop can lead to frustration and to delays in cognitive and social development. Augmentative communication can help children as young as nine to twelve months make choices and express their needs. And, contrary to what some parents fear, it does not prevent children with cerebral palsy from developing speaking skills later on. In fact, research has shown that augmentative communication frequently encourages children to develop verbal skills.

In determining whether a child would benefit from augmentative communication, the critical factor is whether there is a difference or "gap" between how much the child understands (receptive language) and how much she can express (expressive language). For example, if your child understands language at a three-year-old level, but only uses single-word utterances like a

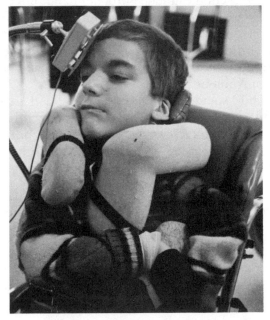

twelve- to fourteen-month-old, she would be an ideal candidate for augmentative communication. Augmentative communication might also be considered if a child cannot speak clearly enough so that unfamiliar listeners such as salesclerks can understand them.

If the SLP decides that your child would benefit from augmentative communication, the next step is to select the most appropriate type of communication system. For example, the SLP might recommend that your child learn to use sign language, a language board, or a voice output talking computer or other computerized device. The SLP would also look at ways to tailor the augmentative communication system to the child's special needs— for example, by using concrete objects such as a real ball or a real cookie instead of abstract symbols for them on a language board, or by using a certain kind of switch to activate the computer.

During this stage of the evaluation, the SLP will consult you and your child to take your preferences into account. For example, she might ask whether you would be willing and able to learn signs or to operate a computer. The SLP should also consult an occupational or physical therapist, because augmentative communication techniques often require work with the whole body. For instance, they generally require optimal seating so the child can point or use eye gaze.

The initial choice of an augmentative communication system will depend on your child's age, motor control, and cognitive abilities. To use manual signs, for example, requires considerable motor control. Frequently, only a small number of signs are taught to children with cerebral palsy, usually during the preschool years. Then, if a child continues to need augmentative communication, she may progress to some kind of two-dimensional language board that requires less motor control to use. Later in the preschool and early elementary school years, the child may begin to use an electronic system. Whatever type of communication system is recommended for your child, the SLP will attempt to teach your child to use it as independently as possible.

How the SLP Treats Your Child

Following your child's evaluation, the SLP will design a treatment program tailored to your child's needs. With your help, she will set both short-term and long-term goals in each area of oral-motor functioning and language development that your child is having trouble with. For example, she may set a long-term goal for your child to be able to use [b] and [p] in any position in a word. To help your child reach that goal, you may set a short-term goal of producing these sounds at the beginnings of words. The SLP will also plan exactly what methods and materials she will use to help your child reach her goals. If the goal, for instance, is for your child to participate in circle time at school, the therapist might recommend the use of a small, voice output, talking computer.

Besides planning how she will treat your child in therapy sessions, the SLP will plan ways for you and your family to help your child with feeding and communication needs. At therapy sessions, the SLP will teach you procedures to do with your child at home. For example, if your child needs a face massage to decrease tactile defensiveness or strengthen the muscles, the SLP will help you place your hands so that you stimulate the proper muscles. Each week, the therapist will write the "home program" down in a notebook, and then follow up the next week to see how it went.

Here are some ways that your SLP might treat your child for specific needs associated with cerebral palsy:

1. Oral-Motor Skills

Feeding. If your child has difficulty sucking, chewing, or swallowing because of muscle tone or sensory integration problems in the face, the SLP will show you how to do a face massage to make feeding easier for her. The SLP will also tell you how much food your child should eat and how much time should be necessary to eat a specific amount of food. In addition, she will explain which temperatures and textures of foods will best stimulate your child's muscles. For example, sucking ice makes certain lip movements easier for some children, and biting and chewing pretzel rods or other foods with dense, scratchy textures can strengthen tongue muscles.

Together with your child's physical therapist, the SLP will determine which positions make it easiest for your child to feed and will help you to order any special positioning equipment your child might need. Together with your child's occupational therapist, the SLP will explain how to offer the cup, spoon, and finger foods to your child, and will recommend adaptations to your child's cup or spoon to make feeding easier. Chapter 4 discusses positioning and special equipment more fully.

Speech. To help your child master troublesome sounds, the SLP will first demonstrate how to prepare your child to use her lips or tongue to make the sounds. For example, the SLP might suggest that your child suck juice pops or blow whistles or bubbles if your child has difficulty with the [b], [p], [m], [w], or [oo] sounds. Next, the SLP will teach you how to help your child make the target sound. For instance, if your child cannot produce a [t], [d], or [n] sound, the SLP might show you how to place peanut butter or honey behind your child's teeth to prompt her to lift the tip of her tongue into the proper position. If necessary, the SLP will also teach you special tongue "warm-up" exercises such as wiggling the tongue to the left and right corners of the mouth.

Because proper breathing is the foundation of good speech, the SLP will help you learn therapeutic handling techniques to encourage more normal breathing patterns. These techniques will largely depend on your learning how to position your child so that her muscle tone is more normal. Using a tape recorder so she can hear herself talk and singing are good follow-up activities if your child is working on respiratory control.

Drooling. If your child drools because of sensory feedback problems, the SLP will show you how to massage your child's face with a washcloth and fabrics with a variety of textures to increase her sensitivity to wetness. She will also show you how to use other techniques to help her learn the difference in feel between wet and dry. If your child drools because of motor problems, the SLP will demonstrate how to position her with her head and trunk aligned so that her muscle tone is as normal as possible. The SLP will also teach you how to stimulate more normal swallowing, which is the key to controlling drooling. Additionally, the SLP may demonstrate how to help your child control her lips so she can keep them closed when she is at rest.

2. Pragmatics/Language Use

Because children with cerebral palsy often have difficulty moving, friends and family members may make a habit of anticipating their needs. They may give a child her favorite stuffed animal before she asks for it at bedtime or interpret her gestures for other children. Unfortunately, if you anticipate all your child's needs, she will have no need to reach out and communicate. As a consequence, her pragmatics may suffer.

The SLP can teach you and your family ways to stimulate your child's development of pragmatics. Often she may show you how to role play with your child. For example, she may set up a tea party with teddy bears as guests to encourage your child to request "more." Or she may give your child a little boy puppet and have her create a conversation with a Grandma puppet. She will also encourage you to work on your child's language use in real-life situations. For instance, the SLP will urge you not to anticipate your child's needs and to encourage her to greet people, ask and answer questions, and make comments.

3. Language

Concepts. Understanding concepts (big/little, high/low, different/same) at an age appropriate level is vital to successful communication. Often, however, it is hard for children to learn concepts relating to activities they have not directly experienced. For example, children with cerebral palsy may have trouble learning the distinction between "under" and "over" if they are physically unable to move under or over an obstacle. If your child is learning concepts at school, the SLP will coordinate her goals with the teacher's to avoid duplication. The SLP will first teach your child concepts by using real objects. For instance, she might have your child touch a heating pad and an ice cube to learn the concepts "hot" and "cold." Later on, she will reinforce the concepts at a more abstract level. She may show your child pictures and ask her to look or point at the hot or cold objects, or to say their names if she can.

Auditory Processing. As Chapter 3 explains, children with cerebral palsy can have hearing problems for a variety of reasons. These problems can interfere with your child's auditory processing, or how her brain is able to respond to sound. As a result, children with cerebral palsy may have trouble with short-term auditory memory skills such as following spoken instructions, retrieving a word already learned, and organizing ideas.

The SLP can use a variety of techniques to help your child improve her auditory processing. Usually she will start by presenting instructions at exactly the length and complexity at which your child has difficulties. If your child is barely able to understand instructions at the sixteen-month level—"give baby a kiss," for example—she would begin at that level. She may make a game out of following instructions—for instance, by playing "Simon Says" with your child—or she may use instructions in a real-life situation—for example, by asking your child to get a knife and fork just before lunch. The SLP may also use commercial cassette tapes or workbooks to help your child strengthen her auditory processing.

Grammar/Syntax. A knowledge of grammar (the rules for using and forming different parts of speech) and syntax (the order in which words are put together to form a phrase or sentence) is essential to effective communication. Children with cerebral palsy can be slower to develop correct grammar usages because they do not have the breath support to produce word endings such as the plural [s], or may have developmental problems that delay learning grammar rules.

The SLP will work with your child on each grammatical structure that gives her trouble—first in isolation, and then during carryover/play activities. For example, if your child has trouble using ['s] to show possession in a sentence such as "It is John's car," the therapist may first have your child practice saying the word "John's." Then she may ask, "Whose car is it?" and help to model the correct response. The therapist might introduce this exercise while playing with toy cars with your child. The SLP will also use special exercises to improve muscle tone in the trunk if your child's delays are due in part to inadequate breath support—for instance, if she doesn't have sufficient breath to pronounce the [s] at the end of plural nouns or the ['s] at the end of possessives.

4. Augmentative Communication

This is an area of treatment in which your participation is vital to your child's success. For your child to get the maximum benefit from her augmentative communication system, everyone needs to use the techniques with her all the time. The goal is to produce a 24–hour-a-day communicator, not a one-hour-a-day one. You and your family must understand that if your child's computer, language board, or signs are left behind or forgotten, it would be the same as if your child had severe laryngitis. You must also understand that it takes a lot of patience to communicate with a child who uses an augmentative communication device because the process can be extremely slow.

Since your support is crucial to the success of your child's augmentative communication techniques, your family needs to feel just as comfortable with the decisions made in this area as they do about decisions to purchase a major piece of equipment such as an electric wheelchair. For example, if your child with cerebral palsy is to learn signs or gestures, you and your other children must also be willing to learn them. You will have to let the SLP know if you would feel more comfortable learning a few signs each week or with learning many signs at once in a course format. Likewise, if your SLP suggests a language board with photos or line drawing symbols, you must be prepared to learn the symbols and to let the SLP know when new symbols are needed—for example, for a trip to Disney World, the beach, or a special restaurant.

Finally, if your child is learning to use a voice output device or computer, you will not only have to learn to operate it, but also learn what to do when it breaks down. And because children who use computer devices are always given language boards to fall back on, you will also need to learn to use a language board. Furthermore, it may be up to you to teach baby sitters, relatives, other therapists, teachers, and others who work with your child how to use the devices.

Getting Involved in Your Child's Speech and Language Program

The previous section pointed out many ways you might be asked to help in your child's home program. Your mere participation, however, does not guarantee the success of your child's therapy. For your child's home program to be effective, you must be honest with the SLP when things don't work out at home. For example, if you are not sure exactly what you are to do, tell the therapist so she can clear up your confusion. Likewise, don't just give up on your child's home program if she won't do as you ask or if the therapist wants you to do something that doesn't fit into your lifestyle. Talk with the therapist, and together you can work out an alternate way to help your child reach the same goal. For example, if the SLP suggests you hold your child's cup hand-over-hand at mealtimes to help improve her sucking and swallowing skills, but you have three other children to feed, it might be better to work on this goal during a quiet snack time.

You, your child, and the therapist should also jointly decide what treats or prizes are appropriate for doing good work at home for Mom and Dad. Although eventually your child should work for praise alone, in the beginning it may help to reward your child with something that interests and motivates her—for example, stickers, model dinosaurs, or baseball cards. At first, you may need to reward your child immediately after every good attempt, but later you should give fewer rewards at greater intervals.

There are a variety of ways your family can reinforce the SLP goals. As mentioned earlier, giving your child a pretzel rod to chew can help her develop better muscle tone in her mouth and face. This technique is called "therapy through food." In addition, it is often convenient to work on therapy goals while riding in a car. You can, for instance, do such breath control exercises as singing along with tapes or naming things you see that begin with a specific sound.

Besides taking part in your child's home program, you might also be asked to help the SLP in therapy sessions. Frequently an extra set of hands is needed to position a child with cerebral palsy while the SLP handles specific muscles. For example, while the therapist positions your child over a therapy ball and tries to stimulate more normal respiration, you might be asked to blow soap bubbles. When your child reaches to pop the bubbles, she will be better positioned for normal breathing.

Especially as your child gets older, there may be times when it is more appropriate for you to leave the treatment room and observe though a screen or from an observation booth. The therapist will want to see how your child communicates independently without a parent hovering nearby. In these cases, the SLP will generally set aside some time at the end of the session to demonstrate new skills and exercises for you and to give homework. For some children with cerebral palsy, this period at the end of the session can be difficult because they are tired, reluctant to share the therapist with their parent(s), or uncomfortable hearing themselves discussed. You and the SLP can sometimes ease these situations by occupying your child with a "treat" for having done a good job—for example, with computer time, stickers, a special toy, a chance to play with the tape recorder, or whatever is appropriate.

Finding a Speech and Language Pathologist for Your Child

Speech and language therapy services are usually a part of early childhood special education programs. You may, however, decide to seek additional SLP intervention on a private basis if you feel your child would benefit from more intensive treatment.

Depending on the size of your community, you may or may not be able to find an SLP with the ideal training to treat your child. Assuming you have several therapists to choose from, however, there are several important professional qualifications you should look for. To begin with, your child's SLP should hold the Certificate of Clinical Competence (C.C.C.) from the American Speech-Language-Hearing Association, and should be licensed by the state where she practices. She should also preferably be NDT certified or have taken workshops in NDT. A specialty in pediatrics and a strong background in the treatment of children with disabilities like your child's are also important. This is because the SLP's ability to handle your child's entire body to normalize muscle tone is so often the key to improving speech skills. As Leslie Davis, my neurodevelopmental speech instructor says, "What you get in the hips is mediated in the lips." That is, as you work to improve the muscle tone and movement patterns throughout the body, you'll see similar positive changes in the respiratory and oral-motor area. Depending on the severity of your child's disability, you may also want to look for an SLP with training in augmentative communication so that she can work with your child on appropriate nonspeech techniques.

Just as important as the SLP's credentials is her ability to create a strong working relationship with your child, your family, and school. When she is working with you, the therapist should give you the feeling that your child is the absolute center of her focus and attention. She should be enthusiastic about your child and her abilities and be able to offer you hope and support. She should also be able to read your family's cues if, for instance, you want her to stop pushing you and your child so hard or to provide extra assistance. Finally, the SLP should help you to integrate your child's private program with her school program. She may do this with phone calls to your child's therapists at school, by observing her school program, or by keeping a notebook of exercises and progress notes.

For help locating a therapist with the right credentials to treat your child, you can contact the ASHA, which maintains a list of SLPs who hold the Certificate of Clinical Competence. You can also consult the directory of the Neurodevelopmental Treatment Association for names of SLPs certified in NDT. For help locating a therapist with the right attitude to treat your child, try asking your pediatrician, other parents of children with cerebral palsy, your state speech and language association, school system therapists, or local hospitals with pediatric diagnostic teams.

WORKING TOGETHER AS A TEAM

As this chapter has pointed out, the work of your child's physical therapist, occupational therapist, and speech and language pathologist may overlap in many ways. Sometimes different therapists may work on identical goals with your child. For example, both the occupational therapist and speech and language pathologist might work on your child's oral-motor control in order to improve her feeding skills. Other times, your child's therapists may deliberately coordinate their goals to enhance your child's development. For example, the SLP might teach your child the concepts of "up" and "down" at the same time the physical therapist is working with your child on standing up and sitting down. Still other times, the progress your child makes with one therapist may lead directly or indirectly to progress with another therapist. For example, the work the physical therapist does with your child on trunk control can make it easier for your child to master the hand movements that the occupational therapist is concerned with; the improvement in your child's muscle tone that both the occupational

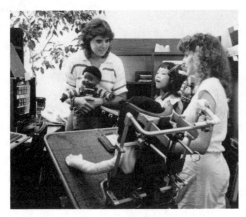

and physical therapists strive for can lay the foundation for important progress with the SLP.

Because there is so much overlap between occupational, physical, and speech and language therapy, it is crucial that your child's therapists work together as a team. They need to communicate with one another regularly to share their goals and their special insights into your child's needs and abilities.

If your child's therapists are all associated with a particular center- or school-based program, they are probably already accustomed to working as a team. The school or center will most likely have assigned your child a *case manager*—a medical, educational, or social work professional who gathers information and ideas from your child's therapists and coordinates their different services.

If you have put together your own team of therapists for your child, you may need to take a more active role in coordinating your child's services. You may want to serve as your child's case manager or ask one of the professionals involved with your child to do so. You may find it helpful to keep a traveling notebook to go from one therapist to the next and also to school for the teacher and school therapists to review. In this notebook, each of your child's therapists can write suggestions for home activities, positions for play and self-care, recommendations for toys, and other pertinent information. They can also attach photographs or line drawings of the exercises they are doing with your child.

As important as it is for each of your child's therapists to keep abreast of what the others are doing with your child, it is perhaps even more important that *you* be kept informed. After all, you know your child's special needs and abilities better than anyone else does and have the most opportunities to work and play with your child. This makes your informed participation vital to the success of your child's therapy programs.

Fortunately, most therapists recognize the importance of working together with parents as part of the treatment team. They will gladly teach you all the special handling techniques, observation skills, and teaching strategies you need to know to help your child get the maximum benefit from her therapy. More importantly, they will listen to your concerns and welcome your input about what works, what doesn't work, and what you would like your child to achieve. If any of your child's therapists do *not* treat you as an equal member of the team, you should seek new therapists. Remember: your child needs and deserves a treatment team where all partners listen to each other and work together to develop ideas that work for you and your child.

Parent Statements

Besides us, his parents, the most important, influential person in our son's life is his physical therapist. We prepare him for life as any parent would, but his PT prepares him for "his" life. . . a way of life we are just beginning to understand.

❧❧❧

When our daughter first started therapy, I thought of it as reaching a goal, not a series of goals.

❧❧❧

First I learned that OT is not just learning how to feed yourself and use a crayon and bend down to pull off your socks. Then I started realizing the tremendous importance of OT.

❀

I do wish the therapists had placed more emphasis on Kelly's pronunciation before now. I would always ask them to, but I didn't have the training to know what sounds should be worked on first and how to help her to learn to make them. Because she's so involved, everyone just kept steering us toward a communication board. I fought it for a long time because I thought she wouldn't try to talk, but thankfully I was wrong.

❀

It's been a lot of hard work finding a communication board, learning it, using it, and continuing to learn more so I can stay one step ahead of her. It's extremely frustrating at times. I stay up all hours of the night trying to learn more about the computer and communication board.

❀

Even at the tender age of twenty-six months, there are parts of herself I think my daughter does not want to deal with. It has taken a while for her to trust her occupational therapist enough to take a chance and go along for the ride—to trust that the benefits would outweigh the physical discomforts and inconvenience of OT.

❀

What worked best for me was to really rely on our physical therapist and our doctor. They were the only two people in my "world." When they said "jump," I said "how high?" I handed things over to them and let them tell us what to do, when to do it, and how to do it. It was very helpful. I had no idea what it means if you have high or low muscle tone in one part of your body or another. If someone had told me a year ago that working on my daughter's trunk muscles would improve her speech (as well as a dozen other things), I would have asked them what cult they belonged to. But seeing is believing, and I have watched the improvements and connections.

❧❧❧

I handed our new baby daughter over to my son's physical therapist and asked, "What do you think? How's her tone?"

❧❧❧

It was very difficult for me to watch our therapists discipline my young son from time to time. I had to step back and realize that he had to learn that there were rules to follow. Most of the time, I just wanted to comfort him and tell him he didn't have to go through this.

❧❧❧

When I watch her in OT, I feel as if she's storing up the future—hopefully one as near normal as possible—long before it happens.

❧❧❧

I think it takes parents longer to adjust to all of the equipment than it does the child. For the child it makes life easier; for the parent it makes life more complicated.

❧❧❧

Carol's world expanded about two feet into another universe after beginning OT. Before OT, her arms were very tight and her balance reactions were uncertain. She would not and could not reach out, much less rotate her trunk in that reaching position.

❧❧❧

Our daughter had two good speech therapists. You can't help but wish that they all had more training, though. There's just so much on the market that they can't know about everything and it's unfair to everyone involved.

❧❧❧

Don't ever say never. It's amazing what a good therapist can teach your child. Progress may be slow, but year after year you realize your child has reached another goal.

❧❧❧

Because I'm the person who spends the most time with Mark, I'm the only one who can really understand what he is saying. I do a lot of translating . . . even for my husband.

❧❧❧

EIGHT

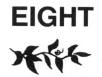

Early Intervention and Special Education

MARIAN H. JARRETT, Ed.D.*

Before you found out that your child had cerebral palsy, you probably thought about his future education. Perhaps you decided that your child would begin preschool as soon as possible so that he could get a head start on reading and counting. Or perhaps you resolved that you would keep your child home until he reached kindergarten age so that he could enjoy just being a kid. Whatever your plans were, they probably changed radically after your child was diagnosed with cerebral palsy.

Most children with cerebral palsy need to begin their formal education much earlier than do children who do not have special needs. They need special educational and therapeutic services to help them function as normally as possible—as soon as possible—within their families and communities. For example, they usually need services to help them improve their motor skills and often need services to help them develop communication skills. Children who have mental retardation or a learning disability also require services designed to help them develop problem-solving and other cognitive skills. Furthermore, when a child has cerebral palsy, the whole family can often benefit from a comprehensive intervention

* Marian H. Jarrett is currently an Infant Development Specialist with Newborn Service, George Washington University Hospital and with Project CAPS, Department of Teacher Preparation and Special Education, at the George Washington University in Washington, D.C.

program that provides support and guidance as they learn the best ways to work and play with their child.

Fortunately, educational opportunities for children with cerebral palsy and their families have never been better. As Chapter 9 explains, in the past twenty-five years Congress has passed several important laws guaranteeing children with cerebral palsy and other disabilities important rights to services. These laws require all states to provide special education services to all children with disabilities from the age of three, and encourage states to provide early intervention services from birth through age two. They also give parents a critical role in planning and monitoring their child's educational program.

To help prepare you for your role in your child's education, this chapter reviews the range of special services usually available for children with cerebral palsy ages birth through five. It explains how the specific services your child will receive are determined and introduces some of the early intervention and special education professionals who will work with you and your child. Finally, the chapter presents some guidelines to help you select the best educational program for your child.

Programs

Depending on your child's age and the extent of his disabilities, he may receive the services he needs in a variety of settings and from a variety of professionals. If he is younger than three, he will receive what are called "early intervention" services, while if he is between three and five, he will receive preschool special education. In either case, the therapeutic and educational services in your child's program will be tailored—with your input—to meet his unique learning needs.

Early Intervention Programs

An early intervention service is one which begins before three years of age and is designed to improve the development of a child with a developmental delay or disability. These services can include physical, occupational, or speech therapy; medical intervention; social services; or infant education.

If your child has motor problems, whether or not he has been diagnosed as having cerebral palsy, it is important that he receive special educational and therapeutic services as soon as possible. Intervention is vital during this very early time because the young brain has a certain degree of *plasticity,* or ability to be molded with appropriate input. At no other stage of life does a child learn and develop as quickly as he does during the first few years of his life. Through early intervention, infants and young children with cerebral palsy can be helped to develop more normal posture, muscle tone, and movement patterns; they can be taught the movements they will later use in feeding, bathing, and dressing themselves and in doing school work; and they can learn through play and teaching experiences that are adapted to their specific needs.

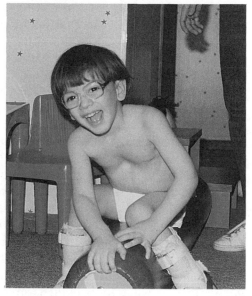

In addition to giving your baby the best chance for optimal development, an early intervention program can provide support and guidance to your family as you learn about your baby and his special needs. The program can help you deal with the disappointment, anger, or sadness you may feel since finding out that your baby has cerebral palsy. It can help you and other family members learn how to make these early days of caring for and playing with your baby easier and more enjoyable. And it can help you begin to learn how you can help your child become the most capable person he can be. Early intervention can help you begin to focus on what your baby *can* do rather than on what he cannot do. Early intervention can help you begin to do something positive to guide your baby down the road of growth and development.

As soon as you know that your baby has a motor delay, you should seek early intervention services. If your baby has mild problems and you begin intervention early, he or she may need services only during the early infant and preschool years. If your child's movement problems are severe or if he has other related disabilities such as mental retardation, he may continue to need special educational and therapeutic services throughout his school years. By beginning intervention early, you can help prevent muscle contractures and deformities that might otherwise develop and that could make it more difficult for your child to move and take care of himself. You can also help alleviate the learning problems your child may have because he cannot handle and relate to toys and objects as other children do.

Early intervention programs for children with cerebral palsy usually have a *family-centered* approach. Because your child depends upon your family for his survival and well-being, his program is designed around the goals that *you* identify as being important for your child and family. For example, you may want your baby to improve his ability to suck and swallow so he can finish his bottle in thirty minutes. Or once your child is slightly older, you may want him to learn the names of his favorite foods so that he can communicate at home and with friends and family. You may want to work on your child's balance in sitting and standing with support so he can learn to walk alone. These types of goals are known as *functional outcomes* because they are intended to help your child function as normally and independently as possible within your family and community.

Occasionally, early intervention is approached as a *child-centered* rather than a family-centered service. You may find a program that resembles a preschool or elementary school program which has just been moved down to a younger level. Goals and objectives for children are determined by the teacher and therapists, and parents get reports of what their child is able to do with each of these professionals. If your child is placed in such a program, try to find ways to show the program staff that you as parents are valuable members of the team. Remember, you have information about your child relevant to the goals of the professionals, and you also have a need to know about adaptive handling, positioning, and learning experiences for your baby. Your child needs your input and support to make the most of his early intervention program.

Preschool Special Education Programs

Special education is instruction specially designed to meet the unique learning needs of children with disabilities. Like early intervention, its goal is to enable children to live the most independent lives possible. Consequently, special education includes more than instruction in traditionally "academic" subjects such as reading, arithmetic, and social studies. It also includes special therapeutic and other services aimed at helping children overcome delays in all areas of development. These services are provided by one or more professionals trained in working with children with disabilities. By law, a child's special education program must include all special services—or "related services," as they are sometimes called—necessary for him to benefit from his educational program. For children with cerebral palsy, services may include occupational, physical, and speech-language therapy; counseling; or the provision of special therapy equipment or computer aids. Depending on the state where you live, your child will first be eligible for special education services at birth or at age three.

Preschool special education differs from special education for school-age children much as regular preschool education differs from regular elementary education. Preschool education programs are frequently half-day rather than whole-day programs. Younger preschoolers may go to school only two or three days a week, while four- and five-year-olds attend five half-days. If your child's special education and therapy needs are great, he may be enrolled in a full-day program for as many as five days a week even at the preschool level. This allows time for him to receive his preschool instruction and to play with other children, as well as to schedule the necessary therapies he requires. Sometimes children with significant needs attend a summer program as well as a regular program during the school year.

Preschool special education and preschool regular education are also alike in requiring more parental involvement than programs for school-age children do. Because of the developmental needs of preschool children and the amount of time they spend learning and growing as members of a family, parents need to carry over learning experiences from the classroom to home. It is also important for parents to share information about their child's motor, cognitive, communication, social, and emotional needs with school staff.

Professionals

Because children with cerebral palsy often have developmental delays in more than one area, they usually need special therapy or instruction provided by a variety of professionals. In both early intervention and preschool special education programs, professionals with different areas of expertise commonly work together as a *multidisciplinary team* to ensure each child's optimal development. Titles and specific areas of responsibility may differ from place to place, but the following types of professionals will likely work with you and your child sometime in his school career.

Special Education Teacher. Depending on your child's program, this professional may be known as a special education teacher or an infant development specialist. Whatever her title, she concentrates on helping your child develop social, self-help, and cognitive or problem-solving skills. She may help your preschool child learn how to hang up his jacket or how to share a toy with a friend. She can show your infant how to find a hidden object or how

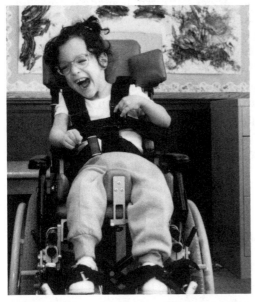

to use a stick to get a toy that is out of reach.

To help your child learn, your child's teacher will focus on how your child interacts with his environment. For example, if she notices that your baby daughter puts blocks in her mouth as soon as she picks them up, the teacher may show her how to bang two blocks together or how to put the blocks in a bucket. Your child's teacher will also work to understand your child's *learning style,* or how she learns best from interactions with people and objects. For example, perhaps your preschooler learns best when she can see something as well as hear it. If so, the teacher can help your daughter follow a story read aloud by showing her the pictures as she reads. Does your child need time to study a task before she begins to work on it? Is she sometimes unable to demonstrate a new skill when asked, but will do it on her own later? With your input about what your child does at home, the infant or special education teacher can begin to describe your child's learning style.

Variations in learning style are common because each child is unique. Your child, like every child, needs to be taught as an individual. Your child may not have mental retardation, but because of his motor problems may need more adaptation of teaching methods and materials than other children do. If your child does have mental retardation, the teacher may need to repeat material many times in the same way for your child to learn. If your child has a short attention span, is easily distractible, or has difficulty correctly perceiving written letters and words, he may need to be taught as a child with learning disabilities. For example, the teacher may need to work with your child in a quiet corner. Or she may need to vary the way she teaches new concepts until she finds the way that makes sense for your child.

As a member of the team working with your child, the special education teacher will especially value the input of the physical, occupational, and speech-language therapists, who can suggest ways she can adapt her teaching to account for your child's motor problems. For example, the OT and PT can explain how to position your child in a chair with good support and good balance so he can draw straight lines. If your child has little speech, the speech-language pathologist can suggest ways he can answer questions with a "yes" or "no" rather than with a sentence.

The special education teacher should also value *your* input about your child's abilities and special problems. As a parent, you need to offer examples of skills your child can do at home but may not be able to show at school. Perhaps he cannot sort cars, blocks, and bears at school, but he can sort socks, underwear, and shirts when he helps you with the laundry at home.

While your baby is young, the infant teacher may need to see him only occasionally to make sure that his learning is on the right track or she may see him for an hour or two a week. When your child enters an early intervention program outside your home or moves into preschool, the special education teacher will likely become an increasingly important member of the team of professionals serving you and your child. Often special education teachers serve as a child's *case manager*—the team leader who maintains communication with a family and coordinates the services all the professionals provide for their child.

Pediatric Physical Therapist. The physical therapist (PT) will work with your child to develop his motor skills and to improve his strength, posture, and range of motion. She usually concentrates on the large muscles, such as those used in rolling, crawling, and walking. The physical therapist will show you how to do special exercises with your child and also how to handle him during daily care and play times.

As an infant, your child will likely see a physical therapist for only one hour a week and as a preschooler, for maybe two or three half-hour sessions a week. This makes it extremely important that you observe the physical therapist and then try out handling and positioning techniques under her direction so that you can exercise and handle your child at home as the therapist recommends. If your child gets appropriate handling and positioning for only that one or one and a half hours per week that he is with the therapist, you can expect to see little change. Ask the therapist to tell you the best ways to work on your child's special motor needs during daily routines such as bathing, dressing, feeding, and playing with your child.

In order to improve your child's muscle tone and ability to develop motor skills, the physical therapist may use special equipment like a large ball or roll when she works with your child. Your child may not like this new activity at first, but most children enjoy therapy sessions once they get used to them. The physical therapist will also be able to advise you on any special equipment your infant or child needs during therapy or to better position him for eating, drinking, playing, or learning. Depending on your child's needs, the special equipment recommended may include an adapted stroller or high chair, a standing table, or a corner chair. Chapter 4 describes many other types of special equipment that can help children with cerebral palsy. Chapter 7 discusses physical therapy in detail, and explains how to choose and work with a therapist.

Pediatric Occupational Therapist. Many of the ways the occupational therapist (OT) works with your baby or child will be similar to those of the physical therapist. However, she may focus more on the functional skills your child needs to be able to play and to feed and dress himself rather than on specific exercises. When the occupational therapist does recommend exercises for your child, she will usually combine them with activities that your child regularly does at home or at school. The occupational therapist will want to see if your child can reach out and grasp objects, how he plays with toys, how he can hold a pencil or crayon, and how he feeds and dresses himself. If your child has difficulty with any activities, the occupational therapist will find ways of positioning him to make movement easier or will adapt toys and feeding utensils to make them easier for him to use.

Besides helping children to move their muscles correctly, occupational therapists can also help children to interpret the sensory signals they receive from their muscles and from senses such as vision and hearing. For example, they can help children overcome over-sensitivities to touch or movement or help them develop better eye-hand coordination.

When your baby is in early intervention, the occupational therapist will concentrate on play and early self-help skills. Because of your baby's reduced strength or coordination, he may not be able to eat independently or to play spontaneously and independently with toys. The occupational therapist may fasten a toy or dish to the table so it does not move when your child uses it. She may build up the handle of a spoon to make it easier to grip. As your child enters preschool, the occupational therapist will become more interested in your child's abilities in pre-academic skills such as drawing and color matching. She may need to build up the handle of a pencil as she did the spoon or she may add knobs to puzzle pieces to enable your child to lift them from their holes.

It is especially important that you tell the occupational therapist how your child is doing at home with the suggestions she has given. That way she can judge the effectiveness of her therapy and change your child's program if necessary. For example, your child may be more dependent on you to dress him at home than when he shows off his dressing abilities at school. Or you may have found a better way to adapt a therapy or classroom activity for your child. For instance, you may have discovered that it is easier for your child to string beads if your wrap tape twice as far as usual around the end of the string.

For more information about occupational therapy and occupational therapists, see Chapter 7.

Speech-Language Pathologist. Many children with cerebral palsy have difficulty controlling the muscles of the mouth, just as they do the muscles in the rest of their body. If your child has this problem, the speech-language pathologist will help your child develop speech and language and learn to communicate.

Like any child, your child will begin communicating with you long before he can talk. The speech-language pathologist will help you identify the facial and body gestures your child uses to let you know what he wants and how he feels. For example, your child may look away when he's tired of playing with you or a toy, or he may stiffen his body when he's angry or stressed. The speech-language pathologist can suggest ways for you to help your child understand language, such as by repeating the name of a toy each time you give it to him or by holding out your arms as you say "Come up." Later, she can suggest ways to get your child to use the words he knows and to expand his vocabulary.

To help your child develop speech, the speech-language pathologist will begin working with your child during feeding and early sound production to ensure that his mouth and respiratory muscles work as well as possible. As your child gets older, the pathologist will work on his articulation so that he will be more intelligible to others.

Sometimes a child's motor problems are so severe or complicated that he is unable to speak clearly enough or quickly enough to be understood. The speech-language pathologist can offer a variety of devices and techniques to aid communication. These include picture boards, hand signs, or computerized communication devices. These devices are adapted to each individual child and can be programmed at any level, from simple one-word responses to the expression of complex thoughts.

While your baby is in early intervention, the speech-language pathologist may not see your child for direct therapy, but instead make recommendations to you and to the other professionals working with him on a regular basis. As your child progresses through the preschool years, the speech-language therapist can work directly with him in improving expressive vocabulary, speech intelligibility, and language comprehension. If your child has motor difficulties in his face and mouth as well as other parts of his body, he may also continue to need help learning to eat independently.

Chapter 7 provides an in-depth discussion of speech and language therapy.

Family Support Professional. Particularly if your child's program uses the family-centered approach, it may include a professional whose role is to focus on the needs of the families of children with handicaps. This professional may be known as a family support person, family coordinator, family counselor, or family resource specialist. The family support professional may be a social worker, psychologist, or counselor, or a special education teacher or therapist who has had additional training and experience working with families.

Whatever his or her title, the family support person can help you and your family work through feelings and problems you may encounter during the process of learning about your child's delay or disability and securing services to meet your child's needs. The family support person can also help you find and use supports such as family, friends, or religion, and help you recognize your family's individual coping style. Additionally, the family support person can assist you by suggesting possible solutions to family problems. Finally, the family support person may offer ideas to help educational and therapeutic staff respond to your family's concerns and wishes.

Depending upon the needs of your child and your family, several other professionals may be members of the team serving your child. These may include a vision specialist, auditory specialist, psychologist, or social worker.

Places

Where is "school" for children in early intervention or preschool special education programs? Because of the variety of services your child may need and the variety of professionals and organizations providing those services, your child may receive services in a private office, a public or private school, a public agency such as the health department, or right in his own home. In some locales, there is a choice of programs serving children with cerebral palsy and other motor problems. In others, there may be only one program serving children with many different special needs or no program at all for the youngest children birth to three. You may even need to do some detective work to find professionals with training in your child's areas of need and put together a program yourself.

The following section describes the types of settings in which early intervention or educational services for children with cerebral palsy are most often provided. The section on "Assessment and Eligibility" later in this chapter explains how to find out which of these types is available in your area and whether your child is eligible for them.

Early Intervention Settings

Home-based Programs. As the name implies, home-based intervention services are provided in a child's home. Few programs, however, are exclusively home-based. Often early intervention programs offer home-based services for children birth to two years of age, then center-based programs from twenty-four months on.

Home-based programs come in many varieties, but in all of them, parents play a crucial role. As a parent, you should expect to participate in each home-based education or therapy session your child receives. You should observe and ask questions about what the teacher or therapist is doing and how this will help your child progress. Especially with your child's physical therapy, you should have "hands on" practice during the session and the therapist should observe and instruct you as you work with your child. For your child to receive the most benefit from the exercises and positioning the therapist shows you, it is important that you and other family members carry them out on a consistent, daily basis.

Because many different forms of home-based services have been developed, it is not possible to describe a "typical" program. However, it is possible to describe some characteristics that differ from program to program. These include program staff, frequency of home visits, and curriculum.

Home-based programs can have many different kinds of staffs. The staff of some programs may be mostly infant special education teachers, or as some are called, infant development specialists. Other programs may offer physical, occupational, and speech therapy as the primary service, with an educator working only with some children. Still other programs may include a social worker or a family support professional. Staff members may visit together in order to give suggestions about how each can best work with your child, but each teacher or therapist will likely come alone most of the time. Since your child has obvious motor needs, the primary person serving him may be the physical therapist. However, his developmental needs probably will span several areas and can best be met by a multidisciplinary team that focuses on all aspects of his development.

The frequency of home visits also differs from program to program. Some programs provide visits weekly, others every two weeks, and others only every few months to monitor development and make recommendations. In some cases, home visits may be combined with regularly scheduled visits to a center to receive therapy or educational services. The type and severity of your child's cerebral palsy should be the main factor that determines how frequently he receives therapy from a physical or occupational therapist.

One final difference among home-based programs is the curriculum they offer. You probably think of curriculum as the course of study offered by an elementary or secondary school. Early intervention programs also have a course of study. Generally, they are designed to teach your child important developmental milestones that he is having difficulty learning on his own—for example, sitting, feeding himself with a spoon, or using two-word phrases. In the past, these skills were usually taught in the order that a normally developing child would learn them (developmentally based skill sequence approach). For instance, children were taught first to roll from their front to their back, then to sit, then to crawl, and finally to walk. The teacher or therapist focused on one skill at a time— analyzing each skill to be learned, breaking it down into a series of teaching steps, instructing the child in these steps, and giving him reinforcement when he did well.

There are several potential problems in using this type of curriculum to teach children with cerebral palsy. First, many children with motor disabilities need to learn skills that are outside of the normal developmental sequence. For example, your child may learn to play with battery-operated toys earlier than usual if this is the easiest way for him to understand the concept of cause and effect. Second, the effects of a child's motor problems on his ability to demonstrate thinking, problem-solving, or other skills may not be taken into account. For example, if your child has poor fine motor skills, he may have difficulty using a stick to retrieve an object out of reach, even if he understands the concept.

Because of these problems, some programs have begun using a different type of curriculum (the interactional or ecological approach). This new approach also teaches children developmental skills such as crawling and stacking blocks, but uses meaningful, naturally occurring situations in your child's own home to do so. For example, if your baby is hungry, his teacher may suggest that you say, "Do you want your bottle?" and then work on his language skills. You might show him the bottle as you repeatedly name it to help him recognize the word "bottle," or help him say "baba" himself. You might also hold the bottle close to your child and encourage him to reach out for it with both hands to develop motor coordination. Likewise, you might encourage him to hold the bottle as he drinks to work on self-help skills. The ultimate goal of this type of curriculum is to teach your child skills that enable him to be as independent as possible. For example, an older child might practice fine motor skills by buttoning his sweater rather than by stringing beads. Parents, too, can benefit from this approach because it lets them take a more active role in choosing goals which fit their child's and their family's world.

Whatever curriculum your child's program uses, you should feel comfortable discussing your child's needs and how you think they can best be met. The staff of any early intervention program should respond to the strengths and needs of each individual infant and family, sometimes serving as teacher or therapist, sometimes serving as counselor or advocate. What the intervention staff does on each home visit should reflect the needs of your infant and family on that particular day, as well as the goals and objectives developed to guide your infant's therapeutic and educational program.

Why Home-based Services? As a parent, you may feel more comfortable if your baby receives early intervention services in your home rather than at a center. This is natural since your baby is still dependent on you and other family members to care for him and to teach him about his world. Many early intervention professionals recognize the importance that the family plays in a child's life during this formative stage. They believe that the only way to have a meaningful impact on a child's life is to work with the whole family. Home visiting gives teachers and therapists more opportunities to involve the whole family in the teaching process. By working one-on-one with your child, they can encourage him to learn in his natural environment. This makes it more likely that he will be able to *generalize* his new skills—that is, to use them in other situations with other people. Teachers and therapists can help you solve the problems you have at home, assess your child's specific needs for equipment, and work with your child's behavior in the context of your family's daily life.

For some families, receiving home-based services may be the only practical option. Home visiting may be the only way to serve a rural area where special-needs infants and families are separated by many miles. And infants with special health care needs may not be able to leave their homes or may find the trip to the center so stressful that they are unable to benefit from therapy or teaching time. Your baby may fall into this category if he was born prematurely or has frequent illnesses.

Center-based Programs. Early intervention services may be provided in a center rather than in your home. The intervention program could be housed in a public health, mental health, or other clinic; a hospital; its own building; or a public or private school. Most likely, there will be children with a variety of developmental delays and disabilities in the program.

As with home-based programs, the types of services and staffs available vary from program to program. How often your child visits the center for education and therapy will also vary. Your two-year-old may go to the center for two or three half-days per week or as many as five full days. Generally, the more severe his motor problems, the more times per week he will require therapy, and the older he gets, the more time he will spend at the center.

In programs that offer center-based services for infants younger than two years, services are generally more individualized. Once a week, you may take your baby to the center, where he will be seen by one or more team members during the visit. Your baby may be seen in a small group of four or five babies with the teacher and therapists moving from infant to infant, working with both parent and child. Alternately, your baby may be scheduled to see each member of the team separately. For example, if your baby's greatest need is for physical therapy, you may take him to see the therapist once or twice per week and to see the infant teacher or speech therapist only once or twice per month.

Some programs have a combination of home- and center-based settings. Your child may go to a center program for a group education program, but continue to receive his physical therapy at home. This home therapy can be especially helpful to you as you learn to deal with your child's problems with movement and muscle tone during daily activities right in your home.

Center-based classrooms usually look very much like any other nursery or preschool classroom, with the addition of special equipment for children with motor problems. Most centers have an area where children can gather for circle time, individual areas or "stations" for children to work alone or in small groups, an area for eating snacks or lunch, a diapering area, and, in full-day programs, a sleeping area. Your child may receive all services in this room if physical, occupational, and speech therapy are a part of classroom activities, or your child may go to a separate room for therapy. The center's curriculum will be similar to those discussed under home-based programs.

If your child had home-based services before entering a center-based program, you will notice you have less contact with his teacher and therapists once he goes to the center. However, most early intervention programs try to maintain communication between the classroom and the family. You may receive a written description of the day's activities with comments about your child's participation in each. Or a "communication book" may be sent home each day or at the end of the week with comments from your child's teacher and therapist. You can then answer their questions and offer your thoughts on what is going on in class or therapy. You can also tell the center staff about events or problems in your child's life at home that may influence his behavior at the center.

If you find that your child's program has no regular means of communication, stress the importance of two-way communication for your family and request that a method of communication be developed. Talk with the staff about what will work best for them and for you. It may be a phone call, a communication book, or a regular visit by you to observe therapy or classroom activities. As a member of your child's early intervention team, you need to give regular input so that your child's needs and performance in all areas can be considered. Additionally, your child will make the most progress when skills learned in the classroom and in therapy can be transferred to the home. You, the parent, are the one who can bridge that gap.

Why a Center-based Program? When your child is in a home-based program and sees the teacher and therapist only one or two times a week, you are your child's primary teacher and therapist. This role certainly has its advantages. However, as your child gets larger and approaches the age of two, you may feel that you do not have the skills to help your child as he should be helped. Or you may find it too stressful or too time-consuming to carry out therapy and teaching activities at home, especially if you work or have other children. Furthermore, your child may not be able to get therapy as often as he needs it if the therapist must travel to your home to see him. In these cases, you may find a center-based program preferable.

At a center, your child can spend a substantial amount of time with teachers and therapists who are trained to use strategies to help him learn and develop. He will probably have more access to the individual therapists who can help him in his areas of need such as motor and communication development. He also has access to a wide variety of appropriate toys and specialized equipment which you do not have at home and which the interventionist cannot easily transport on home visits.

Another important advantage to center-based programs is their impact on your child's social and emotional behavior. Being in a group with other children gives your child the opportunity to play and communicate with his peers. This is particularly important if your child is learning to use an alternate means of communication and can be motivated by communicating with other boys and girls his age who may be using similar communication systems. He may also work harder to crawl, walk, or move around in his wheelchair if he is trying to keep up with his friends.

A center-based program may be less tolerant of your child's misbehavior than you are at home. As a parent, it is sometimes hard not to dismiss your child's behavior because he "gets so frustrated" or he "can't do what the other kids do." Center-based staff can be more objective in dealing with your child. They may also be more familiar with ways to control inappropriate behaviors. It is important that your child, as any child, learn how to behave appropriately both at home and at school. Additionally, your child may need special emphasis on acquiring skills such as attention, participation, endurance, and persistence that he will be expected to have as a preschooler.

Preschool Settings

Once your child reaches preschool age, you can expect that he will receive special education services outside of your home. But exactly where he will attend preschool depends on the public school system in your area. This is because the laws that require states to provide preschool education by 1991 require only that states place children in the *least restrictive environment*—or in the setting that permits maximum contact with normally developing children. Sometimes children with disabilities are "mainstreamed" or placed in classes with normally developing children, and sometimes they are not. The least restrictive environment for one child is not

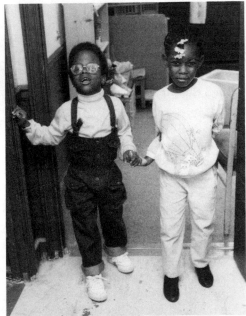

necessarily the least restrictive environment for another.

Because many school systems do not have classes for normally developing three- and four-year-olds, it is often a challenge for schools to find classroom space for preschoolers with disabilities. Some provide special education to young preschoolers by placing children with more severe handicaps with children with milder handicaps. Others engaged in "reverse mainstreaming" by placing normally developing preschoolers into classes for children with special needs. Still others offer preschool special education classes in sites where children with disabilities can be integrated into regular day care programs for part of the day. So, depending on where you live, your preschool child may be taught in either a segregated or an integrated setting. That is, he may spend all of his time with other children with special needs, or he may spend all or part of his time with children who do not have handicaps.

If your child attends preschool in a segregated setting, his classroom might be in a school serving only children with special needs or only children with cerebral palsy or other motor impairments. His classroom could also be in a regular school, in a wing where classrooms for children with special needs are located. These types of classrooms offer children with cerebral palsy several advantages. First, therapists can provide services, and coordinate with teachers, more easily and efficiently. For example, the physical therapist might help position a child in an adaptive chair for classroom circle time and the speech-language pathologist can help a child use his communication board with his classroom friends. Second, a classroom that serves many children with special motor needs is likely to have more therapy equipment available than is a school with only one or two children with cerebral palsy.

Placing children with cerebral palsy or other special needs in classes with peers who do not have disabilities ("mainstreaming") also has its advantages. Most importantly, children in mainstreamed classrooms have the chance to learn from watching and playing with classmates who have more advanced skills in movement, communication, or other areas. By working and playing together with their classmates, children with cerebral palsy, too, can develop better social and communication skills.

If your child does not have mental retardation or special learning problems, he may easily be able to keep up with children his same age in a regular preschool setting. You may, however, need to talk with the teacher or your child's physical therapist about ways to enable your child to participate in classroom activities. For example, he may need to scoot himself from circle time to the play area rather than walk or be carried. He may bat the ball from his wheelchair or be given a head start when walking in from outside play.

A regular classroom setting can also work if your child has special learning and communication needs as well as motor disabilities. He may just need to go to a separate room for his speech and language, physical, or occupational therapy. This type of "pull out" program allows your child to concentrate on his areas of need. It also enables classroom staff to consult with therapists about ways to help your child carry over new skills to the classroom. In addition, the teachers can help select the goals your child needs to participate more fully in the daily classroom routine. A special education teacher may also see your child on a regular basis, either within his classroom or in a separate room to work on individual skills.

Therapists and special education teachers who provide services to children in regular classroom settings are often itinerant—that is, they move from school to school. If your child's therapists or special teachers are not based at your child's school, try to work out some regular means of communicating with them. You may have your child carry a communication book and ask each of his special therapists or teachers, as well as his regular classroom teacher, to regularly give you feedback about his program and suggestions for home activities. Remember, your input about your child's life at home continues to be very important, so be sure to include your feedback in the book. And never hesitate to phone your child's teacher or therapist, ask to observe a therapy session, or arrange a special meeting with school staff.

Once your child enters preschool, his classes may be divided by age. He may begin in a class with other three-year-olds, then move to the fours, then the fives. Other schools mix ages within one classroom. This allows children with a broader range of skills to learn and play together. Here children are likely to be placed according to the skills they need to develop rather than on how old they are. A mixed-age classroom may work best for your child with cerebral palsy because all of his skills probably are not at the same level. He may be able to keep up with the fives during story time, but need to concentrate on four-year-old skills during table activities such as cutting, pasting, and drawing.

Your child's classroom will probably include several special learning areas. You may observe a kitchen area, a block area, a dress-up area, and a quiet area. These areas or stations encourage children to learn and practice necessary skills in a fun and functional way. The instruction that your child receives at this age is often organized into units such as "Community Helpers," "Winter Fun," "Shopping," or "Transportation." By organizing learning experiences around a central theme, the teacher makes them more meaningful for your child. When you know what unit is being studied in your child's classroom, you can offer experiences in the real world to reinforce the concepts being taught at school.

Assessment and Eligibility

As Chapter 9 explains, free early intervention services or preschool special education may be available in your state. If your state offers services for children of your son's or daughter's age, you must follow certain steps before your child is declared "eligible" to begin receiving services at public expense. In particular, you must have your child's abilities and disabilities evaluated to determine which, if any, services he needs.

Eligibility requirements for early intervention and preschool special education services vary from state to state. In general, children diagnosed with cerebral palsy qualify for these services. To find out what the eligibility standards are in your area, call your local elementary school and ask for the person in charge of special education services. You may also contact your state health department, developmental disabilities council, division of mental health/mental retardation, or other agency in charge of early intervention services in your state. In addition, the local or state Child Find Office which is part of the public school system can help you. The Child Find Office is responsible for identifying all children with handicaps in its area. Often the eligibility process begins here. Your child's pediatrician or orthopedic doctor should also be able to refer you to programs available in your area.

The person in charge of early intervention or preschool special education services in your area will tell you what to do next to get your child accepted into a program. If you are seeking early intervention services, the procedure may be fairly informal. For example, someone from the intervention program may schedule an initial visit, either in your home or at the center. During this visit, you may be asked for information about your child's diagnosis and development to help the program staff determine whether or not your child is eligible for the program and what kind of services you and your child need. You might also be asked about your priorities for your child and your family and about how you would like the intervention program to be involved in your family's life. For example, you may want services specifically focused on your child's movement needs. Or as parents, you may want help for yourself and for your other children in adapting your daily lives to accommodate your child with special needs. If the staff determines your child is eligible, services might begin right away.

Eligibility procedures can be somewhat different for preschool special education programs and for early intervention programs with more formal entrance requirements. Your child will need to have a comprehensive *multidisciplinary developmental assessment* to determine his present level of functioning and his unique strengths and needs in all developmental areas. During this assessment, a team of professionals with specialties in many different areas will conduct tests, observe your child, and review his medical history, reports from doctors, and any previous developmental evaluations. Since this assessment should look at the "whole child," and include information about your child's total environment, it is important that you share information about your child at home.

Your child's assessment will be conducted by the designated early intervention agency or the school system providing preschool services. This assessment will be done at no cost to you.

If you believe that the school's assessment of your child is incomplete or inaccurate or for some other reason you want a second opinion, you may ask for an outside specialist to assess your child. If the school is to pay for the assessment, the arrangements must be made through the school. You may also have your child evaluated by another specialist at any time if you pay for it yourself.

Your child will likely be given an assessment not only before he enters an early intervention program, but also before he begins a preschool special education program. Your school system may, however, accept assessment information from your child's early intervention program in making preschool placement decisions. If your child is in an early intervention program, his case manager will help you make the transition into a preschool program. Transition services are a part of both early intervention and preschool programs.

The types of professionals on assessment teams vary, but members of your child's team will probably include a special education teacher, a school psychologist, a physical therapist, an occupational therapist, and a speech-language pathologist. Chapter 7 describes how the occupational and physical therapists and speech-language pathologist test and observe your child to get an idea of his developmental strengths and needs. Here is a summary of what the other professionals may do during your child's developmental evaluation:

Special Education Teacher. The teacher will test your child's cognitive and social-emotional development, as well as his adaptive behavior (his ability to adjust to new environments and apply new skills to new situations). She may look at visual and auditory abilities, pre-academic skills, learning style, and attention to task. To develop a picture of your child's abilities in these areas, the teacher will observe your child and do different types of tests. She will test your child in formal situations, with prescribed sets of materials. She will also test your child informally, often by watching him at play and checking off behaviors she observes on a checklist of behaviors. The special education teacher may be your child's regular classroom teacher or an educational diagnostician who sees your child only for this assessment.

School Psychologist. The psychologist will give your child standardized tests to determine his current level of functioning and his intellectual potential. Because most of these tests are designed for children without disabilities, the psychologist should adapt the testing procedures so they are more appropriate for your child. She should also interpret the results from standardized tests in light of what your child is usually able to do outside of a formal testing situation. The pyschologist should observe your child in the familiar setting of the home or classroom to help her judge the accuracy of test results.

During the assessment process for early intervention services, your child's strengths and needs are not the only things that will be assessed. Your family's strengths and needs as they relate to your goals for your child will also be identified. For example, one of your family's strengths may be older children who can do daily exercises and relieve you of some routine care. On the other hand, you may need help arranging transportation to and from your child's babysitter, help understanding exactly how cerebral palsy affects your child, or help explaining your child's program to his grandparents.

The "family assessment" should include only information that you choose to share with the intervention program. It does not extend to aspects of your family life which do not directly relate to the achievement of your goals for your child. You do not need to discuss your marriage relationship, your problems with your mother-in-law, your financial condition, or how your other children are doing in school.

At the conclusion of your child's assessment, the team leader will review the findings of all the professionals who have examined your child. She will discuss the amount of delay your child has in each developmental area and whether or not these delays are great enough to qualify your child for early intervention or preschool special education services in your community.

If your child is declared eligible for early intervention services, your family will be assigned a case manager. Your case manager can answer your questions and guide you through the process of getting services started and evaluating their appropriateness for your family. Often he or she can also help coordinate the services provided by the teachers and therapists working with your child. Because you have frequent contact with everyone providing services to your child, be sure to let the case manager know your feelings about your child's services and how they are coordinated.

As Chapter 9 explains, once your child is found eligible for preschool services under P.L. 94–142, he will begin receiving special education services free of charge. Your public school system must pay for all services your child needs in order to benefit from his education program. You may want to pay for extra therapy if you and your doctor decide your child needs it.

If your state does not have a statewide program of early intervention services provided at public expense, you may have to pay for your child's program. You may be charged a "sliding scale" fee for some services, so you may need to turn to Medicaid or private insurance to cover some of the costs of your child's program. Scholarships may also be available from some private programs which consider the additional expenses of having a child with special needs, as well as your income. Additionally, you may be able to get funds from religious or community organizations such as the

Kiwanis or Elks, especially if it is to cover a special piece of equipment or a specific period of therapy or intervention.

If you disagree with the assessment and with your child's placement in a public program, you do not have to send him to the program. Until you and the school agree on your child's program, you should not give your permission for him to start the program. Keep the lines of communication open with the school and continue to talk with them and ask questions. Chapter 9 explains how you can appeal the school's decision if you and the staff cannot reach agreement.

Setting Goals for Your Child

Your child's assessment will reveal his general strengths and needs in all developmental areas. But before your child can begin receiving early intervention or preschool special education services, you and the professionals involved in his program must pinpoint the specific skills on which he needs to work. For example, the occupational and physical therapists may have found that your three-year-old has great difficulty controlling his arm and hand movements. These movement problems prevent him from mastering many basic self-help skills, including dressing, brushing his teeth, and feeding himself, and many classroom skills such as completing puzzles, building with blocks, and using the computer. It is up to you and the professionals to decide which of these skills is most important for your child to learn first so you can choose his learning goals accordingly.

Both early intervention and special education programs provide regular opportunities for you to meet with professionals to plan your child's learning goals. In early intervention programs, parents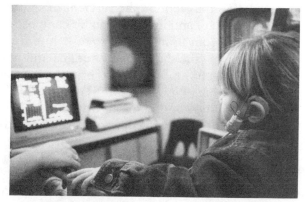

meet with one or more of the team of teachers and therapists to draw up something called an *Individualized Family Service Plan* (IFSP). The IFSP is a written plan detailing your goals for your child and family and the specific early intervention and other services necessary to meet these goals. For example, a goal may be, "Johnny will improve his sucking and swallowing in order to finish his bottle in twenty minutes or less." Services necessary to meet this goal could be physical therapy to improve general motor strength, tone, and coordination; occupational therapy to develop the best positioning for feeding; and speech and language therapy to improve oral-motor coordination. Another goal might be, "In order for Brittany to learn from her environment, she will increase her ability to explore toys on her own." Services to meet this goal could include physical therapy to improve Brittany's ability to roll and crawl, occupational therapy to improve her use of hands for manipulating toys, and special education to encourage her to explore objects by touching and looking at them rather than by mouthing and banging them.

The IFSP must be reviewed at least once every six months, but you can request that it be reviewed and changed at any time as your needs change.

In preschool special education programs—and in special education programs for older children—parents and professionals meet at least once a year to design an *Individualized Education Program* (IEP) for their child. The IEP is a written plan describing the learning goals for your child and listing the services the school system must provide for your child. For example, "Bart will be able to copy a circle, square, and triangle on nine out of ten attempts." To achieve this goal, Bart may require the services of an occupational therapist to adapt his chair and his pencil so he can position his arm to write, and a special education teacher to take him through the process of learning to copy the shapes. Another goal might be, "Elizabeth will use her communication board to communicate her needs at school, home, and in her neighborhood." To meet this IEP goal, Elizabeth might need physical therapy to improve upper body strength for better sitting balance, occupational therapy to improve arm and hand control for pointing, speech and language therapy to teach word concepts and practice use of the board, a special education teacher to teach concepts and guide the use of the board in the classroom, and a parent to oversee use of the board at home. Perhaps a teacher assistant could also make a home visit to observe Elizabeth using the board in her home and neighborhood.

For information about the elements that your child's IEP or IFSP must, by law, include, see Chapter 9.

The intervention or education program developed for your child in IFSP and IEP meetings will be similar. Both can include goals in the developmental areas of gross and fine motor, cognitive, speech-language, social-emotional, and self-help, as well as such services as transportation and counseling. The difference is that the IFSP should be guided by the parents and should contain the goals they have identified for their child and family. The IEP is required to have goals in all areas of delay identified through assessment and classroom evaluation—as well as goals identified by parents. In addition, once your child reaches preschool age, he should begin receiving pre-academic instruction to prepare him for the academic skills of reading, writing, and arithmetic.

How much emphasis your child's program places on academics will depend on his cognitive abilities. For children with cerebral palsy whose disability mainly affects motor skills, pre-academic and academic skills may come easily. Progress will be slower for children with specific learning disabilities that make it difficult to perceive shapes and letters and put them together into words or to understand how to add and subtract. Eventually, they will learn these basic academic skills. Children who have mental retardation can usually learn academic skills, but how far they can go depends on the degree of retardation. Some can learn only basic reading and writing; others can graduate from high school in special education programs. For children who have severe handicaps in addition to cerebral palsy, a functional, rather than an academic program may best meet their needs. Learning centers around the skills a child needs to function in his daily life. These might include eating, dressing, communicating his needs, and finding ways to have fun with classmates or family members.

At your child's IFSP and IEP meetings—or whenever you meet with school or medical personnel—you should always ask questions and offer your opinion about what is being discussed. Do not be intimidated. You are part of the team planning your child's educational program—and an invaluable part—because you know your child and you know what you want for your child. Share your information and your opinions, listen to the professionals, and consider their advice. Work together to build the program which best suits your child's and your family's needs and which offers your child the best educational future.

Choosing a Preschool Program

As discussed earlier, preschool special education programs come in many different forms and can include a wide variety of services and professionals. However, few communities offer every type of preschool program. For example, your community may provide services for children with cerebral palsy only in a segregated setting with other children with cerebral palsy or other disabilities. Or it may only offer special therapy services within a regular preschool class. But you may have a choice. Whatever your choices, remember that these early years are very important for your child. You want him to spend his time in a warm, caring atmosphere that will make him feel good about himself and that will meet his educational and therapeutic needs in all areas.

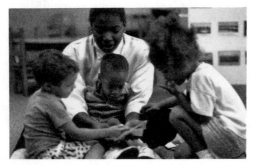

When you look for a preschool program, think of what you would want for your child if he did not have cerebral palsy. Add to this your child's need for specialized teaching, help in learning to communicate, and regular physical therapy to minimize the effects of cerebral palsy. To be sure that you have a clear picture of your child, talk to his teachers and therapists and observe him in school yourself. Discuss his strengths and needs with other family members, with friends, and with professionals. Be clear about your child's educational and therapeutic needs so that you can judge whether or not the class you observe matches his needs. For example, a program that emphasizes free play and outdoor exercise may not match your child's needs for individualized instruction in fine motor and communication skills.

If your child is in an early intervention program or is receiving private therapy, you should ask one of his teachers or therapists to help you identify the kind of program he needs or to go with you to visit programs. Then contact the director of each program you are considering and arrange a time to visit. When you visit programs, take along your child's IFSP or IEP and any other evaluation or therapy reports that will help you and the program staff identify his strengths and needs. You may want to visit once without your child and return later with your child if the program looks like it may meet his needs. This will give the staff a chance to meet your child in person and help them determine if his needs could be met in this program. Be sure to stay long enough to see all aspects of the program, including large and small group work, individual therapy, and transition times.

The following checklist of questions can guide your inquiries and observations about preschool programs. Use your knowledge of your child and the opinions of the professionals working with him to determine the requirements for your child and your family in each area listed. Add to this list as you think about your child and his individual needs for a program.

Program Evaluation Guidelines

1. **To begin with, you might ask staff for some general information about the school and how it operates:**
   - Who does the school serve? Ages of children? Types of needs?
   - How many children and how many classes are in the school?
   - What is the staff-to-child ratio?
   - What kinds of teachers and therapists are on staff?
   - Is transportation to and from school provided?
   - What is the school schedule? What will the day be like for your child?

2. **Ask a general question to get an overall idea or feeling about the program:**
   - What is the philosophy of the program? Child-focused? Parent-focused?

- What type of curriculum is used?

3. After you have gathered some basic information, observe the program in action. While you observe, look for:

- How many adults and children are in the room?
- What are the children doing? (small groups, individual activities)
- Do activities encourage children to develop independence?
- Are activities appropriate to the age level of the children?
- How do the adults interact with the children? Do they talk to them about what they are doing? Do they seem warm and accepting? Dedicated and enthusiastic?
- What types of materials are available? (blocks, books, soft mats for floor play)
- How has the classroom been modified to encourage children with physical disabilities to move around and interact with the environment? Are toys within reach of a crawler? Are there small rugs or obstacles a child could trip over?
- Are classrooms and school grounds clean and well kept?

4. Try to determine whether children are given the individualized attention they need:

- How are individual programs developed and carried out? Ask to see examples of IEPs, therapists' checklists, and other individual plans.
- How often are children's programs re-evaluated?
- Do teachers and therapists regularly communicate with one another about individual students?
- How will the teachers and therapists work with your child? (one-to-one, small group, in the classroom, in a therapy room)

5. Consider how well the therapy services available would meet your child's needs:

- How many physical therapists, occupational therapists, and speech-language pathologists are there?
- How many work on site (in classroom) on a daily basis?

- How many travel from site to site?
- Are they NDT certified/trained?
- How many times per week do children receive therapy?
- Are therapy services integrated into the classroom?
- Are PTs experienced with gait training (or whatever particular need your child has?)
- Are OTs trained in sensory integration?
- Are SLPs experienced with alternate means of communication such as communication boards and computers?
- Do SLPs have oral/motor feeding experience?

6. **Be sure to ask about any other special needs your child might have, for example:**

- Is special equipment available and is the staff trained to operate it?
- Are year-round services available?
- Does the program have a summer camp?

7. **You probably have many questions about how you, as the parent, might fit into the program. Some of these might be:**

- How does staff communicate with parents? By phone calls, communication books, notes home? How might parents let staff know important things or ask questions?
- What are parents' responsibilities for participating in the program?
- What services are offered to parents? (support groups, workshops, training)

8. **Many families work with a number of professionals. You might ask about how this program coordinates with outside professionals:**

- Are program staff willing to act as coordinators?
- Do they prefer that you act as a coordinator and let them know what they need to follow through on?

Once you have found a program for your child, be honest about your child's capabilities and disabilities. Meet with the classroom teacher and let her know what to expect. Get her thoughts on what might make your child's adjustment to the program easy or difficult. Brainstorm together about potential problems and solutions. Let the teacher know that you are available whenever needed to help make your child's preschool experience a pleasant and rewarding one for both your child and the teachers and therapists working with him. If you and your child's teacher establish a good relationship in the beginning, you will be able to rely on one another in the future development of your child's program.

The Parent-Professional Partnership

Over the past few years, the parent-professional relationship in early intervention and preschool special education programs has changed. We have moved from a relationship in which the professional acts as teacher of the parent and decision-maker for the child to a relationship in which professionals and parents jointly consider the needs of the child and the family. The ultimate goal is an equal partnership between parent and professional.

Today collaboration between parents and professionals is becoming increasingly widespread—in part because new laws encourage parents of young children to work in full partnership with professionals. In programs that are seeking to follow this basic philosophy, you will find that you and your child are treated with respect. Your opinion will be solicited and welcomed by the program staff. You will have the opportunity to talk to professionals about the realities of everyday life with a child with cerebral palsy. You will be encouraged to share with the staff and with other parents the knowledge gained from experience with your child. You will be given factual information and professional judgment to help you decide on realistic goals for your child and your family.

Unfortunately, although you have a legal right to be involved in all aspects of your child's educational program, all professionals may not readily accept and respect you as an important member of your child's early intervention or special education team. In this case, you will have to convince the teachers and therapists that your input is vital to ensuring that your child gets the maximum benefits from his program. You will have to work harder to be actively involved in your child's program. You will need to be an advocate for your child and your family. This you would do in any circumstance. Since you have a child with special needs, you must be especially vigilant to make sure that your child's and family's needs are met.

Do not expect to be able to forge a good partnership overnight. Be patient as professionals are required to take on roles that are different than the ones they have played in the past. But also be firm and persistent, open and cooperative. Keep on trying until you have built a relationship in which professionals recognize your rights and responsibilities to make decisions about special services for your child. Chapter 10 provides an introduction to advocacy techniques that can help in getting professionals to come around to your way of thinking.

Conclusion

Your child is a child with cerebral palsy, but first he is a child. He should have the opportunity to grow and develop like any other child. True, playing and learning and communicating will often be more difficult for him than it is for other children. And watching him and helping him will often be more difficult for you. But you can grow and learn together, and you can *enjoy* playing and learning. You can enjoy meeting the challenges of making the world work for your child. These are unique challenges. Not all parents and children have to face them. But there are many people who can help you—people who have taught children with cerebral palsy and people who have helped parents of children with cerebral palsy to learn about their child. They can help. They will help. You and your child can live and learn and grow together.

Parent Statements

The problem with special education is that from the moment the kids enter the classroom until they leave, all that is done is they are tested. If you look at a preschool special ed program compared to a regular preschool program, the difference that's really noticeable is not so much the kids, it's the teachers' constant inquisitions of the children.

❧❧❧

They don't let them be children. They want the kids to perform constantly.

꿏꿏

The best thing I did was to enter my son into a special education program at an early age. The separation was difficult for both of us, but in retrospect we needed to separate in order to grow. We were much too attached to each other, physically and emotionally.

꿏꿏

They may be professionals, but they don't walk a mile in my shoes.

꿏꿏

Ever since Jenny started early intervention, I've been more optimistic—maybe too optimistic. But so far, she's been making great progress and the whole family is getting a lot out of the program.

꿏꿏

I think we have to truly rethink preschool special education so that teachers are there just to assist the kids in doing what the kids want to do.

꿏꿏

In almost every program she's ever been in, I've had to go in and teach everyone about my kid and her equipment.

꿏꿏

Most preschoolers go in and can build blocks; special ed preschoolers go in and have to build blocks in certain ways.

꿏꿏

Train, assess, train, assess. . . . That's what the curriculum is.

꿏꿏

I think most of the staff really cares about my son. It's more than a job to them—they really want to see him progress.

✴✴✴

Separation was extremely hard! I had a child I knew little about, except that she was totally dependent and I loved her very much. The first program she was in was about eleven or twelve miles from home and lasted maybe three hours. We had little money, so in an attempt to save gas money, I'd stay and wait for her. At first I'd wait down the hall and do cross-stitch or something. That was probably the worse thing to do because I could hear her crying. Eventually, I worked my way out of the building to wait and even made some outings in the area.

✴✴✴

I feel it is very important for parents to take a step back and try to see both sides before they criticize or make judgements. We are all in this together and are all trying to do what's best for the child. We just have different perspectives and need to understand each other a little more.

✴✴✴

Finding a teacher who truly cares about your child can make all the difference in the world. When your child is motivated at school, he can make much bigger strides at home.

✴✴✴

When I first heard about early intervention, I couldn't believe all these people would actually come to my house. I still think it's a pretty good deal.

✴✴✴

I sometimes wonder if my child really benefits from state-provided services or if I should push for total mainstreaming and just continue to pay the private therapists.

❀❀❀

When your child has an assessment, it's depressing to see his disability in writing. It's depressing because it's reality.

❀❀❀

NINE

Legal Rights and Hurdles

JAMES E. KAPLAN AND RALPH J. MOORE, JR.*

Introduction

Your child with cerebral palsy has many rights that you should know about. These rights, which include the right to a free appropriate public education, are provided by federal, state, and local laws. They can be essential in helping your child reach her potential by opening doors to education, training, and special services. Cerebral palsy affects every child differently, and the various laws may therefore apply differently. Understanding how these laws work can enable you to ensure that your child receives the services she needs.

There are no federal laws that deal specifically with cerebral palsy. Rather, the rights of children with cerebral palsy are provided in the laws and regulations for people with disabilities generally. In other words, the same laws that protect all children with disabilities also protect your child. To effectively exercise your rights and fully protect your child, you should be familiar with those laws.

* Ralph J. Moore, Jr., is a partner in the law firm of Shea & Gardner in Washington, D.C. James E. Kaplan is a partner in the law firm of Conley, Haley & O'Neil in Bath, Maine. Both are active in the area of the legal rights of children with disabilities. They are the co-authors of "Legal Rights and Hurdles" in *Babies with Down Syndrome: A New Parents' Guide* (Woodbine House, 1986), *Children with Epilepsy: A Parents' Guide* (Woodbine House, 1988), and *Children with Autism: A Parents' Guide* (Woodbine House, 1989). Mr. Moore is the author of *Handbook on Estate Planning for Families of Developmentally Disabled Persons in Maryland, the District of Columbia, and Virginia* (Md. DD Council, 3rd edition, 1989).

In addition to the laws providing for educational services, there are other laws dealing with discrimination, insurance, and government programs that can have an impact on both you and your child. This chapter explains how all of these laws work.

Because cerebral palsy sometimes results in serious lasting disabilities, parents often worry about the future—especially about how to provide for their child when they, the parents, are no longer alive. This chapter also explains the extremely important legal issues that parents must face to protect their child's future well-being. Finally, we summarize briefly the disability benefits generally available from federal and state governments and some related issues that can affect your child with cerebral palsy as an adult.

It would be impossible to discuss here the law of every state or locality. Instead, we provide an overview of the most important legal concepts you need to know. For information about the particular laws in your area, contact the United Cerebral Palsy Association (UCP), the Association for Retarded Citizens (ARC), or your local or state UCP or ARC affiliate.

This chapter is designed to provide accurate and authoritative information about the legal aspects of raising a child with cerebral palsy. The authors and the publisher, however, are not acting as lawyers and are not rendering legal, accounting, or other professional advice. If you need legal or other advice, you should consult a competent professional.

Your Child's Right to an Education

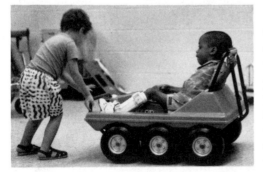

Perhaps nothing has done so much to improve educational opportunities for children with cerebral palsy as The Education for All Handicapped Children Act of 1975, better known as Public Law 94–142 (the "EAHCA"). You may also hear this law referred to as the Individuals with Disabilities Education Act (IDEA). This comprehensive law, along with recent amendments to it, has created vastly improved educational opportunities for almost all children with disabilities. Administered by the U.S. Department of Education and by each state, the law works on a carrot-and-stick basis.

Under Public Law 94–142, the federal government provides funds for the education of children with disabilities to each state that has a special education program that meets a variety of federal standards. To qualify for the federal funds, a state must demonstrate, through a detailed plan submitted for federal approval, that it has a policy assuring all children with disabilities a "free appropriate public education." What this means is that states accepting federal funds under Public Law 94–142 must provide both approved educational services and a variety of procedural rights to children with disabilities and their parents. The lure of federal funds has been attractive enough to induce all states to create special education plans that can truly help children with cerebral palsy.

The EAHCA has its limits. The law only establishes the *minimum* requirements in special education programs for states desiring to receive federal funds. In other words, the law *does not* require states to adopt an ideal educational program for your child with cerebral palsy or a program that you feel is "the best." Because states have leeway under Public Law 94–142, there are differences from state to state in the programs or services available.

States *can* create special education programs that are better than those required by Public Law 94–142, and some have. Parents, organizations, and advocacy groups continually push states to exceed the federal requirements and provide the highest quality special education as early as possible. In addition, these same groups continually urge the federal government to raise the requirements for states under the EAHCA. Check with your local school district to find out exactly what services are available to your child.

What Public Law 94–142 Provides

This section reviews the important provisions of Public Law 94–142.

Coverage. Children with cerebral palsy are covered by Public Law 94–142. The EAHCA applies generally to children who are "orthopedically impaired," "mentally retarded," or learning disabled. A diagnosis of cerebral palsy, developmental or motor delay, central nervous system disorder, or similar condition should be enough to establish that the EAHCA applies to your child. If your child's cerebral palsy hinders her learning, she qualifies for services under the EAHCA.

"Free Appropriate Public Education." At the heart of Public Law 94–142 is the requirement that children with disabilities receive a "free appropriate public education." Like every other child, children with special needs are entitled to receive an education at public expense. They are also entitled to receive an appropriate educational program—one that takes into account their special learning needs and abilities. To help clarify what your child is and is not entitled to, this section examines more precisely what each of the elements of "free appropriate public education" means.

"Free" means just that—regardless of the parents' ability to pay, every part of a child's special education program must be provided at public expense. Often this requirement is satisfied by placing a child in a public school. But if no suitable public program is available, then the school district must place the child in a private program and pay the full cost. In some areas, private schools have programs that are better suited to the needs of children with cerebral palsy. Remember, the EAHCA does not provide for tuition payment for educational services *not* approved by the school district or other governing agency (unless, as explained elsewhere in this chapter, parents are able to overturn the decision of their school district). Parents who place their child in an unapproved program face having to bear the full cost of tuition themselves.

It often is difficult for parents to understand that the "appropriate" education mandated by the EAHCA does not guarantee for their child either the best education that money can buy or even an educational opportunity equal to that given to nondisabled children. The law is more modest; it only requires that children with disabilities be given access to specialized educational services individually designed to benefit the child. A few years ago, the United States Supreme Court decided that a "free appropriate public education" need not enable a child with disabilities to maximize her potential or to develop self-sufficiency. Instead, the basic floor of educational opportunity may be satisfied by a variety of instructional and related services, the extent of which is determined on a child-by-child basis. The law in this area is still evolving.

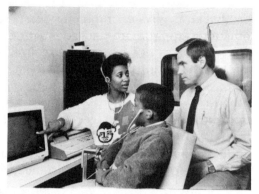

It is the parents' responsibility to make sure that their child receives the most appropriate placement and services. Under the EAHCAA, parents and educators are supposed to work together to design the individualized education program for each child. But to convince a school district to make the best placement for their child, parents must demonstrate to school officials not only that the parents' preferred placement is appropriate, but that other placements the school district might prefer are not. Hopefully in the end there is agreement on the appropriate placement. If not, there are procedures for resolving disputes discussed later in the chapter.

"Special Education and Related Services." Under Public Law 94–142, an appropriate education consists of "special education and related services." "Special education" means specially designed instruction tailored to meet the unique needs of the child with disabilities, including classroom instruction, physical education, home instruction, and—if necessary—instruction in private schools, hospitals, or institutions. "Related services" are defined as transportation and other developmental, corrective, and supportive services necessary to enable the child to benefit from special education.

For children with cerebral palsy, "related services" are a critical part of their special education program. Services provided by a trained occupational therapist, physical therapist, speech therapist, psychologist, social worker, school nurse, aide, or any other qualified person may be required under Public Law 94–142. Some services, however, are specifically excluded. Most important among these exclusions are strictly medical services provided by a licensed physician or hospital.

Because physical problems often result from cerebral palsy, obtaining appropriate and adequate physical, occupational, and speech therapy *as part of your child's special education program* can be critical. In addition, as discussed later, personal assistance services—someone to help with such needs as personal care and mobility—can be an essential related service. Parents should demand that their child receive the related services she needs; this is their child's right under the law. You should make sure your child's education program includes enough physical and occupational therapy and personal assistance, and provides these services appropriately.

"Least Restrictive Environment." Public Law 94–142 requires that children with disabilities must "to the maximum extent appropriate" be educated in the *least restrictive environment* with children who are *not* handicapped. Under Public Law 94–142, there is therefore a strong preference for mainstreaming children with disabilities, including children with cerebral palsy. Some school officials assume that because a child has cerebral palsy, she should be educated in a separate special setting. This generally is not true. Most children with cerebral palsy can be educated with their non-disabled peers, with proper in-classroom supports and therapy.

In practice, the law requires that children with disabilities be integrated into their community's regular schools, if possible. For many children with cerebral palsy, this means full inclusion in regular classes, with special services such as physical or occupational therapy provided outside of class. For some children, this may mean a combination of regular classroom programs and separate special classes, along with physical education, music, assemblies, and other classes taken with the rest of the school. Special services and teaching material can be used to provide extra educational input for children with special needs. The law was intended to end the historical practice of isolating children with disabilities.

The EAHCA also recognizes that regular classrooms may not be suitable for the education of some children with disabilities. In these cases, the law allows for placement in separate classes, separate public schools, private schools, or even residential settings if the school district can demonstrate that this kind of placement is required to meet the individual *educational* needs of the child. When placement within the community's public schools is determined to be not appropriate for a child, the law still requires that she be placed in the least restrictive educational environment suitable to her individual needs. This can include some participation in regular school or regular classroom programs and activities.

When Coverage Begins under Public Law 94–142. Congress recently amended the EAHCA to require states to begin providing educational services at age three. Under Public Law 99–457, states will be required to provide services to all children with disabilities from the age of three, beginning in 1991. In addition, Congress has established a program of grants to support states that offer early intervention services to children from birth. To receive grants under this program, states must have an approved plan of providing early intervention services to infants with disabilities from birth through age two. Each state may decide for itself which agency will provide these early intervention services, so parents need to check with their local school district, the state education agency, or local UCP or ARC about where to go to get them. These services can include physical, occupational, or speech therapy as well as the use of technology to help young children with cerebral palsy maximize their early development. Chapter 7 discusses the types of early intervention services your child may receive.

Under the EAHCA, special education services must continue until children reach age eighteen, and in some cases, age twenty-one.

Length of Services. Currently under Public Law 94–142, states must provide more than the traditional 180–day school year when the unique needs of a child indicate that year-round instruction is a necessary part of a "free appropriate public education." In many states, the decision to offer summer instruction depends on whether the child will regress substantially without summer services. If so, the services must be provided at public expense. Because some children with cerebral palsy can regress without year-round services, their parents should not hesitate to request continuous instruction for the child.

Identification and Evaluation. Because the EAHCA applies only to children with disabilities, your child must be evaluated before she is eligible for special education. Public Law 94–142 requires each state to develop testing and evaluation procedures designed to identify and evaluate the needs and abilities of each child before she is placed into a special education program. All areas of development must be tested: health, vision, hearing, social and emotional status, general intelligence, academic performance, communication ability, and motor skills. On these and other issues, the evaluation procedure is required to take into account the parents' input. This means that parents—who understand their child's developmental needs best—should take an active role in the evaluation. Parents should gather as much information as they can to establish what special educational services their child needs.

"Individualized Education Program." Public Law 94–142 recognizes that each child with disabilities is unique. As a result, the law requires that your child's special education programs be tailored to her individual needs. Based on your child's evaluation, a program specifically designed to address her developmental problems must be devised. This is called an "individualized education program" or, more commonly, an "IEP."

The IEP is a written report that describes:

1. your child's present level of development;
2. both the short-term and annual goals of the special education program;
3. the specific educational services that your child will receive;
4. the date services will start and their expected duration;
5. standards for determining whether the goals of the educational program are being met; and
6. the extent to which your child will be able to participate in regular educational programs.

Under federal regulations, educational placements are supposed to be based on the IEP, not vice versa. That is, the services a child receives, and the setting in which they are delivered, should be determined by the child's individual needs, not by what happens to be currently available in existing programs. Services and placements should be tailored to the child, not the other way around.

A child's IEP is usually developed during a series of meetings among the parents, teachers, and representatives of the school district. Even the child herself may be present. School districts are required to establish committees to make these placement and program decisions. These committees, sometimes called "Admission, Review, and Dismissal" committees (ARD), decide what services your child will receive in addition to deciding where she will receive them.

The effort to write an IEP is ideally a cooperative one, with parents, teachers, and school officials conferring on what goals are appropriate and how best to achieve them. Preliminary drafts of the IEP are reviewed and revised until what hopefully is a mutually acceptable educational program is developed.

IEPs should be very detailed. Although this may seem intimidating at first, detailed IEPs enable parents to closely monitor the education their child receives and to make sure their child is actually receiving the services prescribed. In addition, the law requires that IEPs be reviewed and revised at least once a year (or more often if necessary) to ensure the child's educational program continues to meet her changing needs.

Designing a suitable IEP requires direct parent involvement. You cannot always depend on teachers or school officials to recognize your child's unique needs as you do. To obtain the full range of services, you may need to demonstrate that withholding certain services would result in an education that would *not* be "appropriate." For example, if parents believe that a program using advanced technology available only at a private school is best for their child, they must demonstrate that placement in another program would not be appropriate for their child's specific needs.

Because a child with cerebral palsy has special needs, it is essential that her IEP be written with care to meet those needs. Unless parents request specific services, they may be overlooked. You should make sure school officials recognize the unique needs of your child—the needs that make her different from other children with disabilities, and even from other children with cerebral palsy.

How can parents prepare for the IEP process? First, explore available educational programs, including public, private, federal, state, county, and municipal programs. Observe classes and see for yourself which program is best suited to your child. Local school districts and local organizations can provide you with information about programs in your community. Second, collect a complete set of developmental evaluations to share with school officials—get your own if you doubt the accuracy of the school district's evaluation. Third and most important, decide for yourself what program and services are best for your child, and request that placement.

To support placement in a particular type of program, you should collect "evidence" about your child's special needs. You should support your position that a particular type of placement is appropriate by presenting letters from physicians, psychologists, therapists (physical, speech, or occupational), teachers, developmental experts, and other professionals as the case may be. This evidence may help persuade a school district that it would not be appropriate to deny your child the requested placement. Other suggestions to help parents through the IEP process are:

1. Do not attend IEP meetings alone—you may bring a spouse, physicians, teachers, advocates, and others for support;
2. Keep close track of what everyone involved in your child's case is doing;
3. *Get everything in writing;* and
4. Be assertive. Children with unique developmental challenges need parents to be assertive and persuasive advocates during the IEP process. This does not mean that school officials are always adversaries. It does mean, however, that you are your child's most important advocate; you know her best.

"Individualized Family Service Plan." Parents of children from birth to age two use a plan that is different from the IEP used for older children. Under recent amendments to the EAHCA, states receiving grants to provide early intervention services must draft an "individualized family service plan" (IFSP). These plans are similar to the IEP, but reflect this new law's different focus. Unlike Public Law 94–142, which focuses on the needs of the child, Public Law 99–457 emphasizes services for the family as a whole. The law recognizes that families with children with special needs often need services. For example, IFSPs state what services are provided for: 1) parents learning how to handle and teach their child with cerebral palsy; 2) siblings learning to cope with having a brother or sister with cerebral palsy; and 3) the child with cerebral palsy herself. If your state qualifies for early intervention grants under Public Law 99–457, you will be working with an IFSP. The procedures and strategies for developing a useful IFSP are the same as described above for the IEP.

Resolution of Disputes under Public Law 94–142

It is usually best to resolve disputes with your school district over your child's educational program *during* the IEP (or IFSP) process, before hard positions have been formed. Although Public Law 94–142 establishes dispute resolution procedures that are designed to be fair to parents, it is easier and far less costly to avoid disputes by reaching agreement during the IEP process. Accordingly, you should first try to accomplish your objectives by persuasion. If there is a dispute that simply cannot be resolved with the school district, however, this section discusses how you may use Public Law 94–142 and other laws to resolve that dispute.

Public Law 94–142 establishes a variety of safeguards to protect the rights of children with disabilities and their parents. For instance, written notice is always required before any change is made in your child's identification, evaluation, or educational placement. In addition, parents are entitled to review all of their child's educational records at any time. Further, your school district is prohibited from deceiving you and from making decisions without consulting or notifying you. School officials must state in writing what they plan to do with your child, how, where, when, and why.

Beyond the requirement of prior written notice, the EAHCA allows parents to file a formal complaint locally about *any matter* "relating to the identification, evaluation, or educational placement of the child, or the provision of free appropriate public education to such child." This means that you can make a written complaint about virtually any problem you have with any part of your child's educational (or early intervention) program if you have been unable to resolve that problem with school officials. This is a very broad right of appeal, one that parents have successfully used in the past to correct problems in their children's educational programs.

The process of challenging a school district's decisions about your child's education can be started simply by sending a letter of complaint. This letter, which should explain the nature of the dispute and your desired outcome, typically is sent to the special education office of the school district. For information about starting appeals, you can contact your school district, local advocacy groups, or other parents.

The first step in the appeal process is usually an "impartial due process hearing" before a hearing examiner. This hearing, usually held on the local level, is the parents' first opportunity to explain their complaint before an impartial person who is required to listen to both sides, and then to render a decision. At the hearing, parents are entitled to be represented by an attorney or lay advocate; they can present evidence; and they can examine, cross-examine, and compel the attendance of witnesses. The child has a right to be present at the hearing as well. After the hearing, parents have a right to receive a written record of the hearing and the hearing examiner's findings and conclusions.

Just as with the IEP process, parents must present facts at these due process hearings that show that the school district's decisions about their child's educational program are wrong. To overturn the school district's decision, parents must show that the disputed placement or program does not provide their child with the "free appropriate public education" in "the least restrictive environment" that is required by the EAHCA. Evidence in the form of letters, testimony, and expert evaluations is usually essential to a successful appeal.

Parents or school districts may appeal the decision of a hearing examiner. The appeal usually goes to the state's educational agency. This state agency is required to make an independent decision upon its review of the record of the due process hearing and of any additional evidence presented. The state agency then issues its own decision.

The right to appeal does not stop there. Parents or school officials can appeal beyond the state level by bringing a lawsuit under the EAHCA and other laws in a state or federal court. In this kind of legal action, the court must determine whether there is a preponderance of the evidence (that is, whether it is more likely than not) that the school district's placement is proper for that child. In reaching its decision, the court must give weight to the expertise of the school officials responsible for providing the child's education, but parents can and should also present their own expert evidence.

During all administrative and judicial proceedings, Public Law 94–142 requires that your child remain in her current educational placement, unless you and the local or state agencies agree to a move. Parents who place their child in a different program without agreement risk having to bear the full cost of that program. If, however, the school district is found to have erred, it may be required to reimburse parents for the expenses of the changed placement. Accordingly, you should make a change of program only after carefully considering the potential cost of that decision.

As with any legal dispute, each phase—complaint, hearings, appeals, and court cases—can be expensive, time-consuming, and emotionally draining. As mentioned earlier, it is wise for you to try to resolve problems without filing a formal complaint or bringing suit. For example, you should consult with other parents who have filed complaints and talk to sympathetic school officials. When informal means fail to resolve a problem, however, formal channels should be pursued. Your child's best interests must come first. The EAHCA grants important rights that parents should not be bashful about exercising.

Regarding expenses, parents who ultimately win their dispute with a school district may recover attorneys' fees. Courts have the discretion to award attorneys' fees to prevailing parents. Even if you prevail at the local or state level (without bringing a lawsuit), you likely are entitled to recover attorneys' fees, although this issue is currently under consideration in the federal courts. A word of caution: A court can limit or refuse attorneys' fees if you reject an offer of settlement from the school district, and then do not obtain a better outcome.

The EAHCA is a powerful tool in the hands of parents. It can be used to provide unparalleled educational opportunities to children with cerebral palsy. Using it effectively, however, requires an understanding of how it works. The Reading List at the end of this book includes several good guidebooks to Public Law 94–142 and the special education system. With knowledge of this vital law, you will be able to help your child realize her potential.

Programs and Services
When Your Child Is an Adult

Many children with cerebral palsy grow to live independently as adults. Some, however, will have varying needs for special services depending on how cerebral palsy affects them. These services can be provided through employment and residential or community-based programs. Currently, there are strong local and national movements toward noninstitutional community-based services, practical job training, and supported employment programs. Regrettably, if these kinds of programs are unavailable or filled to capacity, parents are left to provide the necessary support and supervision on their own for as long as possible.

Programs vary from state to state and from community to community. In this age of tight state and federal budgets, these programs typically have long waiting lists and generally are underfunded. After your child reaches age eighteen, her right to a public education may end in many states, even though her needs may continue. Presently, the sad truth is that under Public Law 94–142 thousands of children receive education and training that equip them to live as independently and productively as possible, only to be sent home when they finish schooling with nowhere to go and nothing to do.

Now is the time to work to change this sad reality. The unemployment rate for people with cerebral palsy is appallingly high, especially for young adults. As waiting lists for training programs grow, your child may be deprived of needed services, and, consequently, of appropriate employment opportunities. Programs sponsored by charities and private foundations are limited and most families do not have the resources to pay the full cost of providing employment and residential opportunities. The only other remedy is public funding. Just as parents banded together in the 1970s to demand enactment of the Public Law 94–142, parents must band together now to persuade local, state, and federal officials to take the steps necessary to allow people with disabilities to live in dignity.

Parents of *children* with disabilities should not leave this job to parents of *adults* with disabilities, for children become adults—all too soon. Chapter 10 explains how to become an advocate for your child and for the rights of people with cerebral palsy.

Under a federal law, called the Developmentally Disabled Assistance and Bill of Rights Act, states can receive grants for a variety of programs. Important among them is a protection and advocacy (P&A) system. A P&A system helps protect and advocate for the civil and legal rights of people with developmental disabilities. Because people who are disabled by cerebral palsy may not be in a position to protect their own rights or speak out for themselves, it is important that each state's P&A system offer adequate protection. Consult the Resource Guide at the back of this book for the location of your state's P&A office.

Vocational Training Programs

There is one educational program supported by federal funding that may be available to adults with cerebral palsy. Operating much like Public Law 94–142, several federal laws make funds available to support vocational training and rehabilitation programs for people with disabilities who qualify. Again, as with the EAHCA, states that desire federal funds must submit plans for approval. Federal law provides eligibility for persons who have a physical or mental disability that constitutes a "substantial handicap to employment" and who can be expected to benefit from vocational services. Unlike the EAHCA, however, these laws do not grant people with disabilities enforceable rights and procedures.

In the past, a person whose cerebral palsy was severely disabling was excluded from receiving vocational training services because she likely could not achieve the law's goal of competitive full-time or part-time employment. Recent amendments to the law, however, require services and training to people with severe disabilities even if the most they will achieve is "supported employment." This term means employment in a setting with services such as a job coach or special training which allows an individual to perform work. Now, people with particularly disabling cerebral palsy should no longer be deprived of job training and services just because of their condition.

The state Departments of Vocational Rehabilitation, sometimes called "DVR" or "Voc Rehab," are charged with carrying out these laws. People who apply for Voc Rehab services are evaluated, and an "Individualized Written Rehabilitation Plan" (IWRP) or an "Individualized Habilitation Plan" (IHP), similar to an IEP, is developed. The IHP sets forth the services needed to enable a person with a disability to work productively. Under these programs, adults with cerebral palsy can continue to receive vocational education after they reach age twenty-one. You should contact your state vocational rehabilitation department, the UCP, or local UCP affiliate for specific information on services available to your child. Despite shrinking federal and state budgets, some states and communities offer their own programs, such as group homes, supported employment programs, and life-skills classes. Other parents and organizations will have information about programs available in your area.

Living and Working in the Community

New trends are emerging in the effort to enable people with cerebral palsy to live independently and productively. The focus of these efforts is to help people with cerebral palsy overcome the physical limitations that in the past too often meant lives spent in institutions. One important trend is to provide "personal assistance services" to people with disabilities who need help with daily care and mobility to live in the community. For example, in some programs, a personal assistant can help with cooking meals, cleaning house, and grooming so that a person with cerebral palsy can live independently. In designing an IHP or a residential plan, be sure to ask that personal assistance services be included if they are needed. Because this trend is new, however, availability and funding is spotty. In addition, as discussed below, the extent to which Medicaid will help fund these services varies from state to state and currently is the subject of litigation.

Another current trend is the movement away from caring for people with severe cerebral palsy in large public and private facilities, called "intermediate care facilities" (ICF). Instead, the trend is to provide funding and services for independent living within their community. Under the current law, funding is provided in a way that encourages or even requires care for people in ICFs, despite the experience of many families that shows that even people with severe disabilities lead happier, healthier, and more productive lives in the community. Programs in your state for adults with cerebral palsy *should* provide for a variety of community living and working arrangements. But because this is a relatively new concept, community-based living and working arrangements may not exist in all areas. As discussed below, Medicaid plays a critical role in fostering these types of arrangements. Chapter 10 explains how parents can work to change laws so that these needed services become more available.

Anti-Discrimination Laws

As children with cerebral palsy enter the adult world, protecting their rights to employment and equal opportunity becomes of utmost importance. In 1990, "The Americans with Disabilities Act" (ADA) was enacted to protect people with disabilities from discrimination in employment, public accommodations, transportation, telecommunications, and other areas. This section reviews the highlights of this law and the Rehabilitation Act of 1973, both of which prohibit discrimination against your child with cerebral palsy.

The Americans with Disabilities Act of 1990

The Americans with Disabilities Act (ADA) prohibits discrimination against people with disabilities, including people with cerebral palsy. The law applies to most private employers, public and private services, public accommodations, and telecommunications. Here is what the law provides:

Employment. The ADA states that "no... [employer] shall discriminate against a qualified individual with a disability because of the disability of such individual in regard to job application procedures, the hiring or discharge of employees, employee compensation, advancement, job training, and other terms, conditions, and privileges of employment." This means that private employers cannot discriminate against employees or prospective employees who have a disability. The law defines "qualified individual with a disability" as a person with a disability who, with or without reasonable accommodation, can perform the essential functions of a job. "Reasonable accommodation" means that employers must make an effort to remove obstacles from the job, the terms and conditions of employment, or the workplace that would prevent an otherwise qualified person from working because they have a disability. This can include modifying facilities or equipment to make them accessible, restructuring the job, shuffling schedules, adapting training and policies, and providing readers or interpreters if necessary. Failing to make reasonable accommodations is itself a violation of this law. The law, however, does not *require* employers to hire people with disabilities if doing so imposes an "undue hardship" on the employer. Rather it prohibits employers from refusing to work with people with disabilities simply because of the disability.

Public Services. This part of the ADA prohibits discrimination against people with disabilities by state and local public agencies that provide such services as transportation. It is a violation of the ADA for agencies to purchase buses, rail cars, or other transportation equipment that are not accessible to people with disabilities. Likewise, all architectural barriers in state and local government buildings and facilities must be removed to "the maximum extent feasible," and new buildings and facilities must be constructed without them. The result of this part of the ADA will be to make all public transportation accessible to people with disabilities. And to a person with cerebral palsy this can mean freedom and mobility they never before imagined possible. The ADA also requires that private companies providing transportation services make their buses, trains, or rail cars accessible.

Public Accommodations. One of the most stunning provisions of the ADA is its prohibition of discrimination in public accommodations. Mirroring the approach of the civil rights laws of the 1960s, the ADA bans discrimination against people with disabilities virtually *everywhere*, including: hotels, inns, and motels; restaurants and bars; theaters, stadiums, concert halls, auditoriums, convention centers, and lecture halls; bakeries, grocery stores, gas stations, clothing stores, pharmacies, and other retail businesses; doctor or lawyer offices; airport and bus terminals; museums, libraries, galleries, parks, and zoos; nursery, elementary, secondary, undergraduate, and postgraduate schools; day care centers; homeless shelters; senior citizen centers; gymnasiums; spas; and bowling alleys. The list is practically endless: any place open to the public must be made available to people with disabilities, unless it is not physically or financially feasible to do so. Businesses must make reasonable accommodations and physical alterations to make their places of business accessible to people with disabilities.

The great promise of ADA lies in its provisions that define the failure to make reasonable accommodation as discrimination. For example, if a business refuses to make a doorway accessible to someone in a wheelchair, and it would not impose unreasonable cost on the business to do so, the business can be found to be in violation of the ADA. The end result is that the new law is not simply neutral; it does not merely prohibit active discrimination, but imposes duties to open our society to all people with disabilities.

The ADA has the potential to provide unparalleled freedom and opportunity to people with cerebral palsy. By prohibiting discrimination and requiring reasonable accommodation, the ADA stands as the Bill of Rights for people with disabilities, including people with cerebral palsy.

The Rehabilitation Act of 1973

Before the ADA was enacted, discrimination on the basis of disability was prohibited only in certain areas. Section 504 of the Rehabilitation Act of 1973 continues to prohibit discrimination against qualified people with disabilities in *federally funded programs*. The law provides that "No otherwise qualified individual with handicaps in the United States...shall, solely by reason of his handicap, be excluded from the participation in, be denied the benefits of, or be subjected to discrimination under any program or activity receiving federal financial assistance...."

An "individual with handicaps" is any person who has a physical or mental impairment that substantially limits one or more of that person's "major life activities," which consist of "caring for one's self, performing manual tasks, walking, seeing, hearing, speaking, breathing, learning, and working." The United States Supreme Court has determined that an "otherwise qualified" handicapped individual is one who is "able to meet all of a program's requirements in spite of his handicap." Programs or activities that receive federal funds are required to make reasonable accommodation to permit the participation of people with these kinds of handicaps.

Insurance

For many families with a child with cerebral palsy, finding and keeping insurance that covers their child can be a serious problem. Unfortunately, most insurance companies do not offer health or life insurance at a fair price, or sometimes at any price, to people with cerebral palsy. This is a result of the belief that children and adults with cerebral palsy are likely to submit more insurance claims than others.

About half the states outlaw handicap-based discrimination by prohibiting insurance companies from using a condition such as cerebral palsy as an excuse to deny coverage. The drawback to these laws, however, is that they allow insurance companies to deny coverage if the denial is based on "sound actuarial principles" or "reasonable anticipated experience." Insurers rely on these large loopholes to deny coverage, claiming that people with cerebral palsy are prone to submit more claims. In short, the laws are ineffective in protecting families from insurance discrimination. Even the ADA does not prohibit these same "sound actuary" practices that frequently result in denied coverage.

A few states have begun to lessen the health insurance burdens on families with children with disabilities. Some states offer "shared risk" insurance plans. Under these plans, insurance coverage is offered to people who could not get coverage otherwise. The added cost is shared among all insurance companies (including HMOs) operating in the state. To be eligible, a person must show that she has been recently turned down for coverage or offered a policy with limited coverage. The cost of this insurance is usually higher and

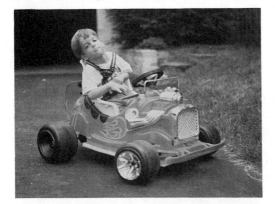

the benefits may be limited, but it is usually better than no health insurance at all. Some laws also cover people who have received premium increases of fifty percent. Check with your state insurance commission, the UCP, or your local

UCP affiliate for information about health insurance programs in your area.

Driver's License

People with cerebral palsy have the same right as everyone else to obtain a driver's license. If they can pass the written test (given verbally if the person is unable to write) and the driving test, people with cerebral palsy can and do obtain licenses. No state is entitled to deny a person with cerebral palsy the opportunity to obtain a driver's license simply because of the condition. A state may, however, require that a driver's vehicle be equipped with manual controls or adaptations such as wheelchair lifts and special pedals. The rules are different for people who have seizures; states can deny a driver's license to a person who has seizures because of the risk posed if she has one while driving.

Planning for Your Child's Future

Although many children with cerebral palsy grow into independent adults, cerebral palsy is a serious lifelong disability for many others. This section of the book is for the parents of children who may need publicly funded services or assistance, or management of funds when they are adults.

The possibility that your child may be dependent all of her life can be overwhelming. To properly plan for your child's future, you need information in areas you may never have thought about before, and you must find inner resources you may not believe exist. In most families, parents remain primarily responsible for ensuring their child's well-being. Consequently, questions that deeply trouble parents include: "What will happen to my child when I die? Who will look after her? How will her financial needs be met? Who will provide the services she will need?"

Some parents of children with cerebral palsy delay dealing with these issues, coping instead with the immediate demands of the present. Others begin to address the future when their child is quite young. They add to their insurance, begin (alone or with grandparents) to set aside funds for their child, and share with family and friends their concerns about their child's future needs.

Whatever the course, parents of children with cerebral palsy need to understand in advance some serious problems that affect planning for the future. Failure to avoid these pitfalls can have dire future consequences for your child and for other family members.

There are three important issues that families of children with cerebral palsy need to consider in planning for the future. These are:

1. the potential for cost-of-care liability;
2. the complex rules governing government benefits; and
3. the child's ability to handle her own affairs.

Of course, there are many other matters that may be different for parents of children with cerebral palsy. For example, insurance needs may be affected, and the important choice of trustees and guardians is more difficult. But these types of concerns face most parents in one form or another. Cost-of-care liability, government benefits, and the inability to manage one's own affairs, however, present issues that are unique to parents of children with serious disabilities.

Cost-of-Care Liability

Some people with cerebral palsy reside in state-run facilities. When a state provides residential services to a person with disabilities, it usually requires her to pay for them if she has the funds to do so. Called "cost-of-care liability," this requirement allows states to tap the funds of the person with disabilities herself to pay for the services the state provides. States can reach funds owned outright by a person with disabilities and even funds set aside in some trusts. A few states go farther. Some impose liability on parents for the care of an adult with disabilities; some impose liability for other services in addition to residential care. This is an area parents need to look into early and carefully.

Parents should understand that payments required to be made to satisfy cost-of-care liability do *not* benefit the person with disabilities. Ordinarily they add nothing to the care and services the individual receives. Instead, the money is added to the general funds of the state to pay for roads, schools, public officials' salaries, and so on.

It is natural for parents to want to pass their material resources on to their children by will or gift. The unfortunate effect of allowing a child with seriously disabling cerebral palsy to inherit a portion of your estate, however, may be the same as naming the state in your will—something most people would not do voluntarily, any more than they would voluntarily pay more taxes than the law requires. Similarly, setting aside funds in your child's name, in a support trust, or in a Uniform Gifts to Minors Act (UGMA) account may be the same as giving money to the state—money that could better be used to meet the future needs of your child.

What, then, can parents do? The answer depends on circumstances and the law of your state. Here are three basic strategies parents can use:

First, strange as it may seem, in some cases the best solution may be to disinherit your child with cerebral palsy, leaving funds instead to siblings in the hope that they will use these funds for their sibling's benefit, even though they will be under *no* legal obligation to do so. The absence of a legal obligation is crucial. It protects the funds from cost-of-care claims. The state will simply have no basis for claiming that the person with disabilities owns the funds. This strategy, however, runs the risk that the funds will not be used for your child with cerebral palsy if the siblings: 1) choose not to use them that way; 2) suffer financial reversals or domestic problems of their own, exposing the funds to creditors or spouses; or 3) die without making arrangements that safeguard the funds.

A preferable method, in states where the law is favorable, is to leave funds intended for the benefit of your child with cerebral palsy in what is called a "discretionary" trust. This kind of trust is created to supplement, rather than replace, state benefits. The trustee of such a trust (the person in charge of the trust assets) has the power to use or not use the trust funds for any particular purpose as long as it benefits the beneficiary—the child with cerebral palsy. In many states, these discretionary trusts are not subject to cost-of-care claims because the trust does not impose any *legal* obligation on the trustee to spend funds for care and support. In contrast, "support" trusts *require* the trustee to use the funds for the care and support of the child and can be subjected to state cost-of-care claims. Discretionary trusts can be created under your will or during your lifetime; as with all legal documents, the trust documents must be carefully written. In some states, to protect the trust against cost-of-care claims, it is necessary to add provisions stating clearly that the trust is to be used to supplement rather than replace publicly funded services and benefits.

A third method to avoid cost-of-care claims is to create a trust, either under your will or during your lifetime, that describes the kind of allowable expenditures to be made for your child with cerebral palsy in a way that excludes care in state-funded programs. Like discretionary trusts, these trusts—sometimes called "luxury" trusts—are intended to supplement, rather than take the place of, state benefits. The state cannot reach these funds because the trust forbids spending any funds on care in state institutions.

In using these estate planning techniques, parents should consult a qualified attorney who is experienced in estate planning for parents of children with disabilities. Because each state's laws differ and because each family has unique circumstances, individualized estate planning is essential.

Government Benefits

There are a wide variety of federal, state, and local programs for people with disabilities. Each of these programs provides different services and each has its own complex eligibility requirements. What parents and grandparents do now to provide financially for their child with cerebral palsy can have important effects on that child's eligibility for government assistance in the future. In addition, the complex rules governing some programs—such as Medicaid—can have far-reaching effects on your child's life.

SSI and SSDI

There are two federally funded income maintenance programs that can provide additional income to people with cerebral palsy: "Supplemental Security Income" (SSI), a public assistance program, and "Social Security Disability Insurance" (SSDI), a disability insurance program. Both are designed to provide a monthly income to qualified people with disabilities.

To qualify as "disabled" for either of these programs, the applicant's cerebral palsy must be so disabling that she cannot engage in "substantial gainful activity." This means that she cannot perform any job, whether or not a suitable job can be found. The

Social Security Administration regulations prescribe a set of tests for making this determination. The test of severity is somewhat different for children and adults. A child with cerebral palsy meets the test of severity if she meets these criteria:

1. She has a severe motor dysfunction (that is, motor disorganization or deficit that interferes with "age-appropriate major daily activities" and disrupts "fine or gross movements" or "gait and station"); or
2. She has a less severe motor dysfunction with:
   a. IQ of 69 or less; or
   b. Seizure disorder (with one major seizure in the year before application); or
   c. Significant interference with communication; or
   d. Significant emotional disorder.

Children with cerebral palsy who also have mental retardation may qualify as disabled if they meet the criteria for that condition.

The eligibility requirements do not end with the above list. Eligibility for SSI is based on financial need, and thus an applicant's resources and other income can disqualify her from receiving SSI. On the other hand, eligibility for SSDI is not based on financial need. It is based on the applicant's own work record prior to disability or on a retired or deceased parent's Social Security coverage in the case of someone disabled before age eighteen. What your child owns in her own name and what income she is entitled to receive under a trust can prevent her from receiving SSI benefits, but not SSDI benefits. Disabled children of deceased federal employees and military personnel may also be entitled to monthly survivor's benefits under the retirement systems for these people.

Many people with cerebral palsy work. In fact, for most parents, finding a job for their child with cerebral palsy is a goal they strive hard to achieve. It is an unfortunate irony, then, that earning a salary can affect eligibility for SSI and SSDI. Under the complex rules governing SSI benefits, earning income can reduce your child's benefits or disqualify her altogether. This is because, as presently administered, SSI is intended to provide income to people whose disabilities prevent them from working. This rule is unfair to people with cerebral palsy who are able to perform some work because it can force a choice between work in the community at reduced pay and needed SSI benefits. People receiving SSI, however, *can*, under the statutory work incentive program, earn up to a certain amount (now $821 per month) and still keep *some* SSI benefits; the benefits will be reduced by the amount of excess income earned. Unfortunately, the work incentive program does not apply to people on SSDI, who lose eligibility if they earn more than a certain amount per month (now $500), because they are deemed not to be disabled. In addition, your child will be ineligible for SSI (but not SSDI) if she has assets in her own name greater than a prescribed level (now $2,000). It is, therefore, vital to properly plan your child's financial future to avoid jeopardizing her right to receive SSI benefits. You should check periodically with the Social Security Administration to determine the current rules that apply to your child.

Medicare and Medicaid

Medicare and Medicaid are also important to people with cerebral palsy, but each has its own eligibility requirements and rules for recipients. Medicaid provides medical assistance to people who are eligible for SSI and to other people with incomes that are insufficient to pay for medical care. Because eligibility is based on financial need, placing assets in the name of a child with cerebral palsy or providing that child with income through a trust can disqualify her. Medicare, however, is not based on financial need. Anyone entitled to receive benefits under Social Security is also entitled to Medicare coverage.

Community-Based Services and Personal Assistance Services. There are two important issues related to Medicaid that seriously affect the lives of people with cerebral palsy:

1. First, under current law, Medicaid will not pay for services for people with disabilities unless they are provided in large Medicaid-certified residential institutions, called "intermediate care facilities" (ICFs). This law is behind the times; most people with disabilities such as cerebral palsy are best served in the *community*, not in institutions. Nevertheless, families today continue to face the prospect of having to institutionalize their child in order for her to receive vital services. Currently, the Secretary of the federal Department of Health and Human Services has the authority to waive the

ICF requirement in a particular case, but nothing requires him to do so. There is legislation before Congress to either allow or require Medicaid to pay for community-based services. If enacted, this legislation will bring Medicaid into the present, and help people with disabilities live as full a community life as possible.

2. The second Medicaid issue affecting people with cerebral palsy involves personal assistance services. Because some people with cerebral palsy need ongoing help with their personal care, personal assistance services are essential to achieve an independent community life. Medicaid, however, does not now pay for personal assistance services. This rule unfairly limits the opportunities of people with cerebral palsy by denying them services—not unlike medical services—aimed at keeping them healthy and out of hospitals and institutions. People with cerebral palsy should not be deprived of the chance to live independently in their community just because they need help bathing, cooking, and grooming. Among the UCP and other organizations concerned with this issue, there is a movement to change this rule. Legislation will shortly be introduced to add personal assistance services to the list of optional Medicaid services or even to establish an entirely new program to provide these essential services directly. Funding personal assistance services will go far to enable people with cerebral palsy to receive the assistance they need to live as independently as possible.

It is important for parents to become familiar with the rules governing SSI, SSDI, Medicaid, and Medicare. It is even more important to avoid an unwitting mistake that could disqualify your child from receiving benefits. If your child may be disabled as an adult, it may not be wise to set aside funds in your child's own name, create a support trust, establish a custodial account under the Uniform Gifts to Minors Act UGMA (discussed below), or allow her to inherit outright under your will. Instead, you should consider following the type of strategies outlined in the section on Cost of

Care Liability. You will need competent professional assistance, of course, because these are quite technical matters.

Competence to Manage Financial Affairs

Even if your child with cerebral palsy may never need state-funded residential care or government benefits, she may need to have her financial affairs managed for her. Care must be exercised in deciding how to make assets available for your child. There are a wide variety of trusts that can allow someone else to control the ways in which money is spent after you die. Of course, the choice of the best arrangements depends on many different circumstances, such as your child's capacity to manage assets, her relationship with her siblings, your financial situation, and the availability of an appropriate trustee or financial manager. Each family is different. A knowledgeable lawyer can review the various alternatives and help you pick the one best suited to your family.

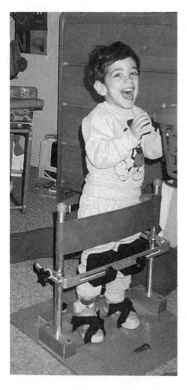

Need for Guardians

Parents frequently ask whether they should nominate themselves or others as guardians for a child with cerebral palsy if a guardian is necessary when the child becomes an adult. The appointment of a guardian costs money and may result in the curtailment of your child's civil rights—the right to marry, to have a checking account, to vote, and so on. Therefore, a guardian should be appointed only if and when needed. If one is not needed during your lifetime, it usually is sufficient to name guardians in your will.

A guardian will be needed if your child inherits or acquires property that she lacks the capacity to manage. Also, a guardian may be required if a medical or service provider refuses to serve your child without authorization by a guardian. Occasionally it is necessary to appoint a guardian to gain access to important records. Unless there is a specific need that can be solved by the appointment of a guardian, however, a guardianship should not be established simply because your child has a disability.

Life Insurance

Parents of children with disabling cerebral palsy should review their life insurance coverage. The most important use of life insurance is to meet financial needs that arise if the insured person dies. Many people who support dependents with their wages or salaries are underinsured. This problem is aggravated by wasting hard-earned dollars on insurance that does not provide the amount or kind of protection that could and should be purchased. It is therefore essential for any person with dependents to understand basic facts about insurance.

The first question to consider is: Who should be insured? Life insurance deals with the financial risks of death. The principal financial risk of death in most families is the danger that the death of the wage earner or earners will deprive dependents of their support. Therefore, life insurance coverage should be considered primarily for the parent or parents on whose earning power the children depend, rather than on the lives of children or dependents.

The second question is whether your insurance is adequate to meet the financial needs that will arise if you die. You should carefully evaluate whether your insurance coverage is adequate. To help you, *Life Insurance*, a book published in 1988 by Consumers Union, provides one useful step-by-step method of calculating the amount of insurance you need.

The next question is: What kind of insurance policy should you buy? Insurance policies are of two basic types: term insurance, which provides "pure" insurance without any significant build-up of cash value or reserves, and other types (called "whole life," "universal life," and "variable life"), which, in addition to providing insurance, include a savings or investment factor. The latter kinds of policies are really a combined package of insurance and investment. The different types of insurance are described in more detail in the Consumers Union book, *Life Insurance*. Whether you buy term insurance and maintain a separate savings and investment program, or whether you buy one of the other kinds of policies that combines them, you should make sure that the insurance part of your program is adequate to meet financial needs if you die. A sound financial plan will meet these needs and will satisfy savings and retirement objectives in a way that does not sacrifice adequate insurance coverage.

Finally, it is essential to coordinate your life insurance with the rest of your estate plan. This is done by designating the beneficiary—choosing who is to receive any insurance proceeds when you die. The beneficiary designation should be reviewed when you make your will. It is frequently desirable to designate a trustee in your will or in a separate revocable life insurance trust as the recipient of insurance proceeds that you intend to make available for the support of your child with cerebral palsy after you die.

Estate Planning for Parents of Children with Cerebral Palsy

More than most parents, the parents of a child with seriously disabling cerebral palsy need to attend to estate planning. Because of concerns about cost-of-care liability, government benefits, and competency, it is vital that you make plans. Parents need to name the people who will care for their child with cerebral palsy when they die. They need to review their insurance to be sure it is adequate to meet their child's special needs. They need to make sure their retirement plans will help meet their child's needs as an adult. They need to inform grandparents of cost-of-care liability, government benefits, and competency problems so that grandparents do not inadvertently waste resources that could otherwise benefit their grandchild's future. Most of all, they need to make a will so that their hopes and plans are realized and the disastrous consequences of dying without a will are avoided.

Proper estate planning differs for each family. Every will must be tailored to individual needs. There are no formula wills, especially for parents of a child with cerebral palsy. There are, however, some common mistakes to avoid. Here is a list:

No Will. If parents die without first making wills, the law generally requires that each child in the family share equally in the parents' estate. The result is that your child with cerebral palsy will inherit property in her own name. Her inheritance may become subject to cost-of-care claims and could jeopardize eligibility for government benefits. These and other problems can be avoided with a properly drafted will. Parents should never allow the state's laws to determine how their property will be divided upon their deaths. Planning can make you feel uneasy, but it is too important to ignore.

A Will Leaving Property Outright to the Child with Cerebral Palsy. Like having no will at all, a will that leaves property to a child with cerebral palsy in her own name may subject the inheritance to cost-of-care liability and may disqualify her from government benefits. Parents of children with cerebral palsy do not just need any will, they need a will that meets their special needs.

A Will Creating a Support Trust for the Child with Cerebral Palsy. A will that creates a support trust presents much the same problem as a will that leaves property outright to the child with cerebral palsy. The funds in these trusts may be subject to cost-of-care claims and jeopardize government benefits. A will should be drafted that avoids this problem.

Insurance and Retirement Plans Naming the Child with Cerebral Palsy as a Beneficiary. Many parents own life insurance policies that name a child with cerebral palsy as a beneficiary or contingent beneficiary, either alone or in common with siblings. The result is that funds may go outright to your child with cerebral palsy, creating cost-of-care liability and government benefits eligibility problems. Parents should designate the funds to pass either to someone else or to go into a properly drawn trust. The same is true of many retirement plan benefits.

Insurance on the Life of the Child with Cerebral Palsy. Some well-meaning parents and grandparents waste money insuring the life of their child with cerebral palsy. This money could be far better used to insure the *parents'* lives. The purpose of life insurance is to protect against the *financial* risks of the death of the insured. If a wage-earning parent dies, the family is deprived of his or her earnings. If a homemaker dies, it may be necessary to hire sitters or household help. In contrast, the death of a child does not have these consequences; typically it creates no financial risk that is appropriate for insurance. As a result, life insurance for your child with cerebral palsy helps no one except the insurance agent, unless your child may someday work, marry, and have children of her own.

Use of Joint Tenancy in Lieu of Wills. Spouses sometimes avoid making wills by placing all their property in joint tenancies with right of survivorship. In joint tenancies, property is owned equally by each spouse; when one spouse dies, the survivor automatically becomes the sole owner. Parents try to use joint tenancies instead of wills, relying on the surviving spouse to properly take care of all estate planning matters. This plan, however, fails completely if both parents die in the same disaster, if the surviving spouse becomes incapacitated, or if the surviving spouse neglects to make a proper will. The result is the same as if neither spouse made any will at all—the child with cerebral palsy shares equally in the parents' estates. As explained above, this may expose the assets to cost-of-care liability and give rise to problems with government benefits. Therefore, even when all property is held by spouses in joint tenancy, it is necessary that both spouses make wills.

Establishing UGMA Accounts for the Child with Cerebral Palsy. Over and over again well-meaning parents and grandparents of children with disabilities open bank accounts under the Uniform Gift to Minors Act (UGMA). When the child reaches age eighteen or twenty-one, the account becomes the property of the child, and may therefore be subject to cost-of-care liability. Perhaps more important, most people with disabilities first become eligible for SSI and Medicaid at age 18, but the UGMA funds will have to be spent before financial eligibility can be established. Parents should *never* set up UGMA accounts for their child with cerebral palsy, nor should they open other bank accounts in the child's name.

Failing to Advise Grandparents and Relatives of the Need for Special Arrangements. Just as the parents of a child with cerebral palsy need properly drafted wills or trusts, so do grandparents and other relatives who may leave (or give) property to the child. If these people are not aware of the special concerns—cost-of-care liability, government benefits, and competency—their plans may go awry and their generosity may be wasted. Make sure anyone planning gifts to your child with cerebral palsy understands what is at stake.

Children and adults with cerebral palsy are entitled to lead full and rewarding lives. Do not shortchange your child's future by failing to plan for it now.

Conclusion

Parenthood always brings responsibilities. But extra responsibilities confront parents of a child with cerebral palsy. Understanding the pitfalls for the future and planning to avoid them will help you to meet the special responsibilities. In addition, knowing and asserting your child's rights can help guarantee that she will receive the education and government benefits to which she is entitled. Being a good advocate for your child requires more than knowledge; you must also be determined to use that knowledge effectively, and, when necessary, forcefully.

Parent Statements

You always wonder whether what you're doing is ultimately going to hurt your child more than help. I don't believe any of the school officials are personally vindictive toward my daughter, but will she fall out of favor with them because of what her parents have chosen to do to assert their legal rights? Will there be retribution?

❧❦❧

They call it a due process hearing but there's really not much that amounts to due process because you have no access to their thinking, their records, anything; you just have access to your own child's records. That really isn't what you need to know sometimes. What you need to know is what is the entire policy for all children, not just yours.

❧❦❧

Public Law 94–142 says my child is entitled to an appropriate education. But who determines what appropriate is?

❧❦❧

I guess we've put off making a will because it's so complicated. You have to be careful that the money is accessible to your child—not the state, not anyone else.

❀❀

I worry about who will care for him. It's easy to just say, "Oh well, I'm sure his sisters will," but that's not fair. We have to really plan for his future now and stop putting it off.

❀❀

I'm not sure just where to start. Are there state services I could seek instead of going to a lawyer? I just don't know.

❀❀

I have found school officials pretty open-minded about Jeff. They seem to care about him. But there are budget limitations that lower the quality and quantity of the services they give him.

❀❀

Sometimes I think my son's rights are just words. When the school district says "appropriate" they mean just that. When I say "appropriate," I mean "best."

❀❀

You can follow all the rules, write a great IEP, and be assertive, but still get stuck with a lousy teacher. All your work goes down the drain, and your kid spends a useless year.

❀❀

My son's teacher is so talented that she does *more* than the IEP requires.

❀❀

I'm really looking forward to the changes the ADA will bring. As my daughter grows, I hope the law really does create the opportunities for her to work and live with dignity and purpose.

❈❈❈

Planning our will so that Jeff is provided for depresses me because it almost assumes he will be incapable of taking care of himself.

❈❈❈

I had to have a long, long talk with Linda's grandparents to make sure their desire to help does not go astray in the future.

❈❈❈

When our son was born, my wife and I had never even thought of making a will. It didn't take us long to realize how dangerous that could be. We called a lawyer who specializes in laws dealing with people with handicaps.

❈❈❈

I feel fortunate that Jeff was born in this era of services and caring for people with cerebral palsy. Services are so much better today than ever before.

❈❈❈

I don't know why we even bother buying health insurance. They won't cover our daughter and don't seem to care beyond their policies and their bottom line.

❈❈❈

I really wish the school program continued year-round. Jeff has mental retardation and really regresses over the summer. He needs the structure school provides. I hope these services come into existence soon. We haven't been able to convince the school to do this.

❈❈❈

Get a good lawyer and ask lots of questions.

TEN

Some Lessons Learned about Advocacy

BY FRAN SMITH*

Over thirty years ago when I learned that my daughter was "cerebral palsied," I was heartsick that she would never be like other girls. At first, I viewed Cheryl's condition as something that would require doctors and therapists to "fix" and I trusted almost anyone in a white coat. I quickly became determined to get the best services for my daughter and vowed that I would do whatever I must to be the best mother to her. Although I had never heard the word "advocacy," already I was committing myself to advocating for my child.

Today, most parents have at least heard of advocacy. Many associate the term with confrontation, and because they are uncomfortable with *that* word, assume that advocacy is not for them. But what advocacy actually means is speaking for or pleading for yourself or others. As parents, we naturally speak for our children. Any time a person or group of people makes a decision about your child, you will want to know about it and should have some say in the decision. I know this for a fact, because I have stood in your shoes.

After Cheryl was born, I became the mother of three other children, one—a son—also with cerebral palsy. Together, Cheryl and Michael taught me a lot about being a parent. And because they

* Fran Smith is the Director of Training and Volunteer Development for United Cerebral Palsy Association.

could not plead their own cases for more and better services, they also inspired me to learn how to advocate on their behalf—and eventually, on behalf of many children, adults, and families.

Through my advocacy work, I have learned that the welfare of children like yours depends on your family being as informed and as strong—as empowered—as it can be. I have often wished that when parents hear the diagnosis of cerebral palsy (or any disability), they could receive a "how-to" manual on everything they should know about the condition, the services their child will need and where to find them, all the laws pertaining to their child, and how to be an effective spokesperson for their child when services are not readily forthcoming. This book is a good start at preparing you to meet the challenges you will face throughout your child's life. Earlier chapters contain a wealth of background information about cerebral palsy, appropriate services, and legal rights and entitlements. This chapter should serve as an introduction to advocacy and provide some practical tips to help you get started speaking out for your child.

The Need for Advocacy

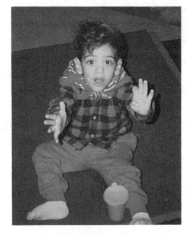

In the best of all situations, you will be told all about your child's cerebral palsy and the medical, therapeutic, and educational services he needs. You will also be told about support groups, parent training programs, and other family supports to help you care for your child. Everything your child needs will be available at the exact time he needs it, and you will be accepted as an equal partner in the planning process for his programs. All the services needed will be adequately funded, and all the professionals who provide them will share your values and love your child and appreciate his uniqueness as you do. You will never have to speak out except to say "Thank you."

In real life, this is rarely the case. To understand why, it helps to know how services for children with cerebral palsy and other disabilities have developed over the past few decades.

Prior to the 1950s, parents either accepted professional advice to place their child with a disability in an institution, or they kept their youngster at home, in many cases hidden from friends and relatives. The Community Services System was started by parents who spurned these customary alternatives. These parents refused to accept that their child was unable to benefit from education, job training, or other services. They banded together, raised money, rented space, and acted as teachers or hired teachers to provide some services. From this grassroots beginning—by parents who believed in their sons and daughters—special education, early intervention, adult developmental services, community living arrangements, and the concepts of increased independence, productivity, and community integration have grown.

Over the years, theory, law, and practice tumbled over each other in the evolution of services—with different results in different parts of the country. In some areas today, we still have services based on the antiquated notion that only some people with disabilities can learn and that the others should be protected from harm in sheltered environments such as special schools, sheltered workshops, and institutions. In other areas, we have services based on the belief that we should respect the dignity and worth of each individual with a disability and give everyone the best possible chance to learn and grow with non-handicapped peers. We have second and third generation federal laws that are ahead of local practice in some places. For example, even though the federal Developmental Disabilities Services Act calls for children and adults to receive services that increase their independence, productivity, and community integration, adult services are nonexistent in many areas. We have *many* medical professionals, educators, therapists, state agency personnel, and local service providers who were trained in earlier decades under old values and laws, and are now encountering parents with different expectations. And we have a declining economy with not enough money for everything currently "on the books" (in law). Worse, the local school board members, county supervisors, state legislators, and congressmen who must decide how to spend these limited funds often lack information about the most promising practices for children, adolescents, and adults with disabilities. Given this patchwork of services, professional attitudes, laws, and funding, you *will* need to speak up on behalf of your child.

Most often when you speak up for your child, you will do so as a parent-advocate—that is, to request a specific service or decision that will benefit your child alone. For example, because you know that children learn a great deal by playing with other children, you might want your child to attend a neighborhood day care center three days a week with physical therapy provided at the day care center. But the administrator of the early intervention program in your area may disagree with you. She may be motivated by the convenience of administering a centralized program and the inconvenience of sending a therapist to the center to serve one child. You could run into a similar conflict in developing your child's IEP, or in planning where he should receive educational services. If you voice your concerns about any aspect of your child's services, you are advocating.

Your advocacy efforts will be guided by the knowledge that you have valuable information about your child that no one else has and that you must share your knowledge to ensure your child's needs are satisfied the best way possible. Remember, you will be the constant in your child's life. Doctors, nurses, therapists, teachers, and other professionals will come and go, but you will be there for a lifetime. You must be ready to participate as an equal partner whenever a decision about your child's future is to be made.

Occasionally, you may find that before your child can receive a particular benefit or right, the system as a whole must be changed so that *all* children are entitled to that right or benefit. System reform requires the coordinated efforts of many individuals. As you talk to other parents, you will learn which ones are willing to work together.

In the past, parent-advocates have played important roles in fighting for and winning universal rights. For example, Public Law 94–142, the federal law that guarantees your child the right to a free, appropriate public education, was adopted in large part because thousands of parents spoke up about their children's right to attend public school. Amendments to the law extending special educational benefits to younger children were also passed at the urging of legions of parent-advocates. Today, further advocacy to enforce and strengthen these provisions is needed. For example, even though Public Law 94–142 has been on the books since 1975, school personnel all too often pay little or no attention to parents' input when making IEP or placement decisions.

It is up to you to decide whether to confine your advocacy to securing the best possible services for your child or to also advocate on behalf of all children with cerebral palsy. But in either case, you will find that the reward—a healthier, happier life for your child— makes your efforts all worthwhile.

Getting Started

Whether you realize it or not, you probably already have some of the basic tools needed to be a successful advocate for your child. No matter how young your child is, you likely have gotten at least some on-the-job training in advocacy. For example, if you spoke up about your concerns about the way your child was developing, you may have gotten your child's cerebral palsy diagnosed sooner than it would have been otherwise. Or if you told the speech-language pathologist that your child needed to increase his vocabulary, she may have added new words to his language board. In fact, the keys to successful advocacy are the same three keys essential to any endeavor: commitment, knowledge, and skill. The sections below explain how to develop each of these vital ingredients.

Commitment

You are the lifelong advocate for your son or daughter. You will always want the very best services for your child. An agency's budget, a staff vacancy, or transportation problems are not your primary concern. It is not your problem if your child's teacher is overworked or if twenty other children need the same services you are requesting for your child. When administrators try to get you to see things their way, you will probably be able to sympathize with them. But your particular and unique role as a parent is to put the interests of your child *first*. Your love for your child and your belief that he deserves the best will fuel this commitment and strengthen your sense of urgency.

Knowledge

Before you can begin advocating for your child, you must know what you are working for. Knowledge about the services your child needs and which services are most appropriate will define your goal. Knowledge about your child's legal rights will strengthen your position in pursuing that goal. And knowledge about where to find services and who has the authority to grant them will tell you where to begin your advocacy efforts.

In my experience, gathering all these different types of knowledge is not the hardest part; figuring out where to find them is. Here are some guidelines to help you get your hands on the information you need:

Appropriate Services for Your Child. Whenever you attempt to obtain appropriate services for your child, consider yourself a consumer. It is critical that you become as informed as you would when purchasing a car or a home. Don't accept the advice of someone who would be providing the service without first talking with other parents, professionals, or advocates. Ask yourself and the potential service provider (therapist, agency, teacher) how their recommendations would benefit your child and your family. You will certainly want to get answers to questions such as: What services does my child need to prepare him to be as independent as possible? How often should he receive these services? What can I do at home to be sure that his routines are consistent with what he does with his teachers and therapists? Are there any other programs or services that we can learn about? What makes one approach better than another? If you gather information from a variety of sources, you will become better informed and will make better decisions. Weigh the benefits described and make your decision based on what sounds best for your child.

Legal Rights. Knowing your child's legal rights will help you determine the course your advocacy should take. Your approach will be very different if you know your child is entitled to a service than if you think you have to depend on the goodwill of someone to "give" you the service. When you know the law is on your side, you do not need to be unduly concerned about how much the service provider likes you or feels that you and your child are worthy. But if you are attempting to obtain a service that is not mandated, you may need to be more diplomatic and obtain support from other parents and professionals. Often, professionals not connected with the agency will want to help your child receive the best services and will help you advocate. When none of these tactics work, the solution may be to change the system. If so, you will need to form or join a group willing to commit to long-range goals of legislation or other kinds of reform.

Every individual with a disability enjoys the same constitutional rights and protection as every other citizen of the United States. Depending on their level of disability, children and adults with cerebral palsy may also be assured certain other rights under federal and state laws. Chapter 9 provides an overview of the most important rights for children with cerebral palsy—to education, to appropriate treatment, to Supplemental Security Income, and to participation in federally funded programs that might benefit them—as well as of the federal laws that guarantee these rights. You will want to familiarize yourself with your child's rights to ensure that he does not miss out on any benefits he is entitled to.

For more specific information about federal laws relating to disabilities, or for information about laws your state may have enacted, you can contact several federally funded agencies. These agencies are listed in the state-by-state listings in the Resource Guide. They include:

1. The Governor's Planning Council on Developmental Disabilities—an agency mandated to plan, coordinate, and advocate for services, and funding for services, for individuals with cerebral palsy and other developmental disabilities. The Planning Council in your state can give you information about locating services such as education, respite care, therapy, and parent or family support for your son or daughter, as well as state laws related to developmental disabilities.

2. The Protection and Advocacy (P&A) System—an agency which protects the rights of, and advocates for, people with developmental disabilities when necessary. Your state P&A office can provide information about the laws in your state and help you if your child has been denied an entitlement or has been discriminated against because of his cerebral palsy.

3. Parent Information and Training Center (PITC)—a program that provides parents with information about the nature of their child's disability, how to locate the appropriate services, and how to advocate on behalf of their child. Most states have a PITC; those that do not are Alaska, Hawaii, Idaho, Iowa, Missouri, Rhode Island, South Carolina, Tennessee, West Virginia, Wyoming, and the District of Columbia.

In addition to the agencies established by federal law, you can contact local and state voluntary agencies and parent groups such as the United Cerebral Palsy Association, the Association for Retarded Citizens, Parent-to-Parent, and Pilot Parents. Your telephone directory usually lists these agencies in the yellow pages under the heading "Social Agencies."

Locating Services. Every state legislature gives the authority for administering disability services to different agencies within that state. To find out which agency to approach for information about a particular service (medical, educational, respite, etc.), you can ask your state Developmental Disabilities Council, as listed in the Resource Guide. Then, when you call the agency, ask for the contact person for the service you want to know about. Every state organizes its services differently, and there is no consistency from state to state or even within the state for eligibility criteria or entry procedures. You will probably have to start at the beginning and turn

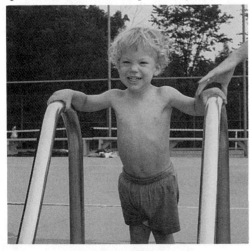

to other parents or advocates when you need help finding services.

Skills

Although you will generally be a stronger advocate the better informed you are, you do not have to wait until you have gathered all possible information about laws and resources before speaking out on behalf of your child. Especially if a service is being withheld or denied to your child, you may not have time to become better informed. For example, if your child has a tendency to develop contractures, yet physical therapy is not included in his early intervention program, you have no time to wait. Especially when your child is young, he cannot recoup the time and opportunities that are lost by waiting.

When time is of the essence, you may have to plunge right into advocacy, learning as you go. Start where you are and do what you need to do, and trust that you will pick up the knowledge and skills that you need. I know from experience how effective this off-the-cuff type of advocacy can be:

When my son was seven years old, he spent one semester in a residential school where the physical therapist rigged a special walker so he could propel himself. For the first time in his life, Michael was able to "walk," and his pride in this new-found independence was beyond measure. Then he returned to his regular special school. There the therapist he had always had very patiently told us why it was not possible for my son to be able to use a walker. For six months I kept asking her to give him a chance. Finally, Michael's orthopedist exploded at the therapist and ordered her to "do what Michael's mother asks. . . All she wants is what's good for her son." I learned two things that day: first, that support from an authority figure enhances anyone's self-esteem, and second, that speaking up for your child just because you feel it's the right thing to do, even when you're tired of hearing how unreasonable you are, can eventually get what you want.

Through the years I've met many parents who have their own stories to tell about how they've spoken up when their feelings compelled them. Love for your child and the knowledge that no one else will do it are the strongest motives.

If your need to advocate is less urgent, you can take the time to plot your strategy more systematically. Because advocacy must often be practiced in situations where you feel some risk if you don't do well, I recommend that you attend training sessions to learn some basic advocacy skills. Training in basic advocacy is offered by United Cerebral Palsy, Parent-to-Parent, and Parent Training and Information Centers. If you can't find any agency that provides training, ask your state Protection and Advocacy Office for help.

Regardless of how much time you have to prepare your case, your goal in advocating should be the same: to obtain a decision based on what is best for your child, not just to explain your position. In advocating for a new or better service for your child, you can use the basic approach that your child needs the service, the agency or organization is established to provide that service, and you don't understand why they are not doing what they should do.

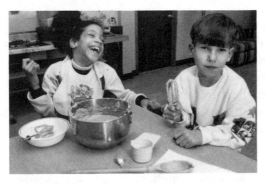

Bear in mind that every service funded with public dollars has, or should have, an appeals procedure for dissatisfied citizens to use. You can find out what this procedure is by asking your P&A office. Keep asking the person (or persons) with authority to make the decision until you get answers. Be persistent. Be assertive. Confrontation need not be hostile to get results. You should certainly never attack anybody on a personal or professional level. For example, don't imply that the special education teacher is incompetent because your child hasn't learned the alphabet yet, or that an administrator is unfeeling because he can't see that your child would learn better communication skills in a preschool with nonhandicapped children. If you maintain your position as asking for what's needed for your child, your motives will be clear and you should be treated fairly.

As important as persistence and diplomacy are in getting your way, there is also another key to effective advocacy: documentation. Your youngster will be seen by an army of professionals in many programs. You, as the parent, are the historian, the keeper of the records. You may be asked over and over again, "When did he first hold up his head?" "When did he first roll over? . . . sit alone?" "Can you tell me how many surgeries he has had and when?" The questions change over time, but you will always be ready with the answers if you keep pertinent information in a journal or notebook. I kept notes about all of the above, plus information on immunizations, illnesses, allergies, etc. I also learned to keep records of telephone calls, the name of the person I talked with, time and date, when the person promised to get back to me. And I collected a thick file of letters and reports from medical, educational, and other professionals. Remember, you never know when you'll need the information, and it's better to have too much than to eventually need something you didn't save.

Getting Help

You do not have to advocate by yourself. Often you will feel more comfortable and confident if a "seasoned" parent or trained advocate accompanies you in formal situations such as IEP planning meetings. That way, you can focus on the needs of your child and the advocate can make sure that the proper procedures are followed. Another approach is to ask the advocate to talk on your behalf because you might become so emotional that you forget what you wanted to say. Or you can ask the advocate just to be present to lend moral support and listen to what you say. Whenever someone accompanies you to a meeting, it's a good practice to discuss what each of you will do and say. Then if something unexpected happens during the meeting, you can cover for each other.

Besides the Parent Training Centers and Protection and Advocacy Agencies mentioned above, many of the parent organizations cited in this chapter can also help you. In addition, there are many types of professional and volunteer advocates who specialize in *case advocacy*—that is, in advocating on a one-on-one basis for a single individual, rather than for a group of individuals (*class advocacy*). They include citizen advocates, ombudsmen, legal advocates, case manager/advocates, and protective service workers. Table 1 provides information about what each of these types of advocates does and about what kinds of agencies you can find them in.

Even if you decide to advocate alone, you may want to ask someone close to you to help you get ready. Ask your spouse, a friend, or another parent to role play the situation so that you can practice presenting your case and answering questions and objections. If you can anticipate major objections far enough in advance, you will be able to gather information documenting your position and better prepare your responses. Remember, you must be absolutely clear on the basic points you want to make and the decision you must have *before* you meet with the person who has the power to grant or deny your request.

Table 1

Definitions of Case Advocacy

Types of Advocates	Purpose	Agency
Citizen Advocate	A capable volunteer who works to defend the rights and interests of a person with developmental disabilities, and provides practical and emotional support for him	Citizen Advocacy Board operated by a private association or agency such as an ARC chapter
Legal Advocate	Someone who represents another in the litigation or legal negotiations process concerning rights, grievances, or appeals	Usually not connected with an agency; usually in private practice as an attorney. May sometimes be associated with the legal services department of an organization or a P&A system
Case Manger/ Advocate ("Personal" Representative)	A trained professional or volunteer who helps an individual with information referral. Also serves as an advocate when there are problems obtaining services	Public or private agencies such as state departments of developmental disabilities, regional service agencies, Catholic Charities, family service agencies
Protective Service Worker	Someone who has authority to investigate alleged abuses, etc., and to initiate action, without the consent or request of a victim	Usually a public "protective" agency such as a state department for child protective services

(Adapted from a chart prepared by Marie L. Moore, National Advocacy Coordinator, United Cerebral Palsy, New York, NY, 1976, for use by states in developing Protection & Advocacy Systems.)

In short, when you are unable to obtain satisfaction with the basic approach to parent advocacy, seek help. Do not assume that you have failed, rather that the system—or someone within it—is unresponsive. The welfare of your child depends upon results, and you should use all possible sources of assistance.

An Introduction to Class Advocacy

If services for your child are not available, there will certainly be other parents seeking similar services. And if you are angry and upset because your child is denied an important right, other parents will surely share your outrage. You will want to do what parents before you have done, and join forces with others to create services and win new rights.

Again, there are many organizations that can help you and your fellow parents plead your case. These include UCP and ARC chapters, Independent Living Centers, and state Developmental Disability Planning Councils. But remember, a dedicated group of parent-advocates can also accomplish a great deal on its own. Provided you know how to phrase your message, when you talk, officials will certainly listen.

If you feel hesitant to approach a public figure about your child's problems, bear in mind that legislators depend on their constituents to keep them informed about issues. You, as a parent, have a role in keeping your elected officials informed about whatever affects your child and your family. They hear from paid lobbyists and other vested interests on hundreds of issues. But they simply can't keep up with all the issues that affect children with cerebral palsy and other disabilities unless they also hear from parents. For instance, today many parents of adults with severe cerebral palsy would like their children to live independently in the community rather than in an "Intermediate Care Facility" (ICF). But under present laws, funding often encourages or requires care in ICFs. Since this is a fairly esoteric issue, you can't assume that your legislator understands or is even aware of the need to change the laws.

The first time I ever "advocated" before a legislative committee in the California Assembly was a learning experience. I had no preparation, had never attended a training course on advocacy, and was not part of an organized group. I did, however, have an urgent need to speak up. The program that my daughter attended was going to close due to inadequate funding. A legislator had developed a bill to provide supplemental funding for this program and all others like it in the state. The senator was going to introduce the bill before the Ways and Means Committee and asked for a parent to testify on behalf of the young people with disabilities. Someone told me that no one else would testify, so I should. I spoke from the heart and talked about what would happen to this group of young people if the only program that they had were to close. When the senator and I were through speaking, a member of the Committee made a motion to pass the bill, and everyone voted "aye." Suddenly, I was a legislative advocate. The first time was the hardest. After that, I learned how a bill becomes a law, the best way to present testimony, and how to influence legislators.

There are many ways to acquaint your legislator with the issues that concern *you*. You can use a letter to introduce yourself and to discuss what is on your mind. You can make an appointment to visit your legislator either back home where you live, or in the city where his or her office is located. You can invite your legislator to attend a parent meeting in someone's home or at a program site. You can attend a town hall meeting—alone or with other parents—and speak your mind. You can talk with other parents and together

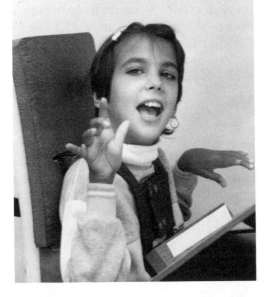

devise a strategy to approach your elected officials. Keep in mind that America has a representative form of government. In order for an elected official to represent you, he or she must hear from you.

Conclusion

Over the years, parents of children with disabilities have witnessed and experienced many changes in the services offered, the settings in which they are provided, and even the fundamental values underlying the services. We no longer accept the premise that our children with disabilities are a burden and will do best "with their own kind." We know they are precious, bringing joy and love not just to us but to everyone they meet. We know they will thrive in warm, nurturing environments, just as any other child will do, and that their families and their non-disabled peers *are* "their own kind."

When we insist on the best for our own child, we can turn for inspiration to the successes of thousands of children who have benefitted from appropriate services. We no longer need to rely on the "charity" approach to services, because we have many federal and state laws that declare it is good public policy to serve our children. And we no longer need feel that we are "just a parent" and that professionals know best what to do for and with our children. Parent involvement in developing service plans for their son or daughter, in designing and implementing services, and in monitoring services and the agencies providing services has demonstrated the critical role parents can play—and must play—in the lives of their children.

Your world holds both promise and challenge. Resolve to capture every possible opportunity for your child. You probably know your youngster better than anyone else does, and you certainly love him better. Trust that your knowledge and feelings will prepare you to begin advocating. You will learn as you go. Your child's future depends on the work of a few, or a lot, of advocates. Be one.

Parent Statements

I usually am an active advocate for my child, but sometimes I wonder if I should be spending more time with my kid and less time with the issues.

❊❊❊

I feel all parents should be trained in parent advocacy. They need to know what the laws and their rights are. They also need classes in assertiveness training if they aren't already assertive. It's very important to make these people listen and to get your point across where your child is concerned.

✵✵✵

If you don't know the laws or your rights, how do you know what is being done is the most that's possible? Just because a school tells you that's how it is, doesn't mean it's the truth.

✵✵✵

Parents of children with CP need so much training in so many areas. It's unbelievable how much we're supposed to know.

✵✵✵

I was really nervous the first time I disagreed with the school about my daughter's IEP. But they were really pretty open minded about the whole thing, and we were able to work out a compromise. Now I don't hesitate to speak up when I think something's not right.

✵✵✵

I was amazed when I wrote to my Senator and he—or at least, somebody in his office—actually wrote back. Now I'm waiting to see if anything comes of it.

✵✵✵

My husband and I have each developed our own advocacy roles. I basically do all the research into the issues and our son's rights, and then my husband handles the confrontation. Parents need to know what they are entitled to by law in order to demand it.

✵✵✵

The services must continue to improve. Technology is so advanced that more and more at-risk infants are surviving, but surviving with injuries—often brain damage. I think we are going to see the handicapped population increase in the next decade.

✵✵✵

It can be pretty overwhelming if you think about everything your child should be entitled to. I have to remind myself that I'm not a crusader, but just a concerned parent protecting his child's future.

❧❧❧

Keep looking and digging. The resources are out there.

❧❧❧

Glossary

Abduction—The outward movement of a limb away from the body.

Absence seizures. *See* Petit mal seizures.

Acuity—The ability to see clearly.

Adaptive behavior—The ability to adjust to new environments, tasks, objects, and people, and to apply new skills to those new situations.

Adaptive equipment—Equipment offering special support which is adapted to your child's special needs (corner chair, prone board, etc.).

Adduction—The inward movement of a limb towards the body.

Advocacy—The act of supporting or promoting a cause. Speaking out.

Advocacy groups—Organizations that work to protect the rights and opportunities of children with disabilities and their families.

AFO (Ankle foot orthoses)—A short leg brace worn inside the shoe which extends up to the calf. Made of lightweight plastic.

Agnosia. *See* Sensory impairments.

Akinetic seizure. *See* Atonic seizure.

Amblyopia (lazy eye)—Partial loss of sight due to suppression of central vision in the cortex when both eyes do not have the same acuity.

Ambulatory—Having the ability to walk.

Anticonvulsant—A drug used to control seizures. Even though all seizures are not convulsions, this term is commonly used.

Applied behavior analysis—A method of teaching designed to change behavior in a precisely measurable and accountable manner. Also called **behavior modification.**

ARD Committee (Admission, Review, and Dismissal Committee)—This committee is made up of teachers and other professionals. It is responsible for the admission of children to special education, review of the progress of children in special education programs, and dismissal of children from special education.

Articulation—Sound production.

Asphyxia—Lack of sufficient oxygen and circulation of the blood resulting in possible brain damage and a loss of consciousness.

Aspirate—To suck or draw in, as by inhaling.

Assessment—Process to determine a child's strengths and weaknesses. Includes testing and observations performed by a team of professionals and parents. Usually used to determine special education needs. Term is used interchangeably with **evaluation.**

Asymmetrical—When one side of the body differs from the other.

Astigmatism—Blurry vision caused by abnormal curvature of the cornea.

Ataxic—Having unbalanced, jerky movements.

Ataxia—A condition in which damage to the cerebellum results in an unbalanced gait.

Athetoid—Having involuntary or uncontrolled writhing movements.

Atonic—Relating to lack of normal muscle tone.

Atonic (akinetic) seizure—A sudden loss of muscle tone which may cause the child to fall.

Atrophy—Deterioration of muscle tissue.

Attention—The ability to concentrate on a task.

Attention span—The amount of time one is able to concentrate on a task. Also called **attending** in special education jargon.

Audiometry—The testing of hearing.

Auditory—Relating to the ability to hear.

Auditory sequential memory—Ability to hear and repeat a sequence of words or numbers.

Augmentative communication—The use of non-speech techniques such as signs, gestures, or pictures to supplement a child's speech abilities.

Behavior modification—*See* Applied behavior analysis.

Beneficiary—The person indicated in a trust or insurance policy to receive any payments that become due.

Bilateral—Relating to both sides.

Bite reflex—A reflex which causes an infant to close his mouth tightly, for example, when his gums or teeth are touched.

Bivalved casts—Removable plaster casts worn to improve toe walking, stretch out tight muscles, or improve wrist or elbow flexion and other abnormalities.

Bradycardia—Very slow heart rate.

Brain stem—Portion of the brain between the cerebellum and the spinal cord.

Bruxism—Grinding of teeth repeatedly.

Case manager—The person responsible for coordinating services and information from the members of a multidisciplinary team.

Cause-and-effect—The concept that actions create reactions.

Cataracts—Clouding of the lens in the eye, which blocks the visual images from entering the retina.

Central nervous system—The brain and spinal cord. The part of the nervous system primarily involved in voluntary movement and thought processes.

Cerebellum—Part of the brain that helps coordinate muscle activity and control balance.

Cerebral palsy—A movement and posture disorder resulting from a nonprogressive defect of the brain (brain damage).

Chorea—Abrupt, quick, jerky movements of the head, neck, arms, or legs.

Choreoathetosis—A form of cerebral palsy which causes variable muscle tone and involuntary movements of the limbs.

Clonus—Rapid, rhythmic movements (alternate muscle relaxation and contractions) which result from spastic muscles.

Cognition—The ability to know and understand the environment.

Conductive hearing loss—A loss of hearing due to ear infections (middle ear disease) or anatomic abnormalities such as cleft lip or palate.

Congenital—Present at or before birth.

Contraction—Momentary tightening or shortening of a muscle.

Contracture—Shortening of muscle fibers resulting in a decrease of joint mobility.

Convulsion—Involuntary contractions of the muscles due to abnormal electrical activity of the brain. A seizure.

Cortical blindness—Total or partial blindness resulting from injury to the brain's visual centers in the cerebral cortex. The child is able to pick up visual information with his eyes, but his brain cannot process and interpret the information.

Cost-of-care liability—The right of a state providing care to someone with disabilities to charge for the care and to collect from that person's assets.

Craniofacial—Pertaining to the area of the skull and the bones of the face.

Cue—Input that prompts a person to perform a behavior or activity.

Depakene—Valproic acid. An antiepileptic seizure medication.

Development—The process of growth and learning during which a child acquires skills and abilities.

Developmental disability—A handicap or impairment beginning before the age of eighteen which may be expected to continue indefinitely and which causes a substantial disability. Such conditions include pervasive developmental disorders, autism, cerebral palsy, and mental retardation.

Developmental milestone—A developmental goal such as sitting or using two-word phrases that functions as a measurement of developmental progress over time.

Developmentally delayed—Having development that is slower than normal.

Digit—Toe or finger

Dilantin—Phenytoin. An antiepileptic seizure medication.

Diplegia—A type of cerebral palsy in which spasticity primarily affects the legs.

Diplopia—Double vision.

Discretionary trust—A trust in which the trustee (the person responsible for governing the trust) has the authority to use or not use the trust funds for any purpose, as long as funds are expended only for the beneficiary.

Disinherit—To deprive someone of an inheritance. Parents of children with disabilities may do this to prevent the state from imposing cost-of-care liability on their child's assets.

Dispute resolution procedures—The procedure established by law and regulation for the fair resolution of disputes regarding a child's special education.

Dorsiflexion—Upward motion of the foot toward the body.

Due process hearing—Part of the procedures established to protect the rights of parents and special-needs children during disputes under Public Law 94-142. These are hearings before an impartial person to review the identification, evaluation, placement, and services by the educational agency.

Dysarthria—Impaired articulation due to problems in muscle control.

Dyskinesia—A general term for involuntary movements.

Dyspraxia—Difficulty planning movements and putting them into sequence.

Dystonia—Slow, rhythmic, twisting movements.

EAHCA—*See* Education for All Handicapped Children Act.

Early development—Development during the first three years of life.

Early intervention—The specialized way of interacting with infants to minimize the effects of conditions that can delay early development.

Echolalia—A parrot-like repetition of phrases or words just heard (immediate echolalia), or heard hours, days, weeks, or even months ago (delayed echolalia).

Education for All Handicapped Children Act—The federal law that guarantees all children with disabilities the right to a free approrpriate public education. It is Public Law 94–142.

EEG. *See* Electroencephalogram.

Efferent—Originating from the central nervous system, a nerve impulse which travels to a nerve or muscle.

Electroencephalogram (EEG)—The machine and test used to determine levels of electrical discharge from nerve cells. Often used in seizure diagnosis.

Electromyogram—A test which measures electrical levels in muscles, used in diagnosing muscle and nerve disorders.

Engagement—The ability to remain focused on, and responsive to, a person or object.

Epilepsy—A recurrent condition in which abnormal electrical discharges in the brain cause seizures.

Equilibrium—Balance.

Equinus—Walking on toes due to a shortening of the calf muscles.

Esophagus—The tube through which food travels from the pharynx to the stomach.

Estate planning—Formal, written arrangements for handling the possessions and assets of people after they have died.

Esotropia—A condition in which the eye(s) turns inward.

Etiology—The study of the cause of disease.

Eversion—When a body part turns out away from the body.

Evaluation. *See* Assessment.

Expressive language—The ability to use gestures, words, and written symbols to communicate.

Extension—Limbs or trunk becoming straight or extended. The opposite of **flexion.**

Exotropia—A condition in which an eye turns outward.

Facilitation—Helping to move, making movements easier.

Febrile seizures—Generalized tonic-clonic seizures brought on by a sudden rise of temperature to 102 degrees or higher.

Femoral bone—The long, heavy bone extending from the knee to the hip.

Fine motor—Relating to the use of the small muscles of the body, such as those in the face, hands, feet, fingers, and toes.

Flexion—The bending of joints.

Flexion deformity—Abnormal flexion at a joint.

Flexor—A muscle controlling joint flexion.

Floppy—Having weak posture and loose movements.

Fluctuating tone—Having a combination of low and high muscle tone.

Focal motor seizures—Jerking of a few muscle groups without an initial loss of consciousness.

Form perception—The ability to perceive a pattern of parts making up a whole.

Free Appropriate Public Education—The basic right to special education provided at public expense. This right is guaranteed by P.L. 94-142.

Gag reflex—A reflex that causes a child to gag or choke when his palate or tongue is touched.

Gastroenterologist—A specialist in digestive disorders.

Gastroesophageal reflux—A condition in which stomach contents are forced back up into the esophagus and sometimes the mouth.

Genetic—Inherited.

Generalization—Transferring a skill taught in one place, or with one person, to other places and people.

Goniometer—An instrument used to measure joint range of motion.

Grand mal seizure. *See* Tonic-clonic seizure.

Gross motor—Relating to the use of the large muscles of the body, such as those in the legs, arms, and abdomen.

Habilitation—Teaching new skills to children with developmental disabilities.

Handicapped—Having some sort of disability, including physical disabilities, mental retardation, sensory impairments, behavioral disorders, learning disabilities, or multiple handicaps.

Head control—The ability to control the movements of the head.

Hemiplegia—A type of cerebral palsy in which only the right or left side of the body is affected.

Hepatitis—An inflammation of the liver.

High tone—A tightness or spasticity of the muscles.

Hyperactivity—A specific nervous-system-based difficulty which makes it hard for a person to control muscle (motor) behavior and results in restlessness, fidgeting, overactive movements.

Hyperextensible—Overly flexible.

Hyperopia—Farsightedness; a condition in which distant objects can be clearly seen, but nearby objects appear blurred.

Hyperplasia—Excessive growth of tissue—for example, of gum tissue.

Hypertonia—An increased tension or spasticity of the muscles. High tone.

Hypotonia—Decreased tension of a muscle. Low tone.

Identification—The determination that a child should be evaluated as a possible candidate for special education services.

IEP—Individualized Education Program. The written plan that describes what services the local education agency has promised to provide your child.

IFSP—Individualized Family Service Plan. The written document that describes what services your child will receive through his early intervention program.

Imitation—The ability to observe the actions of others and to copy them in one's own actions. Also known as **modeling.**

Incontinence—Lack of bladder or bowel control.

Infantile myoclonic seizures—Sudden, brief, involuntary muscle contractions involving one or several muscle groups.

Inhibition—Movements and positioning which discourage muscle tightness.

Inhibitive casts—Casts fitted with a sole and a raised ledge under the toes; used to inhibit muscle tightness and produce more normal tone.

Input—Information that a person receives through any of the senses (vision, hearing, touch, taste, smell) that helps that person develop new skills.

Integration. *See* Mainstreaming.

Interdisciplinary team—A team of professionals from different fields of expertise who evaluate your child and then develop a comprehensive summary report of his or her strengths and needs.

Interpretive—The session during which parents and teachers review and discuss the results of a child's evaluation.

Intracerebral—Within the brain.

Intracranial—Within the skull.

In utero—Referring to the period during fetal development.

Inversion—When a part of the body turns in.

Involuntary movements—Uncontrolled movements.

I.Q. (Intelligence Quotient)—A measure of cognitive ability based on specifically designed standardized tests.

KAFO (Knee ankle foot orthoses)—A long-leg brace of lightweight plastic with hinges at the knee joint which offers support to the whole leg.

Kinesthetic—Relating to the ability to perceive movement.

Kyphosis—Rounded back; a deformity of the upper spine.

Labyrinth—The inner ear.

Language—The expression and understanding of human communication.

Laterality—A motor awareness of both sides of the body.

Learning disability—Difficulty processing certain types of information in a child with normal intelligence.

Least restrictive environment—The requirement under Public Law 94-142 that children receiving special education must be made a part of a regular school to the fullest extent possible.

Local Education Agency (LEA)—The agency responsible for providing educational services on the local (city, county, and school district) level.

Long-leg sitting—Sitting with legs extended straight out in front of the body.

Lordosis—Sway back; a deformity of the lower spine.

Low tone—Decreased muscle tone.

Lower extremities—The legs.

LRE. *See* Least restrictive environment.

Lumbar—Relating to the lower back.

Luxury trust—A trust that describes the kind of allowable expenses in a way that excludes the cost of care in state-funded programs in order to avoid cost-of-care liability.

Mainstreaming—The practice of involving children with disabilities in regular school and preschool environments.

Malnutrition—Nutritional intake that is insufficient to promote or maintain growth and development.

Malocclusions—Faulty bites such as overbites or underbites.

Mandible—Lower jaw bone.

Maxilla—Upper jaw bone.

Medicaid—A joint state and federal program that offers medical assistance to people who are entitled to receive Supplementary Security Income.

Medicare—A federal program that provides payments for medical care to people who are receiving Social Security payments.

Mental retardation—Below normal mental function. Children who are mentally retarded learn more slowly than other children, but "mental retardation" itself does not indicate a specific level of mental ability. The level of mental function may not be identifiable until a much later age.

Midline—an imaginary reference line down the center of the body separating left from right.

Modeling—*See* Imitation.

Monoplegia—Type of cerebral palsy in which only one limb is affected.

Motor—Relating to the ability to move oneself.

Motor delay—Slower than normal development of movement skills.

Motor patterns—The ways in which the body and limbs work to make sequenced movement.

Motor planning—The ability to think through and carry out a physical task.

Muscle facilitation—To encourage a muscle to work harder through techniques such as proper positioning, special equipment, sensory input, etc.

Muscle tone—The amount of tension or resistance to movement in a muscle.

Multidisciplinary team. *See* Interdisciplinary team.

Multihandicapped—Having more than one handicap.

Myopia—Nearsightedness; a condition in which close objects can be seen clearly but distant objects are blurry.

Nerve Block—An injection of medication into nerves to the muscles to impair the conduction of impulses along the nerve and reduce spasticity.

Neurodevelopmental treatment (NDT)—A specialized therapy approach that concentrates on encouraging normal movement patterns and discouraging abnormal reflexes, postures, and movements. Used by physical, occupational, and speech therapists.

Neuroleptic—Medicine which produces changes in functioning of the nervous system.

Neurologist—A physician specializing in medical problems associated with the brain and spinal cord.

Neuromotor—Involving both nerves and muscles.

Neurotransmitter—The chemical substance between nerve cells in the brain which allows the transmission of an impulse from one nerve to another.

Nystagmus—A jerky, involuntary movement of the eyes.

Occupational therapist (OT)—A therapist who specializes in improving the development of fine motor and adaptive skills.

Ophthalmologist—a physician who specializes in treating the eye and diseases of the visual system.

Optokinetic—Relating to movement of the eyes when visually following a moving object.

Optometrist—A professional who performs eye examinations and prescribes glasses.

Oral motor—Relating to the movement of muscles in and around the mouth.

Oral tactile defensiveness—An over-sensitivity to touch around the mouth.

Orthodontist—A dentist who specializes in correcting irregularities of teeth and/or jaw alignment.

Orthopedic—Relating to the bones, joints, or muscles.

Orthopedist—A physician specializing in bones and joints.

Orthotics—Lightweight devices made of plastic, leather, or metal which provide stability at the joints or passively stretch the muscles.

Osteotomy—An operation to cut and realign the bones; for example, to change the angle of the femoral bone and the hip joint.

Otitis media—Inflammation of the middle ear due to bacterial infection or other causes.

Palatal—Relating to the back portion of the roof of the mouth.

Palmar grasp—Using only fingers, not the thumb, to grasp an object in the palm of the hand.

Parent-professional partnership—The teaming of parents and teachers (or doctors, nurses, or other professionals) to work together to facilitate the development of babies and children with special needs.

Periodontal—Relating to the gums and bones that surround the teeth.

Petit mal (absence) seizures—Brief, abrupt loss of consciousness (5 to 10 seconds) followed by a rapid, complete recovery; also associated with staring or repetitive eye blinking.

Phalanges—The bones of fingers or toes.

Phenobarbital—An anticonvulsant medication.

Phonation—Voice production.

Phoneme—Smallest unit of sound found in speech.

Phonetic—Relating to articulated sounds.

Physical therapist (PT)—A therapist who works with motor skills.

Pincer grasp—The use of the thumb and forefinger to grasp small objects.

Placement—The selection of the educational program for a child who needs special education programs.

Plantar surface—Sole of the foot.

Posture—Positioning or alignment of the body.

Pragmatics—Understand how and why language is used.

Primitive reflexes—Early reflexes that usually disappear after about six months of age.

Prompt—Input that encourages a child to perform a movement or activity. *See* Cue.

Prone—Lying on the stomach.

Pronation—Turning inward of a hand or foot.

Psychomotor (complex partial) seizures—Seizures which cause decreased alertness and changes in behavior.

Public Law 94–142. *See* Education of Individuals with Disabilities Act.

Pulmonary—Relating to the lungs.

Quadriplegia—A type of cerebral palsy in which the whole body is affected.

Range of motion (ROM)—The degree of movement present at a joint.

Receptive language—The ability to understand spoken and written communication as well as gestures.

Reciprocal motion—The alternate movements of arms and legs.

Reflex—An involuntary movement in response to stimulation such as touch, pressure, or joint movement.

Reinforcement—Providing a pleasant consequence (positive reinforcement) or removing an unpleasant consequence (negative reinforcement) after a behavior in order to increase or maintain that behavior.

Related services—Services that enable a child to benefit from special education. Related services include speech, occupational, and physical therapies, as well as transportation.

Respiration—Breathing.

Respite care—Skilled adult- or child-care and supervision that can be provided in your home or the home of a care-provider. Respite care may be available for several hours per week or for overnight stays.

Retina—The lining of the back portion of the eye which receives visual images.

Retinopathy of Prematurity (R.O.P.)—A condition in which high concentrations of oxygen received while a baby is on a respirator damages capillaries in the eye, leading to myopia or a detached retina.

Retraction—Drawing back a part of the body.

Rhizotomy, selective dorsal—A neurosurgical procedure involving selective cutting of the nerves of the spine to reduce the spasticity of muscle groups.

Rigidity—Extremely high muscle tone in any position, combined with very limited movements.

Rooting—A newborn reflex in which babies turn their mouths toward the breast or bottle to feed.

R.O.P. *See* Retinopathy of Prematurity.

Scoliosis—Curvature of the spine.

Screening test—A test given to groups of children to sort out those who need further evaluation.

SEA—The State Education Agency.

Seizure—Involuntary movement or changes in consciousness or behavior brought on by abnormal bursts of electrical activity in the brain.

Self-help—Relating to skills such as eating, dressing, bathing, and cleaning which enable a person to care for himself.

Sensorineural hearing loss—Hearing loss resulting from damage to the inner ear, the auditory nerve, or both, which is present at birth or acquired later in childhood from meningitis, high fever, or medications.

Sensory ability (integration)—The ability of the central nervous system to process and learn from sensations such as touch, sound, light, smell, and movement.

Sensory impairments—Problems handling information relayed to the brain from the senses. *See also* Dyspraxia; Tactile defensiveness.

Sensory seizures—Seizures which produce dizziness or disturbances in vision, hearing, taste, smell, or other senses.

Side sitting—Sitting with both knees bent and to one side of the body.

Scissoring—Crossing legs together when standing or being held upright.

Social ability—The ability to function in groups and to interact with people.

Soft tissue releases—Operations on the muscles, tendons, or ligaments to correct deformities or improve movement.

Spastic—Having increased muscle tone (stiff muscles) resulting in difficult movements.

Special education—Specialized instruction based on educational disabilities determined by a team evaluation. It must be precisely matched to educational needs and adapted to the child's learning style.

Special needs—Needs generated by a person's handicap.

Speech/language pathologist—A therapist who works to improve speech and language skills, as well as to improve oral motor abilities.

Splints—Devices made of molded, rigid plastic used to stretch the soft tissues or to hold a limb in a position that makes movement easier.

S.S.D.I.—Social Security Disability Insurance. This money has been paid into the Social Security system through payroll deductions on earnings. Disabled workers are entitled to these benefits. People who become disabled before the age of twenty-two may collect S.S.D.I. under a parent's account, if the parent is retired, disabled, or deceased.

S.S.I.—Supplemental Security Income is available for low-income people who are disabled, blind, or aged. S.S.I. is based on need, not on past earnings.

Sternum—The breast plate.

Stimulus—A physical object or environmental event that may have an effect upon the behavior of a person. Some stimuli are internal (earache pain), while others are external (a smile from a loved one).

Strabismus—Lack of coordinated eye movement resulting in crossing and/or wandering eyes.

Subluxation—Partial dislocation.

Supine—Back-lying position.

Support trust—A trust that requires that funds be expended to pay for the beneficiary's expenses of living, including housing, food, and transportation.

Sutures—Stitches, used to close a wound.

Symptomatic—Having a cause that is identified.

Tactile—Relating to touch.

Tactile defensiveness—Abnormal sensitivity to touch.

Tailor sitting (Indian style)—Sitting cross-legged on the floor.

Thalamus—A portion of the brain involved in refining movement of the muscles.

Therapist—A trained professional who works to overcome the effects of developmental problems.

Tongue protrusion reflex—A reflex that causes the tongue to forcefully push food out of the mouth.

Tonic—Having continuous increased muscle tone.

Tonic-clonic (grand mal) seizure—A type of seizure which causes a sudden loss of consciousness followed immediately by a generalized convulsion in which extremities become stiff, then jerk rhythmically.

Trachea—Windpipe.

Tympanometer—An electrical instrument which measures changes in pressure and mobility of the eardrum to detect middle ear fluid.

Uniform Gifts to Minors Act (UGMA)—A law that governs gifts to minors. Under the UGMA, gifts become the property of the minor at age eighteen or twenty-one.

Unilateral—One-sided.

Urologist—A physician who specializes in urinary diseases.

Vestibular—Pertaining to the sensory system located in the inner ear that allows the body to maintain balance and enjoyably participate in movement such as swinging and roughhousing.

Vision therapist—A therapist who assesses and enhances useful vision.

Visual sequential memory—The ability to remember a sequence of pictures one sees.

Vocational training—Training for a job. Learning skills to perform in the work place.

Reading List

This Reading List is designed to help parents of children with cerebral palsy learn more about the topics discussed in each chapter of the book. It includes only those publications that are especially readable, informative, and helpful from a parent's standpoint. To find out about other useful titles for parents *and* professionals, try checking with your library or bookstore, as well as with the parents' groups listed in the Resource Guide.

Chapter 1

Batshaw, Mark L. and Yvonne M. Perret. *Children with Handicaps: A Medical Primer.* 2d ed. Baltimore: Paul H. Brookes, 1986. This textbook clearly answers a range of technical medical questions. Includes informative descriptions of mental retardation; visual impairments; hearing, speech, and language problems; attention deficit disorders; learning disabilities; cerebral palsy, epilepsy; and other disabilities. Illustrations and graphs in the cerebral palsy section are especially helpful.

Finnie, Nancie R. *Handling the Young Cerebral Palsied Child at Home.* New York: E.P. Dutton, 1975. This informative, illustrated reference clearly describes abnormal movements and postures, and explains how to cope on a daily basis with the management and development of a child with cerebral palsy. Considered a classic among parents as well as professionals.

Harrison, Helen with Ann Kositsky. *The Premature Baby Book.* New York: St. Martin's Press, 1981. If your child's cerebral palsy has been linked to premature birth, this guide may help you understand your child's disability. Explains many problems which are a result of prematurity and offers an abundance of support for parents of preemies.

Schleichkorn, Jay. *Coping with Cerebral Palsy: Answers to Questions Parents Often Ask.* Austin: Pro-Ed, 1983. Answers questions parents often have about the nature and causes of cerebral palsy, medical problems, surgery, educational concerns, and therapies. It is a compilation of material from parent interviews.

Chapter 2

Dickman, Irving with Sol Gordon. *One Miracle at a Time: How to Get Help for Your Disabled Child - From the Experience of Other Parents.* New York: Simon & Schuster, 1985. A collection of experiences written by parents of disabled children. Very helpful.

Featherstone, Helen. *A Difference in the Family: Life with a Disabled Child.* New York: Penguin, 1982. Drawing on her personal experiences as well as interviews with parents and professionals, the author movingly shares what life is like when a child in the family has disabilities.

Friedberg, Joan Brest, June B. Mullins, and Adelaide Weir Sukiennik. *Accept Me As I Am: Best Books of Juvenile Nonfiction on Impairments and Disabilities.* New York: R.R. Bowker, 1985. As the title suggests, this book contains detailed reviews of the best books of juvenile nonfiction on impairments and disabilities.

Good, Julia Darnell and Joyce Good Reis. *A Special Kind of Parenting: Meeting the Needs of Handicapped Children.* Franklin Park, Ill.: La Leche League International, 1985. A book that deals with family issues such as coping, acceptance, strengthening your marriage, and medical crises. It is based on firsthand experience of one of the authors and responses to a questionnaire answered by other parents.

Moore, Cory. *A Reader's Guide for Parents of Children with Mental, Physical, or Emotional Disabilities.* Rockville, Md.: Woodbine House, 1990. A must! A description of more than 1,000 books, magazines, and other types of literature on various disabilities for parents as well as children of all ages. Includes ordering information.

Thompson, Charlotte E. *Raising a Handicapped Child: A Helpful Guide for Parents of the Physically Disabled.* New York: William Morrow, 1986. A great book for new parents of a child with cerebral palsy. Dr. Thompson explores the many emotions parents experience following a diagnosis, and offers strategies and practical advice for coping with the many challenges confronting parents.

Chapter 3

Batshaw, Mark L. and Yvonne M. Perret. *Children with Handicaps: A Medical Primer.* 2d ed. Baltimore: Paul H. Brookes, 1986. The chapter on cerebral palsy discusses a range of medical concerns, including surgery and orthotics. There are also helpful chapters on visual and hearing impairments, epilepsy, and other disabilities.

Prensky, Arthur and Helen Palkes. *Care of the Neurologically Handicapped Child.* New York: Oxford University Press, 1982. This book describes seven common neurological problems, including cerebral palsy, epilepsy, learning disabilities, hyperactivity, and mental retardation, and explains how they affect development.

Reisner, Helen. *Children with Epilepsy: A Parents' Guide.* Rockville, Md.: Woodbine House, 1988. Valuable reading for parents of children with cerebral palsy who also have seizures. The chapter on medical concerns thoroughly explains the types of seizures and discusses medications and other treatments.

Schleichkorn, Jay. *Coping with Cerebral Palsy: Answers to Questions Parents Often Ask.* Austin: Pro-Ed, 1983. Among the questions answered in this useful book are some about medical and surgical problems and dealing with medical and dental professionals.

Chapter 4

Adams, Ronald C., Alfred H. Daniel, and Lee Rullman. *Games, Sports, and Exercises for the Physically Handicapped.* 3d ed. Philadelphia: Lea & Febiger, 1982. Explains the importance of physical activity for people with physical disabilities and describes appropriate activities for people with different types of disabilities. Primarily for teachers, but also useful for parents.

Finnie, Nancie R. *Handling the Young Cerebral Palsied Child at Home.* New York: E.P. Dutton, 1975. The emphasis in this practical, classic work is on holding, positioning, and other day-to-day problems parents of children with cerebral palsy face.

Jones, Monica Loose. *Home Care for the Chronically Ill or Disabled Child.* New York: Harper & Row, 1980. A comprehensive guide to meeting your child's needs at home.

Murphy, Judy. *Home Care of Handicapped Children: A Guide. Orthopedic Handicaps.* Lyons, Colo.: Carol L. Lutey Publishing, 1982. This book includes guidelines for lifting, lowering, carrying, and properly positioning your child and offers self-help activities. A good guide for all aspects of care giving.

Perske, Robert, Andrew Clifton, Barbara M. MccLean, and Jean Ishler Stein, eds. *Mealtimes for Persons with Severe Handicaps.* Baltimore: Paul H. Brookes, 1986. Parents and professionals talk about what makes mealtimes more successful for children with cerebral palsy or other disabilities.

Russell, Philippa. *The Wheelchair Child: How Handicapped Children Can Enjoy Life to Its Fullest.* New York: Prentice Hall, 1985. Covers many issues parents face when their child uses a wheelchair.

Chapter 5

Dickman, Irving with Sol Gordon. *One Miracle at a Time: How to Get Help for Your Disabled Child - From the Experience of Other Parents.* New York: Simon & Schuster, 1985. A collection of experiences written by parents of children with disabilities. Very helpful.

Garber, Stephen W. *The Good Behavior Book*. New York: Villard Books, 1987. This book is not written specifically for children with cerebral palsy, but is a wonderful guide to dealing with childhood stages and behavior management issues. A must for *all* parents.

Hecker, Helen. *Travel for the Disabled: A Handbook of Travel Resources and 500 Worldwide Access Guides*. Vancouver, Wash.: Twin Peaks Press, 1985. A useful guide to help families find accessible accommodations when planning their vacations.

Lindemann, James E. and Sally J. Lindemann. *Growing Up Proud: A Parents' Guide to the Psychological Care of Children with Disabilities*. New York: Warner Books, 1988. A psychologist husband-and-wife team offer guidelines to help parents help their children with disabilities "grow up proud." A wide range of disabilities and ages are covered.

Meyer, Donald J., Patricia F. Vadasy, and Rebecca R. Fewell. *Living with a Brother or Sister with Special Needs: A Book for Sibs*. Seattle: University of Washington Press, 1985. An introduction to disabilities written for siblings. Covers basic information about many disabilities, deals with siblings' feelings, and offers solutions to common problems.

Schleifer, Maxwell J. and Stanley D. Klein, eds. *The Disabled Child & the Family: An Exceptional Parent Reader*. Boston: The Exceptional Parent Press, 1985. An anthology of articles about family issues for parents of children with disabilities. The articles were originally published in *The Exceptional Parent* magazine. Includes useful resources.

Stein, Sara Bonnett. *About Handicaps: An Open Family Book for Parents and Children Together*. New York: Walker, 1974. This book was written for parents and children with or without handicaps. Provides a frank look at the relationship between two boys, one of whom has cerebral palsy. Includes separate text for adults and children. Highly recommended.

Chapter 6

Caplan, Frank, ed. *The Parenting Advisor*. Garden City, N.Y.: Anchor Press/ Doubleday, 1977. Presents the views of experts on the development of infants and children. For all parents.

Mollan, Renee. *Yes They Can! A Handbook for Effectively Parenting the Handicapped*. Buena Park, Calif.: Reality Productions, 1981. Practical advice for parents on how to promote independence and responsibility.

Morris, Lisa Rappaport and Linda Schulz. *Creative Play Activities for Children with Disabilities: A Resource Book for Teachers and Parents*. 2d ed. Champaign, Ill.:

Human Kinetics, 1989. This book has two hundred and fifty games and activities designed to encourage the development of children with disabilities. Activities are appropriate for infants to eight-year-olds. Good resource section included.

Musselwhite, Caroline Ramsey. *Adaptive Play for Special Needs Children: Strategies to Enhance Communication and Learning.* Boston: College-Hill Press, 1987. Written for professionals as well as parents, this book explains how to teach developmental skills through play and promotes the use of play in all settings. Clearly a textbook, but has valuable information for parents.

Prensky, Arthur and Helen Palkes. *Care of the Neurologically Handicapped Child.* New York: Oxford University Press, 1982. This book describes seven common neurological problems, including cerebral palsy, epilepsy, learning disabilities, hyperactivity, and mental retardation, and explains how they affect development.

Schwartz, Sue and Joan E. Heller Miller. *The Language of Toys: Teaching Communication Skills to Special-Needs Children.* Rockville, Md.: Woodbine House, 1988. A parents' guide to using toys to help children develop language skills. Includes clear explanations of developmental stages.

White, Burton L. *The First Three Years of Life.* Rev. ed. New York: Prentice Hall Press, 1985. One of the classics on child development, covering the first three years.

Chapter 7

Ayres, A. Jean. *Sensory Integration and the Child.* Los Angeles: Western Psychological Services, 1979. Explains how Dr. Ayres uses occupational therapy to help some children who have sensory processing problems. Includes ways parents can reinforce therapy goals at home.

Finnie, Nancie R. *Handling the Young Cerebral Palsied Child at Home.* New York: E.P. Dutton, 1975. Helpful drawings and explanations of handling and positioning techniques can help parents in carrying out home therapy programs.

The Helping Hand: A Manual Describing Methods for Handling the Young Child with Cerebral Palsy. National Clearing House of Rehabilitation Training Materials (115 Old USDA Building, Oklahoma State University, Stillwater, OK 74078). Describes, with illustrations, the basic principles of Neurodevelopmental Treatment. Also includes background information on cerebral palsy.

Musselwhite, Caroline Ramsey. *Adaptive Play for Special Needs Children: Strategies to Enhance Communication and Learning.* Boston: College-Hill Press, 1987. Written for professionals as well as parents, this book explains how to teach developmental skills through play and promotes the use of play in all settings. Clearly a textbook, but has valuable information for parents.

Schwartz, Sue and Joan E. Heller Miller. *The Language of Toys: Teaching Communication Skills to Special-Needs Children.* Rockville, Md.: Woodbine House, 1988. Describes how parents can use homemade and commercially made toys to stimulate their child's language development. Includes background information on language development and delays. Activities are appropriate for children up to the developmental age of sixty months.

Chapter 8

Anderson, Winifred, Stephen Chitwood, and Deidre Hayden. *Negotiating the Special Education Maze: A Guide for Parents and Teachers.* 2d ed. Rockville, Md.: Woodbine House, 1990. A practical, step-by-step guide to obtaining an appropriate education for your child. Includes helpful information about special education laws, meeting with school officials, planning IEPs, choosing a program, and resolving conflicts.

Healy, Alfred, Patricia D. Keesee, and Barbara S. Smith. *Early Services for Children with Special Needs: Transactions for Family Support.* Baltimore: Paul H. Brookes, 1989. Focuses on P.L. 99-457, the amendment that requires states to provide early intervention services for children birth to two. Describes ways for families and professionals to work together to reach children's goals.

Orelove, Fred P. and Dick Sobsey. *Educating Children with Multiple Disabilities: A Transdisciplinary Approach.* Baltimore: Paul H. Brookes, 1987. Explains how teachers, therapists, medical professionals, and parents can work as a team to enhance the learning of children with multiple disabilities.

Shore, Kenneth. *The Special Education Handbook: A Comprehensive Guide for Parents and Educators.* New York: Teachers College Press, 1986. In a readable style, guides parents through the special education process from their child's first referral up through placement in a program. This books helps parents feel comfortable advocating for their child's education program.

Chapter 9

Anderson, Winifred, Stephen Chitwood, and Deidre Hayden. *Negotiating the Special Education Maze: A Guide for Parents and Teachers.* 2d ed. Rockville, Md.: Woodbine House, 1990. Provides a clear explanation of the educational rights of children with disabilities and explains how parents can help obtain an appropriate education for their child.

Budoff, Milton and Alan Orenstein. *Due Process in Special Education: On Going to a Hearing.* Cambridge, Mass.: Brookline Books, 1982. An examination of due process procedures in special education.

Moore, Ralph J., Jr. *Handbook on Estate Planning for Families of Developmentally Disabled Persons in Maryland, the District of Columbia, and Virginia.* Baltimore: Maryland State Planning Council on Developmental Disabilities, 1981. An estate planning guide for parents of children with disabilities. Although the emphasis is on the laws of Maryland, Virginia, and the District of Columbia, the general legal principles are usually applicable to other states.

Russell, L. Mark. *Alternatives: A Family Guide to Legal and Financial Planning for the Disabled.* Evanston, Ill.: First Publications, 1983. Although some information in this book is outdated, it still contains valuable suggestions on estate planning for parents of children with disabilities. Includes information on taxes, wills, trusts, insurance, and financial planning.

Chapter 10

Biklen, Douglas. *Let Our Children Go: An Organizing Manual for Advocates and Parents.* Syracuse, N.Y.: Human Policy Press, 1974. Although written before the passage of P.L. 94-142, this manual still has some useful pointers about advocating for better education and treatment of children with special needs.

Des Jardins, Charlotte. *How to Get Services by Being Assertive.* Chicago: Coordinating Council for Handicapped Children (20 E. Jackson Blvd., Room 900, Chicago, IL 60604), 1980. A practical guide to advocating for services for your child.

Markel, Geraldine Ponte and Judith Greenbaum. *Parents Are to Be Seen and Heard: Assertiveness in Educational Planning for Handicapped Children.* Explains how parents can use their knowledge to get educational services for their child. Includes suggestions for dealing with school personnel assertively.

Shields, Craig V. *Strategies: A Practical Guide for Dealing with Professionals and Human Service Systems.* Richmond Hill, Ontario: Human Services Press; distributed by Paul H. Brookes, 1987. Discusses common problems parents have with professionals and human service systems and suggests methods for resolving these problems.

Suggested Children's Literature

Cross, Molly. *Wait for Me!* New York: Random House in conjunction with the Children's Television Workshop, 1987. It's hard for Elmo to keep up with his friends because he is so much younger and smaller. But Elmo finds a way to make his own fun, and when his older friend Grover arrives home, Elmo realizes that it is Grover who has missed out on the fun. This book can help children deal with the feeling of being left out and left behind.

Exley, Helen. *What It's Like to Be Me.* 2d ed. New York: Friendship Press, 1984. A beautifully illustrated and written book by young people with disabilities. The authors explain what it feels like to be treated differently from others and how they would like very much to be like all able-bodied people.

Fassler, Joan. *Howie Helps Himself.* Niles, Ill.: Albert Whitman, 1975. A story for young children about Howie, a little boy with cerebral palsy who wants to learn to operate his wheelchair independently. Howie deals with frustrations as well as successes in coming to terms with his disability.

Piper, Watty. *The Little Engine That Could.* New York: Platt & Munk, 1954. This book is a great motivation tool to read to a child with cerebral palsy. Remember, "I think I can, I think I can."

Sadler, Marilyn. *It's Not Easy Being a Bunny.* New York: Random House, 1983. P.J. Funnybunny is not happy being a bunny. In his search for another identity, P.J. tries living with many different animals until he decides it really isn't so bad being just a bunny after all. A good book for helping children explore their feelings about being different and coming to terms with who they are. . . instead of who they'd like to be.

Southall, Ivan. *Let the Balloon Go.* New York: Bradbury Press, 1968. The story of a young boy with a physical disability who deals with the frustrations involved in his struggle for more freedom.

Stein, Sara Bonnett. *About Handicaps: An Open Family Book for Parents and Children Together.* New York: Walker, 1974. This book was written for parents and children with or without handicaps. Provides a frank look at the relationship between two boys, one of whom has cerebral palsy. Includes separate text for adults and children. Highly recommended.

Whinston, Joan Lenett. *I'm Joshua and "Yes I Can."* New York: Vantage Press, 1989. Joshua has cerebral palsy and is being mainstreamed into first grade. His family and teachers help him cope with his worries about the transition.

Periodicals

Augmentative Communication News, c/o Sunset Enterprises, One Surf Way, Suite 215, Monterey, CA 93940. Bimonthly newsletter about augmentative communication products, research, and policy.

Closing the Gap, P.O. Box 68, Henderson, MN 56044. A bimonthly newsletter that focuses on technology in special education and rehabilitation. Publishes a comprehensive resource guide annually.

The Exceptional Parent, P.O. Box 3000, Dept. EP, Denville, NJ 07834-9919. A long-respected source of information and guidance for families of children with disabilities. This magazine not only has wonderful articles, but also has an annual tax guide, annual resource guide, and an abundance of advertisements for special equipment, clothing, and toys. A must!

Newsletter, NICHCY, Box 1492, Washington, DC 20013. A newsletter on issues of importance to people living or working with children with special needs. Free subscription.

Pacesetter Newsletter, Parent Advocacy Coalition for Educational Rights (PACER), 4826 Chicago Ave., Minneapolis, MN 55417. A quarterly newsletter focusing on special education issues.

Parenting, Box 52424, Boulder, CO 80321–2424. Although your child has special needs, it is very helpful to also read a magazine directed at parents of "normal" children. This general parenting magazine often includes information and articles relating to children with special needs.

Special Equipment Suppliers

There are dozens of suppliers of adaptive equipment, toys, and clothing in the United States today. The companies below are only a representative sampling of suppliers whose equipment is especially suited for children with cerebral palsy. For the names of additional suppliers, check *The Exceptional Parent* magazine, which is usually overflowing with advertisements for special toys, equipment, clothing, and educational materials. And remember, always check with your child's doctor or therapist before investing in any special equipment.

Adaptive Equipment

Equipment Shop
P.O. Box 33
Bedford, MA 01730
617/275–7681
Offers quality products, including strollers, seats, adaptations, balls, prone standers, etc. Also see listing under "Toys."

Kaye Products Inc.
535 Dimmocks Mill Road
Hillsborough, NC 27278
919/732–6444
Adaptive equipment and therapy products exclusively for children. Products are durable, easily adjusted to size, and well constructed.

Ortho-Kinetics
P.O. Box 1647
Waukesha, WI 53187
414/542–6060; 800/824–1068
Prone standers, standing frames, adaptive chairs, travel chairs, bath seats, and other adaptive equipment for children with physical disabilities.

J.A. Preston Corporation
60 Page Road
Clifton, NJ 07012
201/777–2700; 800/631–7277
Offers a wide variety of well-made equipment for children and adults with disabilities. They also offer some toys.

Rifton
Equipment for the Handicapped
Route 213
Rifton, NY 12471
914/658–3141
Has good quality wedges, baby and toddler chairs, swings, potty chairs, bath and shower chairs, adaptive tables, rolls, and wedges. See also listing under "Toys."

Wheelchairs

Listed below are some of the major manufacturers of wheelchairs. Most of these companies produce a variety of wheelchairs, one of which may be right for your child. Since each child with cerebral palsy has unique needs, it's impossible to recommend a specific wheelchair that is ideally suited for all children. In buying a wheelchair, it's best to do your research, consult with your doctor and therapist, and *then* make your purchase decision.

ETAC USA, Inc.
2325 Parklawn Drive, Suite P
Waukesha, WI 53186
800/678–3822

Everst & Jennings
3233 West Mission Oaks Blvd.
Camarillo, CA 93012
805/987–6911

Sunrise Medical Quickie Designs
2842 Business Park Avenue
Fresno, CA 93727
209/292–2171

Wheelring, Inc.
199 Forest Street
Manchester, CT 06040
203/647–8596

Communication/Technical Equipment

AT&T National Special Needs Center
800/233–1222
AT&T offers telephone-related devices for people with hearing impairments as well as those with speech and motion impairments. These devices will be of interest once your child has telephone communication needs.

Apple Computer, Inc.
Apple Office of Special Education
20525 Mariani Boulevard
Mail Stop 23D
Cupertino, CA 95014
Sells a variety of Apple-compatible computer accessories and software for children with special needs. For an authorized Apple dealer near you, call 800/538–9696.

IBM Corporation
IBM National Support Center for Persons with Disabilities
Box C–1030
Atlanta GA 30055
Offers IBM-compatible computer accessories and software for children with special needs.

Toys

The following companies carry adaptive as well as regular toys that may meet your child's needs. Some can supply adaptive switches. These companies are by no means your only choices. Many appropriate toys can be found at your local toy store or through other companies that specialize in adaptive toys.

Equipment Shop
P.O. Box 33
Bedford, MA 01730
617/275–7681
The Equipment Shop offers tricycle adaptations as well as two different hand-powered vehicles.

Hals Pals
P.O. Box 3490
Winter Park, CO 80482
These wonderful dolls have special needs too. Dolls with a variety of handicaps are available. They can be a special someone for your child to play with.

Kaye's Kids
1010 E. Pettigrew Street
Durham, NC 27701–4299
919/683–1051
Kaye's Kids offers a variety of toys for a range of skills. Kaye Products designs and manufactures adaptive equipment; therefore Kaye's Kids seem to know just what toys will work for your child.

The Nintendo Hands-Free Controller
800/422–2602
This Nintendo controller straps to a child's chest so that the game is controlled by the child's breathing. Can be adapted to various physical disabilities.

J.A. Preston Corporation
60 Page Road
Clifton, NJ 07012
J.A. Preston offers toys ranging from puzzles to tricycles for children with special needs. They also manufacture a wide range of adaptive equipment.

Rifton
Equipment for the Handicapped
Route 213
Rifton, NY 12471
This company manufactures a variety of adaptive tricycles. They include a tricycle for the small child, a chain tricycle available in small or large for the older child, and a hand-driven tricycle in a variety of sizes. They also offer an adaptive easel and manufacture adaptive equipment.

Salco
11445 150th Street East
Nerstrand, MN 55053
507/645–8720
Salco has a very appealing selection of puzzles equipped with knobs and rounded edges in order to make handling easier for children who have difficulty with their grasp. They also offer "puzzle switches" which activate when the correct piece or color has been inserted.

Toys for Special Children
385 Warburton Avenue
Hastings, NY 10706
914/478–0960
Not only does this company offer interesting toys, it has many delightful adaptive ones as well. Best of all, they offer a wide variety of capability switches. Their 24–page printed catalog is $3.00 and their 60 minute video catalog is $6.50.

Clothing

Here are several companies that specialize in adaptive clothing. Special clothing is not by any means a necessity for the very young child, but as your child grows older she may benefit from these garments, depending on her limitations. Once again, remember that these companies are not your only choices. Check listings or advertisements in publications for children with disabilities and their families.

Special Clothes
P.O. Box 4220
Alexandria, VA 22303
703/683–7343
These adaptive garments are attractive as well as functional. Everything from undergarments to winter wear is available. They also carry footwear. Sizes from toddlers (sizes 3–4) to young adults.

Exceptionally Yours
60 Joseph Road
P.O. Box 3246
Framingham, MA 01701
508/877–9757
Great looking, casual clothes designed with plenty of room, Velcro-like closures, large-ring heavy-duty zippers, elastic waistbands, ankle cuffs, and knee pads. Sizes from 2T to adult extra large (42–44).

Resource Guide

National Organizations

The national organizations listed below provide a variety of services that can be of help to you and your child with cerebral palsy. For further information about any of these organizations, call or write and request a copy of their newsletter or other publications.

Accent on Information
P.O. Box 700
Bloomington, IL 61702
309/378–2961
For a nominal fee, this organization will perform information searches on topics such as daily care and products and devices for people with disabilities. They also offer useful publications, including a *Buyer's Guide* that lists equipment and devices as well as their manufacturers. Write and request information on Accent Special Publications.

Alexander Graham Bell Association for the Deaf
3417 Volta Place, NW
Washington, DC 20007
202/337–5220 (Voice/TDD)
Their Children's Rights Program conducts educational advocacy for deaf children and has consulting services for legal rights. The organization answers questions from families of hearing impaired children and publishes a journal and newsletter.

American Academy for Cerebral Palsy and Developmental Medicine
1910 Byrd Ave., Suite 118
P.O. Box 11086
Richmond, VA 23230–1086
804/282–0036
The Academy can refer families to physicians with expertise in treating cerebral palsy.

American Association of University Affiliated Programs
   for Persons with Developmental Disabilities
8630 Fenton St., Suite 410
Silver Spring, MD 20910
301/588–8252
Many universities offer programs and services for children with disabilities and their families. Most University Affiliated Programs offer diagnosis and treatment of disabilities and conduct research on handicapping conditions and methods of teaching. You can obtain a list of all University Affiliated Programs by writing to the AAUAP at the above address.

American Council for the Blind
Suite 1100
1010 Vermont Avenue, NW
Washington, DC 20005
202/393–3666; 800–424–8666 (1–5 pm)
The ACB serves people with blindness, visual impairments, and deaf-blindness. They advocate for civil rights, national health insurance, rehabilitation, eye research, technology, and other issues that concern blind citizens. You can call the toll-free number for information and referrals.

American Foundation for the Blind
15 West 16th Street
New York, NY 10011
212/620–2000; 800/232–5463
The Foundation is a national clearinghouse for information on all aspects of visual impairment. They can also refer you to services for your child and offer useful publications.

American Physical Therapy Association
1111 N. Fairfax Street
Alexandria, VA 22314
703/684–2782
The APTA has a free list of publications, "Publications of Interest to Parents and Educators of Handicapped Children." They can also direct you to the APTA chapter in your area. Call and ask for Information Central.

American Occupational Therapy Association
P.O. Box 1725, 1383 Piccard Drive
Rockville, MD 20850
301/943–9626
The AOTA is a professional organization for occupational therapists. It can refer you to a qualified OT in your area.

American Society for Deaf Children
814 Thayer Avenue
Silver Spring, MD 20910
301/585–5400 (Voice/TDD)
The ASDC provides parents with general information about deafness and raising children with hearing impairments and can refer you to other parents of deaf children in your area. The organization publishes a newsletter, available to members, which covers educational and legislative issues as well as aids for deaf children.

American Speech-Language-Hearing Association
10801 Rockville Pike
Rockville, MD 20852
301/897–5700 (Voice/TDD)
ASHA researches communication disorders. It has fifty state affiliates that can provide information about services available locally. The organization offers brochures on speech/hearing disorders and information on computer software and augmentative communication.

Association for the Care of Children's Health
7910 Woodmont Ave., Suite 300
Bethesda, MD 20814
301/654–6549
Through education, advocacy, and research programs, ACCH meets the psychological and developmental needs of children and families in the health care setting. They offer a bi-monthly newsletter and a Parent Resource Guide, as well as other publications.

ARC
500 E. Border St., Suite 300
Arlington, TX 76010
817/261–6003
A grassroots national organization of people with mental retardation and their advocates. Publishes information on all types of developmental delays and supports an extensive network of local associations.

Center for Special Education Technology
Council for Exceptional Children
1920 Association Dr.
Reston, VA 22091–1589
703/620–3660
The Center provides information on technology, equipment companies, and special education issues. Write or call with your specific questions.

Children's Defense Fund
25 E St., NW
Washington, DC 20001
202/628–8787
CDF is a legal organization that lobbies and brings test cases to court to expand the rights of children, including children with cerebral palsy.

Clearinghouse on Disability Information
Office of Special Education and Rehabilitative Services
U.S. Department of Education
400 Maryland Avenue, SW
Room 3132, Switzer Building
Washington, DC 20202–2524
202/732–1241; 732–1245; 732–1723
This federal organization offers information on civil rights, federal benefits, medical services, education, and support organizations. It publishes *OSERS News in Print,* a newsletter regarding federal activities affecting people with disabilities, and *Pocket Guide to Federal Help for Individuals with Disabilities,* a summary of services and benefits available to individuals who qualify.

Council for Exceptional Children
1920 Association Drive
Reston, VA 22091–1589
703/620–3660
This organization focuses on the educational needs of exceptional children. It conducts computer searches for information and publishes journals.

Epilepsy Foundation of America
4351 Garden City Drive
Landover, MD 20785
301/459–3700; 800/EFA–1000
The EFA answers questions and provides information on seizure disorders and medications. The professionals on staff can also refer you to other organizations and agencies depending on your needs. The toll free number can be reached from all area codes except 301.

IBM National Support Center for Persons with Disabilities
P.O. Box 2150
Atlanta, Georgia 30055
800/IBM–2133
This is a clearinghouse for information on adaptive as well as technical equipment.

International Institute for Visually Impaired
230 Central Street
Auburndale, MA 02166
617/332–4014
The IIVI is an information and resource center for parents of blind children, birth to 7 years old.

Kids on the Block
9385 C Gerwig Lane
Columbia, MD 21046
410/290-9095; 800/368-KIDS
Kids on the Block is a performing arts puppet show that gears its show to children. The characters have a variety of handicaps. KIDS is organized in 49 states.

Learning Disability Association of America
4156 Library Road
Pittsburgh, PA 15234
412/341-1515
The LDA is a grassroots national organization with over five hundred local offices to meet the needs of those with learning disabilities. They can provide information on school program development, legislative action, advocacy, and publications.

March of Dimes Foundation
1275 Mamaroneck Avenue
White Plains, NY 10605
914/428-7100
The March of Dimes is dedicated to preventing birth defects and publishes many brochures and pamphlets of interest to parents of children with special needs.

National Association for Parents of Visually Impaired
P.O. Box 180806
Austin, TX 78718
512/459-6651
This national organization of parents promotes the development of parent groups, provides information and publications about visual impairments, and sponsors workshops.

National Association of Private Schools for Exceptional Children
1625 I St., Ste. 506
Washington, DC 20006
202-223-2192
This association publishes a newsletter and a directory of private schools for children with special needs.

National Association for Visually Handicapped
305 East 24th Street
New York, NY 10010
212/889-3141
A national non-profit organization which serves partially sighted/low vision children and adults, this association distributes public education materials.

National Braille Press
88 St. Stephen Street
Boston, MA 02116
617/266–6160
The National Braille Press offers print-braille books through a Children's Braille Book-of-the-Month Club (no obligation to buy).

National Easter Seal Society
70 East Lake Street
Chicago, IL 60601
312/726–6200
The National Easter Seal Society is dedicated to helping people with disabilities and their families by offering screening, advocacy, public education, and other services. The society also publishes many valuable booklets and pamphlets. Through its Fun and Fitness Club, it helps children integrate physical therapy into organized fitness activities. See state listings for the chapter nearest you.

The National Foundation of Dentistry for the Handicapped
1600 Stout Street
Suite 1420
Denver, CO 80202
303/573–0264
This organization can supply publications relating to dental care for people with handicaps, and also answer specific questions.

National Head Injury Foundation
333 Turnpike Road
Southborough, MA 01772
508/485–9950; 800–444–NHIF (Family Help Line)
The foundation has information available on resources and facilities for care. They publish a quarterly newsletter as well as the *National Directory of Head Injury Rehabilitation Services,* which lists over 350 facilities and programs.

National Information Center for Children
    and Youth with Disabilities
P.O. Box 1492
Washington, DC 20013
202/884–8200; 800/695–0285
This clearinghouse provides free information on educational programs and other special services to parents of children with handicaps. You may call or send in questions. NICHCY also produces fact sheets, information packets, and "State Sheets" which list each state's resources for people with disabilities.

National Information Center on Deafness
Gallaudet University
800 Florida Avenue, NE
Washington, DC 20002
202/651–5051 (Voice); 202/651–5052 (TDD)
The NICD provides information and printed materials about deafness, and referrals to other resources. It also offers reading lists on topics in education of deaf children. Information services and single copies of publications are free.

National Lekotek Center
2100 Ridge Avenue
Evanston, IL 60204
The Lekotek Centers provide toy lending services, play sessions, and support for children with special needs and their family. There are 48 centers in the U.S.

National Library Service for the Blind and
    Physically Handicapped
Library of Congress
1291 Taylor Street, NW
Washington, DC 20542
202/287–5100; 800/424–8567 or 8572
Through this service, the Library of Congress provides free equipment and recorded and braille books for preschoolers, children, and adults. They also publish the reference circular "Parent's Guide to the Development of Pre-School Handicapped Children: Resources and Services."

The Newington, Connecticut ABELDATA Resource Service
800/344–5405
This service provides listing of manufacturers of specialized toys and equipment.

Neuro-Developmental Treatment Association (NDTA)
P.O. Box 70
Oak Park, IL 60303
708/386–2454; 800/869–9295
The NDTA is a professional organization for physical, occupational, and speech therapists; teachers; and physicians who are certified in NDT techniques. A membership directory may be purchased from the national office.

Sibling Information Network
1776 Ellington Rd.
South Windsor, CT 06074
203/648–1205
The Network is an organization for siblings of people with disabilities. Its quarterly newsletter contains resource information and addresses family issues.

Siblings for Significant Change
105 E. 22nd St.
New York, NY 10010
212/420–0430
This national sibling organization provides information and referral services, access to legal aid, counseling programs, and community education.

Specialnet
GTE Education Services, Inc.
2021 K Street, NW
Suite 215
Washington, DC 20006
202/835–7300
Through a computer network, Specialnet offers support for families of children with disabilities.

United Cerebral Palsy Associations
Seven Penn Plaza
Suite 804
New York, NY 10001
212/268–6655; 800/USA–1UCP
UCP is a national organization for people with cerebral palsy and their families. Through its local chapters, it provides a variety of services, including information and referral, parent support, advocacy, and educational and work programs for people with cerebral palsy. A subscription to its *Family Support Bulletin* is free. Other publications are also available. See the state listings for the affiliate nearest you.

Local Organizations

The following list contains addresses, phone numbers, and names of contact people for public and private agencies in each state that provide certain kinds of assistance to people with special needs and their families. We wish to thank the National Information Center for Children and Youth with Handicaps (NICHCY) for contributing much of this information.

Here are brief descriptions of the types of organizations this list includes:

The State Department of Education is the agency responsible for providing education to school-aged children, including special education services to children with cerebral palsy. In many states, the Department of Education also administers early intervention programs for special-needs children aged 0–2, and preschool programs for those aged 3–5. If it does not, it can refer you to the agency that does.

The State Vocational Rehabilitation Agency provides medical, therapeutic, educational, counseling, training, and other services needed to prepare people for work. The state agency can refer you to the local office nearest you.

The State Mental Retardation Program provides funding, in some states, for residential and day programs for children and adults with mental retardation. In other states, the State Mental Retardation Program can direct you to the appropriate funding agency.

The Developmental Disabilities Council provides funding for direct services for people with developmental disabilities. Most provide services such as diagnosis, evaluation, information and referral, social services, group homes, advocacy, and protection.

The Protection & Advocacy Agency is a legal organization established to protect the rights of people with disabilities. It can supply information about the educational, health, residential, social, and legal services available for children with cerebral palsy in your state.

United Cerebral Palsy (UCP) chapters are local affiliates of the national organization that provide support and information to children with cerebral palsy and their families, and direct them to resources and people in the community who can help them.

Association of Retarded Citizens (ARC) chapters and their many programs are essential resources for parents whose children with cerebral palsy also have mental retardation. Each state's ARC is listed below, but there are also many local branches. To locate the branch nearest you, contact your state ARC or check your telephone book under "Association for Retarded Citizens" or "ARC," or look under the name of your city, county, region, state, or state capital (e.g., "Montgomery County ARC").

Parent Programs include privately and publicly funded groups that offer support, information, and referral services to parents of children with special needs.

State Easter Seal Societies carry out the work of the national society on a local level. State Societies offer a variety of services for children with disabilities and their families, including information and referral, advocacy, and support.

ALABAMA

Program for Exceptional Children &
Youth
50 N. Ripley St.
Montgomery, AL 36130–3901
205/242–8114
Contact: Anne Ramsey, Coordinator

Div. of Rehab. and Crippled Children's
Services
Dept. of Education
2129 E. South Blvd.
Montgomery, AL 36111
205/281–8780
Contact: Lamona Lucas, Dir.

Assoc. Commissioner for Mental
Retardation
Dept. of Mental Health
200 Interstate Park Dr.
P.O. Box 3710
Montgomery, AL 36193
205/271–9295
Contact: Larry Latham

Alabama DD Planning Council
200 Interstate Park Dr.
P.O. Box 3710
Montgomery, AL 36193–5001
205/271–9278
Contact: Joan B. Hannah, Director

Alabama Disabilities Advocacy Program
The University of Alabama
P.O. Drawer 2847
Tuscaloosa, AL 35487–2847
205/348–4928

UCP of Greater Birmingham
2430 11th Ave., North
Birmingham, AL 35234
205/251–0165
Contact: Gary Edwards, Exec. Dir.

ARC/Alabama
444 S. Decatur
Montgomery, AL 36104

205/262–7688
Contact: Douglas Sanford, Exec. Dir.

Special Education Action Committee
(SEAC)
P.O. Box 161274
Mobile, AL 36616–2274
205/478–1208; 800/222–7322 (in AL)
Contact: Carol Blades, Dir.

Alabama Easter Seal Society
P.O. Box 20320
Montgomery, AL 36120–0320
205/288–8382
Contact: Barry Cavan, Exec. V.P.

ALASKA

Office, Special Services
Dept. of Education
P.O. Box F
Juneau, AK 99811
907/465–2970
Contact: William S. Mulnix, Administrator

Div. of Vocational Rehab.
Dept. of Education
Pouch F, Mail Stop 0581
State Office Building
Juneau, AK 99811
907/465–2814
Contact: Keith Anderson, Dir.

Dev. Disabilities Section
Div. of Mental Health and DD
Dept. of Health and Social Services
Pouch H–04
Juneau, AK 99811
907/465–3372
Contact: Christine Hagmeier, Acting
Dir.

DD Planning Council
600 University Ave., Ste. B
Fairbanks, AK 99709–3651
907/474–2440
Contact: Dorothy Truran, Exec. Dir.

Advocacy Services of Alaska
615 E. 82nd, #101
Anchorage, AK 99518
907/344–1002
Contact: David Maltman, Dir.

Alaska Assn. for Retarded Citizens
22112–A Arca Dr.
Anchorage, AK 99506
907/277–6677
Contact: Mary Jane Starlings

Alaska Parent Coalition
7530 Blackberry
Anchorage, AK 99502

Special Education Parent Team
  (SEPT)
210 Ferry Way, Ste. 200
Juneau, AK 99801
907/586–6806
Contact: Linda Griffith

Easter Seal Society of Alaska
3231 Spenard Road
Anchorage, AK 99503
907/561–SEAL

ARIZONA

Special Education
Dept. of Education
1535 W. Jefferson
Phoenix, AZ 85007–3280
602/542–3183
Contact: Kay Lund, Asst. Commissioner

Rehabilitation Services Bureau
Dept. of Economic Security
1300 W. Washington St.
Phoenix, AZ 85007
602/542–3332
Contact: James B. Griffith, Admin.

Div. of Dev. Disabilities
Dept. of Economic Security
P.O. Box 6123
Phoenix, AZ 85005
602/258–0419
Contact: Lyn Rucker, Asst. Director

Governor's Council on DD
1717 W. Jefferson St.
Box 6123 (074Z)
Phoenix, AZ 85005
602/542–4049
Contact: Rita Charron, Director

Arizona Center for Law in the Public
  Interest
363 N. First Ave., Ste. 100
Phoenix, AZ 85003
602/252–4904; 602/327–9547
Contact: Pat Brown, Interim Director

UCP of Central Arizona
7337 N. 19th Ave.
Phoenix, AZ 85021
602/864–1300
Contact: Carol Parks-Sherer, Exec. Dir.

Assn. for Retarded Citizens/AZ
5610 South Central
Phoenix, AZ 85040
602/243–1787
Contact: Patricia Brown, Exec. Dir.

Pilot Parent Partnerships
2150 E. Highland Ave., #105
Phoenix, AZ 85016
602/468–3001
Contact: Mary Slaughter, Exec. Dir.

Easter Seal Society of Arizona
903 N. Second Street
Phoenix, AZ 85004
602/252–6061
Contact: Del Black, Exec. Dir.

ARKANSAS

Special Education/Dept. of Education
Education Bldg., Room 105–C
No. 4 Capitol Mall
Little Rock, AR 72201
501/682–4221
Contact: Diane Sydoriak, Assoc. Dir.

Div. of Rehabilitation Svcs.
Dept. of Human Services

7th and Main Sts.
300 Donaghey Plaza, N.
Little Rock, AR 72203
501/682–6708
Contact: Bobby Simpson, Deputy Dir.

Div. of DD Services
Dept. of Human Services
P.O. Box 1437, Waldon Bldg.
7th and Main Sts., 5th Fl.
Little Rock, AR 72203–1437
501/682–8662
Contact: Ann Majure, Deputy Dir.

Governor's DD Planning Council
Ariz. Health Planning & Dev. Agency
4815 W. Markham St.
Little Rock, AR 72201–3866
501/661–2399
Contact: Patsy Fordyce, Dir.

Advocacy Services, Inc.
1120 Marshall St., Ste. 311
Little Rock, AR 72202
501/371–2171
Contact: Nan Ellen East, Exec. Dir.

UCP of Central Arkansas
10400 W. 36th St.
Little Rock, AR 72204
501/224–6067
Contact: Edmond A. Benton, Exec. Dir.

Assn. for Retarded Citizens/AR
Union Station Square, S–406
Little Rock, AR 72201
501/375–4464
Contact: Nancy Sullivan, Exec. Dir.

Arkansas Disability Coalition
519 E. Capitol
Little Rock, AR 72202
501/376–3420
Contact: Bonnie Johnson, Dir.

FOCUS, Inc.
2917 King St., Ste. C
Jonesboro, AR 72401
501/935–2750
Contact: Barbara Semrau

Parent-to-Parent
Union Station Square, Ste. 412
Little Rock, AR 72201
501/375–4464
Contact: Sheri Cobb, Coordinator

Arkansas Easter Seal Society
2801 Lee Avenue
P.O. Box 5148
Little Rock, AR 72225
501/663–8331
Contact: James Butler, Exec. Dir.

CALIFORNIA

Special Education
Dept. of Education
P.O. Box 944272, Room 610
Sacramento, CA 95814
916/323–4768
Contact: Patrick Campbell, Dir.

Dept. of Rehabilitation
Health and Welfare Agency
830 K St. Mall
Sacramento, CA 95814
916/445–3971
Contact: P. Cecilio Fontanoza, Dir.

Dept. of Developmental Services
Health and Welfare Agency
1600 9th St., N.W., 2nd Fl.
Sacramento, CA 95814
916/323–3131
Contact: Gary Macomber, Dir.

State Council on Dev. Disabilities
200 O St., Room 100
Sacramento, CA 95814
916/322–8481
Contact: James Bellotti, Exec. Dir.

CA Protection & Advocacy
100 Howe St., Ste. 185N
Sacramento, CA 95825
916/488–9950; 800/952–5746 (in CA)

UCP of California
1507 21st St., Room 204
Sacramento, CA 95814

415/348–1641
Contact: Lou Kuehner, Exec. Dir.

Assn. for Retarded Citizens/CA
1510 J St., Ste. 180
Sacramento, CA 95814
916/441–3322
Contact: Frederic Hougardy, Exec. Dir.

Team of Advocates for Special Kids
(TASK)
18685 Santa Inez
Fountain Valley, CA 92708
714/962–6332
Contact: Joan Tellefsen, Dir.

Parents Helping Parents
535 Race St., Ste. 220
San Jose, CA 95126
408/288–5010
Contact: Florene Poyadue

Easter Seal Society of the Bay Area
6221 Geary Street
San Francisco, CA 94121
415/752–4888
Contact: Stan Hutton, Exec. Dir.

COLORADO

Special Education Services Unit
Dept. of Education
201 E. Colfax Ave.
Denver, CO 80203
303/866–6694
Contact: Brian McNulty, Exec. Dir.

Division of Rehabilitation
Dept. of Social Services
1575 Sherman St., 4th Fl.
Denver, CO 80203
303/866–2866
Contact: Anthony Francavilla, Dir.

Division for Dev. Disabilities
3824 West Princeton Circle
Denver, CO 80236
303/762–4550
Contact: Sheila Aderman, Acting Dir.

Colorado Dev. Disabilities Council
777 Grant St., Ste. 410

Denver, CO 80203–3518
303/894–2345
Contact: William L. Gorman, Exec. Dir.

The Legal Center
455 Sherman St., Ste. 130
Denver, CO 80203
303/722–0300
Contact: Mary Anne Harvey, Exec. Dir.

UCP of Denver
2727 Columbine St.
Denver, CO 80205
303/355–7337
Contact: Raymond Baldwin, Exec. Dir.

Assn. for Retarded Citizens/CO
4155 E. Jewell Ave., Ste. 916
Denver, CO 80222
303/756–7234
Contact: Jeff Strully, Exec. Dir.

PEAK Parent Center
6055 Lehman Dr., Ste. 101
Colorado Springs, CO 80918
719/531–9400; 800/284–0251 (in CO)
Contact: Judy Martz & Barbara Buswell, Co-Directors

Colorado Easter Seal Society
5755 W. Alameda Avenue
Lakewood, CO 80226
303/233–1666

CONNECTICUT

Bureau of Special Educ. & Pupil Personnel Svcs.
Dept. of Education
25 Industrial Park Rd.
Middletown, CT 06457
203/638–4265
Contact: Tom B. Gillung, Bureau Chief

Div. of Rehabilitation Services
Board of Education
10 Griffin Rd. North
Windsor, CT 06195
Contact: Marilyn Cambell, Division Dir.

Dept. of Mental Retardation
90 Pitkin St.
East Hartford, CT 06108
203/528–7141
Contact: Brian Lensink, Commissioner

DD Council
90 Pitkin St.
East Hartford, CT 06108
203/725–3829
Contact: Edward T. Prenata, Dir.

Office of Protection & Advocacy for
Handicapped & DD Persons
60 Weston St.
Hartford, CT 06120–1551
203/297–4300; 800–842–7303 (in CT)
Contact: Eliot J. Dober, Exec. Dir.

UCP of Connecticut
130 Hunting St.
Bridgeport, CT 06606
203/229–3351
Contact: Barry Buxbaum, Exec. Dir.

Assn. for Retarded Citizens/CT
45 S. Main St.
West Hartford, CT 06107
203/233–3629
Contact: Margaret Dignoti, Exec. Dir.

Conn. Parent Advocacy Center (CPAC)
P.O. Box 579
East Lyme, CT 06333
203/739–3089; 800/445–2722 (in CT)
Contact: Nancy Prescott, Dir.

Parent-to-Parent
Univ. of CT/Dept. of Pediatrics
The Exchange
Farmington, CT 06032
203/674–1485
Contact: Molly P. Cole

WeCAHR
11 Lake Ave. Ext.
Danbury, CT 06811
203/792–3540
Contact: Pat Tompka, Coord.

Easter Seal Society of Connecticut
P.O. Box 100
147 Jones St.
Hebron, CT 06248-0100
203/228–9438
Contact: John Quinn, Pres.

DELAWARE

Exceptional Children Special Programs
Division
Dept. of Public Instruction
P.O. Box 1402
Dover, DE 19903
302/736–5471
Contact: Carl M. Haltom, State Dir.

Div. of Vocational Rehabilitation
Dept. of Labor
321 E. 11th St.
Wilmington, DE 19801
302/571–2851
Contact: Anthony Sokolowski, Dir.

Division of Mental Retardation
Dept. of Health & Social Svcs.
Robins Building
802 Silver Lake Blvd., Walker Rd.
Dover, DE 19901
302/736–4386
Contact: Thomas Pledgie, Dir.

DD Planning Council
Priscilla Bldg.
156 S. State St.
Dover, DE 19901
302/736–4456
Contact: James F. Linehan, Administrator

Disabilities Law Program
144 E. Market St.
Georgetown, DE 19947
302/856–0038
Contact: Christine Long, Administrator

UCP of Delaware
240 N. James St., Ste. B–3
Newport, DE 19804

302/996–9494
Contact: William McCool III, Exec.
   Dir.

Assn. for Retarded Citizens/DE
Tower Office Park
240 N. James St.
Suite B–2
Wilmington, DE 19804
302/996–9400
Contact: Rita Mariani, Exec. Dir.

Parent Info. Center of Delaware (PIC)
700 Barksdale Rd., Ste. 6
Newark, DE 19711
302/366–0152
Contact: Marie-Anne Aghazadian,
   Exec. Dir.

Easter Seal Society of Del-Mar
Tower Office Park
240 N. James St., Ste. 100
Wilmington, DE 19804
302/998–8090
Contact: Sandra Kother, Exec. Dir.

DISTRICT OF COLUMBIA

Div. of Special Education & Pupil Personnel Services
DC Public Schools
10th & H Sts., NW
Washington, DC 20001
202/724–4018
Contact: Doris A. Woodson, Asst. Su-
   perintendent

Vocational Rehab. Svcs. Admin.
Dept. of Human Resources
605 G St., NW
Washington, DC 20001
202/727–3227
Contact: Katherine Williams, Admin.

Dept. of Human Services
Dev. Disabilities Admin.
409 O St., NW
Washington, DC 20001
202/673–7678
Contact: Reginal Wells, Administrator

D.C. DD Planning Council
605 G St., NW, Room 1120
Washington, DC 20024
202/727–4034
Contact: Les Bernard, Acting Dir.

Information, Protection & Advocacy
   Center for Handicapped Individuals
   (IPACHI)
300 I St., NE, Ste. 202
Washington, DC 20002
202/547–8081
Contact: Yetta W. Galiber, Exec. Dir.

UCP of Washington, DC/Northern VA
3135 8th St., NE
Washington, DC 20017
202/269–1500
Contact: Stanley Pryor, Exec. Dir.

ARC/DC
900 Varnum St., NE
Washington, DC 20017
202/636–2950
Contact: Vincent Gray

Parents Reaching Out Services
Shaw-Terrell Community Ctr.
1st & Pierce St., N.W.
Washington, D.C. 20003
202/727–5404
Contact: Gloria Stokes, Dir.

Easter Seal Society
The Children's Center
2800 13th St., NW
Washington, DC 20009
202/232–2342
Contact: Nancy Marconi, Exec. Dir.

FLORIDA

Bureau of Education for Exceptional
   Students
Dept. of Education
Knott Bldg.
Tallahassee, FL 32399
904/488–1570
Contact: Bob Connors, Director

Div. of Vocational Rehabilitation
Dept. of Labor & Employment Security
1709–A Mahan Dr.
Tallahassee, FL 32399
904/488–6210
Contact: Calvin Melton, Dir.

Dept. of Health & Rehab. Svcs.
1311 Winewood Blvd.
Building 5, Room 215
Tallahassee, FL 32301
904/488–4257
Contact: Kingsley Ross, Asst. Secretary

Florida DD Planning Council
1317 Winewood Blvd.
Building 1, #309
Tallahassee, FL 32301
904/488–4180
Contact: Joseph Krieger, Dir.

Advocacy Center for Persons with Disabilities
2661 Exec. Center, Circle W.
Clifton Bldg., Ste. 209
Tallahassee, FL 32301
904/488–9070
Contact: Jonathan Rossman, Exec. Dir.

UCP of Florida
1605 E. Plaza Dr., Ste. 8
Tallahassee, FL 32308
Contact: Heather Moore, State Coordinator

Assn. for Retarded Citizens/FL
411 E. College Ave.
Tallahassee, FL 32301
904/681–1931
Contact: Chris Schuh

Parent Education Network of FL
  (PEN)
1211 Tech Blvd., Ste. 105
Tampa, FL 33619–7833
813/623–4088; 800/825–5736
Contact: Janet Jacoby, Project Manager

Parent to Parent of Florida
3500 E. Fletcher Ave., Ste. 225
Tampa, FL 33612

813/974–5001
Contact: Susan Duwa

Florida Easter Seal Society
1010 Executive Center Dr.
Suite 101
Orlando, FL 32803
407/896–7881
Contact: Robert Griggs, Exec. Dir.

GEORGIA

Program for Exceptional Students
Dept. of Education
1970 Twin Towers East
205 Butler St.
Atlanta, GA 30334
404/656–2425
Contact: Joan A. Jordan, Director

Div. of Rehabilitation Services
Dept. of Human Resources
878 Peachtree St., NE, Rm. 706
Atlanta, GA 30309
404/894–6670
Contact: Darlene Taylor, Dir.

Mental Retardation Services
Div. of Mental Health/Mental Retarda-
  tion
Dept. of Human Resources
878 Peachtree St., NE
Atlanta, GA 30309
404/894–6313
Contact: Charles Kimber, Deputy Dir.

Governor's Council on Dev. Disabilities
878 Peachtree St., NE, Rm. 620
Atlanta, GA 30309–3917
404/894–5790
Contact: Zebe Schmitt, Exec. Dir.

Georgia Advocacy Office
1708 Peachtree St., NW, Ste. 505
Atlanta, GA 30309
404/885–1234; 800/537–2329
Contact: Pat Powell, Exec. Dir.

UCP of Greater Atlanta
1687 Tullie Circle, NE
Suite 112

Atlanta, GA 30329
Contact: Barbara Sachs, Exec. Dir.

Assn. for Retarded Citizens/GA
1851 Ram Runway, Ste. 104
College Park, GA 30337
404/761–3150
Contact: Pat Smith, Exec. Dir.

Parents Educating Parents (PEP)
Georgia ARC
1851 Ram Runway, Ste. 102
College Park, GA 30337
404/761–2745
Contact: Cheryl Knight, Project Dir.

Parent to Parent of Georgia
1644 Tullie Circle, NE
Atlanta, GA 30329
404/451–5484
Contact: Cathy Spraetz, Exec. Dir.

Georgia Easter Seal Society
2030 Powers Ferry Road
Suite 140
Atlanta, GA 30339
404/980–9033
Contact: J. Douglas Hillhouse, Exec.
Dir.

HAWAII

Special Education Section
Dept. of Education
3430 Leahi Ave.
Honolulu, HI 96815
808/737–3720
Contact: Margaret Donovan, Administrator

Vocational Rehab. & Svcs. for the Blind
Dept. of Social Services
P.O. Box 339
Honolulu, HI 96809
808/548–4769
Contact: Toshio Nishioka, Administrator

Developmentally Disabled Division
741A Sunset Ave.
Honolulu, HI 96816

808/732–0935
Contact: Ethel Yamane, Chief

State Planning Council on Developmental Disabilities
500 Ala Moana Blvd.
Honolulu, HI 96813
808/548–8482
Contact: Diana Tizard, Dir.

Protection and Advocacy Agency
1580 Makaloa St., Ste. 1060
Honolulu, HI 96814
808/949–2922
Contact: Patty Henderson, Exec. Dir.

UCP of Hawaii
245 N. Kukui St.
Suite 207
Honolulu, HI 96817
Contact: Donna Fouts, Exec. Dir.

Assn. for Retarded Citizens/HI
3989 Diamond Head Rd.
Honolulu, HI 96816
808/737–7995
Contact: Ahmad Saidin, Exec. Dir.

Assisting with Appropriate Rights in
Education (AWARE)
200 N. Vineyard Blvd., Ste. 103
Honolulu, HI 96817
808/536–9684
Contact: Ivalee Sinclair, Project Director

Special Parent Information Network
335 Merchant St., Rm. 353
Honolulu, HI 96813
808/548–2648

Easter Seal Society of Hawaii
710 Green Street
Honolulu, HI 96813
808/536–1015
Contact: P. Lee Mason, Chief Exec. Officer

IDAHO

Special Education
Dept. of Education

650 W. State St.
Boise, ID 83720–0001
208/334–3940
Contact: Vickie Simmons, Supervisor

Div. of Vocational Rehabilitation
State Board for Vocational Education
650 W. State St., Rm. 150
Boise, ID 83720
208/334–3390
Contact: George J. Pelletier, Administrator

Bureau of Developmental Disabilities
Div. of Community Rehabilitation
Dept. of Health and Welfare
450 W. State, 10th Fl.
Boise, ID 83720
208/334–5531
Contact: Paul Swatsenbarg, Chief

Idaho State Planning Council on DD
450 W. State
Boise, ID 83720–0001
208/334–5509
Contact: John D. Watts, Exec. Dir.

Idaho's Coalition of Advocates for the
  Disabled
1409 W. Washington St.
Boise, ID 83702
208/336–5353
Contact: Brent Marchbanks, Dir.

UCP of ID
5530 Emerald Rd.
Boise, ID 83706
Contact: Janet Atkinson, Exec. Dir.

Idaho Parents Unlimited (IPUL)
1365 N. Orchard, #107
Boise, ID 83706
208/377–8049
Contact: Martha Gilgen

ILLINOIS

Special Education
State Board of Education
Mail Code E–216
100 N. First St.

Springfield, IL 62777–0001
217/782–6601
Contact: Gail Liberman, Director

Dept. of Rehabilitation Services
State Board of Vocational Education
  and Rehabilitation
623 E. Adams St.
P.O. Box 19429
Springfield, IL 62794
217/785–0218
Contact: Philip C. Bradley, Director

Dept. of Mental Health & DD
402 Station Office Building
Springfield, IL 62706
217/782–7395
Contact: William Murphy, Deputy Dir.

Illinois Council on DD
State of IL Center
100 W. Randolph 10–601
Chicago, IL 60601
312/814–2080
Contact: Cathy Ficker Terrill, Dir.

Protection & Advocacy
175 W. Jackson Blvd., Ste. A–2103
Chicago, IL 60604
312/341–0022
Contact Zena Naiditch, Dir.

UCP of Illinois
3 W. Old State Capital Plaza
Springfield, IL 62701
217/789–0390
Contact: Barbara Esela, Exec. Dir.

Assn. for Retarded Citizens/IL
Printer's Square
700 S. Federal St., Ste. 123
Chicago, IL 60605
312/922–6932
Contact: Steven Laubacher, Exec. Dir.

Coordinating Council for Handicapped
  Children
20 E. Jackson Blvd., Rm. 900
Chicago, IL 60604
312/939–3513
Contact: Charlotte Des Jardins, Director

Designs for Change
220 S. State St., Rm. 1900
Chicago, IL 60604
312/922–0317
Contact: Donald Moore, Director

Direction Service of Illinois
730 E. Vine, Room 107
Springfield, IL 62703
217/523–1232; 800/634–8540 (in IL)
Contact: Merle Wallace

Illinois Alliance for Exceptional
   Children and Adults
2005 Clover Lane
Champaign, IL 61821
217/359–5345
Contact: Alice Kelly, President

Illinois Easter Seal Society
2715 S. 4th St.
Springfield, IL 62705
217/525–0398
Contact: Jim Gray, Exec. Dir.

INDIANA

Div. of Special Education
Dept. of Education
Room 229, State House
Indianapolis, IN 46204
317/232–0570
Contact: Paul Ash, State Director

Div. of Vocational Rehabilitation
Dept. of Human Services
251 N. Illinois St.
P.O. Box 7083
Indianapolis, IN 46207
317/232–1139
Contact: Gary Mott, Acting Dir.

Div. of Developmental Disabilities
Dept. of Mental Health
117 E. Washington St.
Indianapolis, IN 46204–3647
317/232–7836
Contact: Josef Reum, Commissioner

Governor's Planning Council on DD
143 W. Market St., Ste. 404

Indianapolis, IN 46204
317/232–7770
Contact: Suellen Jackson-Boner, Dir.

Indiana Advocacy Services
850 N. Meridian St., Ste. 2–C
Indianapolis, IN 46204
317/232–1150; 800/622–4845
Contact: Mary Lou Haynes, Exec. Dir.

UCP of Indiana
445 N. Pennsylvania St.
Indianapolis, IN 46204
Contact: Michael Gallagher, Exec. Dir.

Assn. for Retarded Citizens/IN
110 E. Washington St., 9th Fl.
Indianapolis, IN 46204
317/632–4387
Contact: John Dickerson, Exec. Dir.

Task Force on Education for the Handicapped
833 Northside Blvd., Bldg. #1 REAR
South Bend, IN 46617
219/234–7101; 800/332–4433 (in IN)
Contact: Richard Burden, Exec. Dir.

Indiana Parent Information Network
2107 E. 65th St.
Indianapolis, IN 46220
317/232–2291
Contact: Donna Olson

Indiana Easter Seal Society
3816 E. 96th Street
Indianapolis, IN 46240
317/844–7919
Contact: Richard Janishewski, Pres.

IOWA

Special Education Director
Dept. of Public Instruction
Grimes State Office Building
Des Moines, IA 50319–0146
515/281–3176
Contact: Frank Vance

Div. of Vocational Rehab. Services
Dept. of Public Instruction
510 E. 12th St.

Des Moines, IA 50319
515/281–4154
Contact: Jerry Starkweather, Administrator

Div. of Mental Health Resources
Dept. of Social Services
Hoover State Office Building
Des Moines, IA 50319
515/281–6003
Contact: Sally Cunningham, Acting Dir.

Governor's Planning Council for DD
Dept. of Human Services
Hoover State Office Bldg., 5th Fl.
Des Moines, IA 50319–0001
515/281–7632
Contact: Karon Perlowski, Council
    Coordinator

Iowa Protection and Advocacy Service
3015 Merle Hay Rd., Ste. 6
Des Moines, IA 50310
515/278–2502
Contact: Mervin L. Roth, Dir.

UCP of Iowa
Shops Building, Ste. 306
Des Moines, IA 50309
Contact: Jane I. Butler, Exec. Dir.

Assn. for Retarded Citizens/IA
715 E. Locust
Des Moines, IA 50309
515/283–2358
Contact: Mary Etta Lane, Exec. Dir.

Iowa Exceptional Parents Center
    (IEPC)
33 N. 12th St.
P.O. Box 1151
Fort Dodge, IA 50501
515/576–5870
Contact: Carla Lawson, Dir.

Easter Seal Society of Iowa
Highland Park Station
P.O. Box 4002
Des Moines, IA 50333
515/289–1933
Contact: Rolfe Karlsson, Exec. Dir.

KANSAS

Special Education
Dept. of Education
120 E. 10th St.
Topeka, KS 66612
913/296–4945
Contact: James E. Marshall, Director

Rehabilitation Services
Dept. of Social and Rehab. Svcs.
300 SW Oakley, 2nd Fl.
Topeka, KS 66606
913/296–3911
Contact: Gabriel Faimon, Commissioner

Community Programs
Dept. of Social and Rehab. Svcs.
State Office Bldg., 5th Fl.
Topeka, KS 66612
913/296–3471
Contact: Rick Schults, Director

Kansas Planning Council on DD Svcs.
Dept. of Social & Rehab. Svcs.
State Office Bldg., 5th Fl. North
Topeka, KS 66612
913/296–2608
Contact: John Kelly, Exec. Dir.

Kansas Advocacy & Protection Svcs.
513 Leavenworth St., Ste. 2
Manhattan, KS 66502
913/776–1541; 800/432–8276
Contact: Joan Strickler, Exec. Dir.

UCP of Kansas
P.O. Box 8217
Wichita, KS 67208
Contact: Dave Jones, Exec. Dir.

Assn. for Retarded Citizens/KS
P.O. Box 676
Hays, KS 67601

Families Together
3601 Sw 29th St., Ste. 127
Topeka, KS 66614
913/273–6343
Contact: Patricia Gerdel, Director

Family Together
1111 W. 59th Terrace
Shawnee, KS 66203
913/268–8200
Contact: Brent Glazier, Exec. Dir.

Goodwill Industries/Easter Seal Society
   of Kansas
P.O. Box 8169
Wichita, KS 67208
316/744–9291
Contact: Marie Abney, Exec. Dir.

KENTUCKY

Dept. of Education
Office of Education for Exceptional
   Children
Capitol Plaza Tower, Rm. 820
Frankfort, KY 40601
502/564–4970
Contact: Linda Hargan, State Dir.

Office of Vocational Rehab.
Dept. of Education
Capitol Plaza Tower, 9th Fl.
Frankfort, KY 40601
502/564–4566
Contact: Carroll Burchett, Assoc. Super-
   intendent

Div. of Mental Retardation
Dept. for Mental Health & Mental
   Retardation Svcs.
275 E. Main
Frankfort, KY 40621
502/564–7700
Contact: Charlie Bratcher, Director

Kentucky DD Planning Council
Dept. for Mental Health & Mental
   Retardation Svcs.
275 E. Main St.
Frankfort, KY 40621–0001
502/564–7841
Contact: Prudence Moore, Dir.

Office for Public Advocacy
Division for P&A
Perimeter Park West
1264 Louisville Rd.

Frankfort, KY 40601
502/564–2967; 800/372–2988 (in KY)
Contact Gayla Peach, Dir.

UCP of Eastern Kentucky
Diniaco Ct., P.O. Box 413
Ashland, KY 41105–0413
Contact: Mary Lou Strait, Exec. Dir.

Assn. for Retarded Citizens/KY
833 E. Main
Frankfort, KY 40601
502/875–5225
Contact: Patty Dempsey, Exec. Dir.

Kentucky Special Parent Involvement
   Network (KY-SPIN)
318 W. Kentucky St.
Louisville, KY 40203
502/589–5717; 800/525–7746
Contact: Paulette Logsdon, Dir.

Directions Service Center
Blue Grass Area Chapter
1450 Newtown Pike
Lexington, KY 40511
606/233–9370
Contact: Jenny Mayberry, Director

Kentucky Easter Seal Society
233 E. Broadway
Louisville, KY 40202
502/584-9781
Contact: Guion Miller, Exec. Dir.

LOUISIANA

Dept. of Education
Special Education Services
P.O. Box 94064, 9th Fl.
Baton Rouge, LA 70804–9064
504/342–3633
Contact: Walter Gatlin, Dir.

Division of Vocational Rehab.
Office of Human Development
1755 Florida Blvd.
P.O. Box 94371
Baton Rouge, LA 70804
504/342–2285
Contact: Alton Toms, Director

Office of Mental Retardation
Office of Human Service
Box 3117, Bin 21., Rm. 308
Baton Rouge, LA 70821–3117
504/342–0095
Contact: Jerry Vincent, Deputy Asst.
Sec.

State Planning Council on DD
P.O. Box 3455
Baton Rouge, LA 70802–6029
504/342–6804
Contact: Anne L. Farber, Exec. Officer

Advocacy Center for the Elderly & Disabled
210 O'Keefe, Ste. 700
New Orleans, LA 70112
504/522–2337; 800/662–7705 (in LA)
Contact: Lois Simpsom, Exec. Dir.

UCP of Louisiana
2380 Barataria Blvd., Ste. 5
Marreno, LA 70072
Contact: John Paul Gustin, Exec. Dir.

Assn. for Retarded Citizens/LA
658 St. Louis St.
Baton Rouge, LA 70802
504/383–0742
Contact: Ben Brooks, Exec. Dir.

Project PROMPT
1500 Edwards Ave., Suite O
Harahan, LA 70123
504/734–7736
Contact: Sharon Duda, Dir.

Parent Linc
200 Henry Clay Ave.
New Orleans, LA 70118
504/896–9268
Contact: John Hill

Easter Seal Society of Louisiana
4937 Hearst Plaza
Suite 2L
Metairie, LA 70001
504/455–5533
Contact: Daniel Underwood, Exec. Dir.

MAINE

Div. of Special Education
Dept. of Education & Cultural Services
State House, Station 23
Augusta, ME 04333
207/289–5953
Contact: David Noble Stockford, Dir.

Bureau of Rehab. Services
Dept. of Health and Welfare
32 Winthrop St.
Augusta, ME 04330
207/289–2266
Contact: Pamela Tetley, Dir.

Dept. of Mental Health & Mental
Retardation
411 State Office Bldg., Station 40
Augusta, ME 04333
207/289–4220
Contact: Ron Welch, Assoc. Commissioner

Maine Dev. Disabilities Council
Nash Bldg., Station 139
Capitol & State Sts.
Augusta, ME 04333
207/289–4213
Contact: Peter Stowell, Exec. Dir.

Maine Advocacy Services
One Grand View Place, Ste. 1
P.O. Box 445
Winthrop, ME 04364
207/377–6202; 800/452–1948
Contact: Laura Petovello, Exec. Dir.

UCP of Northeastern Maine
103 Texas Ave.
Bangor, ME 04401
207/241–2885
Contact: Ruth Shook, Exec. Dir.

Special Needs Parent Information Network (SPIN)
P.O. Box 2067
Augusta, ME 04338–2067
207/582–2504; 800/325–0220 (in ME)
Contact: Deborah Guimont, Director

Easter Seal Society of Maine
84 Front St.
P.O. Box 518
Bath, ME 04530
207/443–3341
Contact: William Haney, Exec. Dir.

MARIANA ISLANDS

Special Education
Lower Basin
Saipan, Mariana Islands 96950
670/322–9956
Contact: Margaret Dela Cruz,
  Coordinator

Vocational Rehabilitation Svcs.
Dr. Torres Hospital
Saipan, Mariana Islands 96950
Contact: Manuel Villagomez, Chief

Developmental Disabilities Council
P.O. Box 2565
Saipan, Mariana Islands 96950
670/322–3014

Catholic Social Services
P.O. Box 745
Saipan, Mariana Islands 96950
670/234–6981

MARYLAND

Division of Special Education
Dept. of Education
200 W. Baltimore St.
Baltimore, MD 21201–2595
301/333–2400
Contact: Richard J. Steinke, State Dir.

Div. of Vocational Rehab.
Dept. of Education
200 W. Baltimore St.
Baltimore, MD 21201
301/333–2294
Contact: James Jeffers

Developmental Disabilities Admin.
Dept. of Health & Mental Hygiene
201 W. Preston St.
O'Connor Bldg., 4th Fl.
Baltimore, MD 21201

301/225–5600
Contact: Lois M. Meszaros, Director

Maryland State Planning Council on
  DD
One Market Place, Box 10
201 W. Preston St.
Baltimore, MD 21201–2323
301/333–3688
Contact: Susan Elrod, Dir.

Maryland Disability Law Center
2510 St. Paul St.
Baltimore, MD 21218
301/333–7600
Contact: Steven Ney, Dir.

UCP of Maryland
1616 Forest Dr.
Annapolis, MD 21403
301/263–9600
Contact: Charlene Hughins-Uhl, Exec.
  Dir.

Assn. for Retarded Citizens/MD
5602 Baltimore Natl. Pike
Suite 200
Baltimore, MD 21228
301/744–0255
Contact: Christine Boswell, Exec. Dir.

Parent Support Network
Infants and Toddlers Program
118 N. Howard, Ste. 608
Baltimore, MD 21201
301/225–4190
Contact: Carol Ann Baglin, Director

Information & Referral
MD State Dept. of Education
200 W. Baltimore St.
Baltimore, MD 21201
301/333–2478; 800/383–6523
Contact: Marjorie Shulbank, Information Specialist

Easter Seal Society of Maryland
3700 4th St.
Baltimore, MD 21225
301/355–0100
Contact: Carol Hudson, Pres.

MASSACHUSETTS

Division of Special Education
Dept. of Education
1385 Hancock St., 3rd Fl.
Quincy, MA 02169–5183
617/770–7468
Contact: Mary Beth Fafard, State Dir.

Mass. Rehab. Commission
Fort Point Place
27–43 Wornwood St.
Boston, MA 02210
617/727–2172
Contact: Elmer C. Bartels, Commissioner

Dept. of Mental Retardation
160 N. Washington St.
Boston, MA 02114
617/727–5608
Contact: Mary McCarthy, Commissioner

Mass. DD Planning Council
600 Washington St., Room 670
Boston, MA 02111–1704
617/727–4178
Contact: Jody Shaw, Exec. Dir.

Disability Law Center
11 Beacon St., Ste. 925
Boston, MA 02108
617/723–8455
Contact: Richard Howard, Exec. Dir.

UCP Assn. of Metropolitan Area
71 Arsenal St.
Watertown, MA 02172
617/926–5480
Contact: Mike Ripple, Exec. Dir.

Assn. for Retarded Citizens/MA
217 South St.
Waltham, MA 02154
617/891–6270
Contact: Philip Campbell, Exec. Dir.

Federation for Children with Special
Needs
95 Berkeley St.

Boston, MA 02116
617/482–2915; 800/331–0688 (in MA)
Contact: Artie Higgins, Director

Parent-to-Parent
1249 Boylston St.
Boston, MA 02215
617/266–4520
Contact: Cindy Politch, Coordinator

Massachusetts Easter Seal Society
Denholm Building
484 Main Street
Worcester, MA 01608
508/757–2756
Contact: Richard LaPierre, Pres.

MICHIGAN

Special Education Services
Dept. of Education
P.O. Box 30008
Lansing, MI 48909–7508
517/373–9433
Contact: State Director

Bureau of Rehabilitation
Dept. of Education
101 Pine St., 4th Fl.
P.O. Box 30010
Lansing, MI 48909
517/373–3391
Contact: Peter P. Griswold, Dir.

Bureau of Residential Svcs. & Center
for Persons with Developmental Disabilities
Dept. of Mental Health
Lewis Cass Bldg., 6th Fl.
Lansing, MI 48913
517/373–6440
Contact: George Garland, Director

Michigan Dev. Disabilities Council
Lewis Cass Bldg., 6th Fl.
Lansing, MI 48926
517/373–0341, 0342
Contact: Elisabeth J. Ferguson, Exec.
Dir.

Michigan P&A Service
109 W. Michigan Ave., Ste. 900
Lansing, MI 48933
517/487–1755
Contact: Elizabeth W. Bauer, Exec. Dir.

UCP of Michigan
320 N. Washington Square, Ste. 60
Lansing, MI 48933
517–482–9496
Contact: Terry Hunt, Exec. Dir.

Assn. for Retarded Citizens/MI
313 S. Washington, Ste. 310
Lansing, MI 48933
517/487–5426
Contact: Marjorie Mitchell, Exec. Dir.

Citizens Alliance to Uphold Special
  Education (CAUSE)
313 S. Washington Sq., Ste. 040
Lansing, MI 48933
517/485–4084; 800/221–9105 (in MI)
Contact: Cheryl Chilcote, Exec. Dir.

Parents Are Experts
17000 West 8 Mile Rd., Ste. 380
Southfield, MI 48075
313–557–5070
Contact: Edith Sharp, Project Coord.

Peer Support Project
530 W. Ionia St., Ste. C
Lansing, MI 48933
517/487–9260
Contact: Mary Marin

Easter Seal Society of Michigan
4065 Saladin Drive, SE
Grand Rapids, MI 49546
616/94–2081
Contact: Susan Quinn, Exec. Dir.

MINNESOTA

Special Education Section
Dept. of Education
812 Capitol Square Bldg.
550 Cedar St.
St. Paul, MN 55101–2233

612/296–1793
Contact: Norena A. Hale, Manager

Div. of Vocational Rehabilitation
Dept. of Jobs and Training
390 N. Robert St., 5th Fl.
St. Paul, MN 55101
612/296–1822
Contact: David Schwartzkopf, Asst.
  Commissioner

Div. for Persons with Dev. Disabilities
Dept. of Human Services
444 Lafayette Rd.
St. Paul, MN 55155–3825
612/296–9139
Contact: Edward Skarnulis, Dir.

Governor's Planning Council on DD
658 Cedar St., Room 300
St. Paul, MN 55101
612/296–4018
Contact: Colleen Wieck, Exec. Dir.

Legal Aid Society of Minneapolis
222 Grain Exchange Bldg.
323 Fourth Ave., South
Minneapolis, MN 55415
612/332–7301
Contact: Steve Scott, Director

UCP of Minnesota
1821 University Ave., Ste. S–233
St. Paul, MN 55104
612/646–7588
Contact: Joan Brintnall, Exec. Dir.

Assn. for Retarded Citizens/MN
3225 Lyndale Ave. South
Minneapolis, MN 55408
612/827–5641
Contact: Sue Aberholden, Exec. Dir.

PACER Center, Inc.
4826 Chicago Ave. South
Minneapolis, MN 55417–1055
612/827–2966; 800/53–PACER (in MN)
Contact: Marge Goldberg, Paula
  Goldberg, Co-Directors

Pilot Parents
201 Ordean Bldg.
Duluth, MN 55802
218/726-4745
Contact: Lynne Frigaard

Goodwill Industries/Easter Seal Society
of Minnesota
2543 Como Avenue
St. Paul, MN 55108
612/646-2591
Contact: James Dreiling, Pres.

MISSISSIPPI

Bureau of Special Services
Dept. of Education
P.O. Box 771
Jackson, MS 39205–0771
601/359–3490
Contact: Carolyn Black, State Director

Dept. of Vocational Rehab.
P.O. Box 1698
Jackson, MS 39215
601/354–6825
Contact: Morris Selby, Director

Bureau of Mental Retardation/Dept. of
Mental Health
1100 Robert E. Lee Bldg.
239 N. Lamar St.
Jackson, MS 39201
601/359–1288
Contact: Roger McMurtry, Dir.

Miss. Dev. Dis. Planning Council
1101 Robert E. Lee Bldg.
Jackson, MS 39201
691/359–1290
Contact: Ed C. Bell, Director

Miss. P&A System for DD
4793 B McWillie Dr.
Jackson, MS 39206
601/981–8207
Contact: Rebecca Floyd, Exec. Dir.

Assn. for Retarded Citizens/MS
2727 Old Canton Rd., Ste. 173
Jackson, MS 39216

601/362–4830
Contact: Linda Bond, Exec. Dir.

Mississippi Parent Advocacy Center
(MS-PAC)
332 New Market Dr.
Jackson, MS 39209
601/922–3210; 800/231–3721 (in MS)
Contact: Anne Presley, Director

Mississippi Parent Network
425 Louisa St.
Pearl, MS 39208
601/932–7743
Contact: Kathy Odle, Director

Mississippi Easter Seal Society
P.O. Box 4958
3226 N. State
Jackson, MS 39216
601/982–7051
Contact: Patricia Weir, Exec. Dir.

MISSOURI

Coordinator of Special Education
Dept. of Elementary and Secondary
Education
P.O. Box 480
Jefferson City, MO 65102
314/751–4909
Contact: John Heskett

Div. of Vocational Rehab.
Dept. of Education
2401 E. McCarty St.
Jefferson City, MO 65101
314/751–3251
Contact: Don L. Gann, Asst. Commissioner

Division of MR/DD
P.O. Box 687
1915 Southridge Dr.
Jefferson City, MO 65102
314/751–4054
Contact: Gary Sluyter, Dir.

MO Planning Council for DD
Dept. of Mental Health
P.O. Box 687

1915 Southridge Dr.
Jefferson City, MO 65102
314/751–4054
Contact: Kay Conklin, Coordinator

MO Protection & Advocacy Service
925 S. Country Club Dr., Unit B–1
Jefferson City, MO 65109
314/893–3333; 800/392–8667 (in MO)
Contact: Cynthia N. Schloss, Director

UCP of Kansas City
106 E. 31st Terrace
Kansas City, MO 64111

UCP of Missouri
925 S. Country Club Dr., Ste. A1
Jefferson City, MO 65101
Contact: Joyce Wardenburg, Exec. Dir.

Missouri Parents Act-MPACT
1722W South Glenstone, Ste. 125
Springfield, MO 65804
417/882–7434; 800/666–7228 (in MO)
Contact: Marianne Toombs, Director

Missouri Parents Act-MPACT
625 Euclid, Ste. 225
St. Louis, MO 63108
314/361–1660; 800/284–6389 (in MO)
Contact Pat Jones, Director

Missouri Easter Seal Society
5025 N. Northrup Ave.
St. Louis, MO 63110
314/664–5025
Contact: Barbara Robinson, Exec. Dir.

MONTANA

Director of Special Education
Office of Public Instruction
State Capitol, Room 106
Helena, MT 59620
406/444–4429
Contact: Robert Runkel

Rehabilitative Svcs. Division
Dept. of Social & Rehab. Svcs.
P.O. Box 4210
Helena, MT 59601
406/444–2590
Contact: Margaret Bullock, Administrator

Dev. Disabilities Planning Council
25 S. Ewing, Rm. 506
Helena, MT 59620
406/449–8325
Contact: Greg Olsen, Director

Montana Advocacy Program
1410 8th Ave.
Helena, MT 59601
406/444–3889
Contact: Kris Bakula, Exec. Dir.

Parents, Let's Unite for Kids (PLUK)
EMC/IHS
1500 N. 30th St.
Billings, MT 59101–0298
406/657–2055
Contact: Kathy Kelker, Director

Northern Rocky Mountain Easter Seal
  Society
4400 Central Avenue
Great Falls, MT 59401
406/761–3680
Contact: Sally Cerny, Pres.

NEBRASKA

Director of Special Education
Dept. of Education
P.O. Box 94987
Lincoln, NE 68509–4987
402/471–2471
Contact: Gary M. Sherman

Div. of Rehabilitation Services
Dept. of Education
P.O. Box 94987
301 Centennial Mall, 6th Fl.
Lincoln, NE 68509
402/471–3645
Contact: Jason D. Andrew, Director

Office of Mental Retardation
Dept. of Public Institutions
P.O. Box 94728
Lincoln, NE 68509
402/471–2851, ex. 5110
Contact: David Evans, Director

Governor's Planning Council on DD
301 Centennial Mall S.
PO. Box 95007
Lincoln, NE 68509
402/471–2330
Contact: Mary Gordon, Director

Nebraska Advocacy Services
522 Lincoln Center Bldg.
215 Centennial Mall South
Lincoln, NE 68508
402/474–3183
Contact: Timothy Shaw, Exec. Dir.

Assn. for Retarded Citizens/NE
521 S. 14th St., Ste. 211
Lincoln, NE 68508
402/475–4407
Contact: Ginger Clubine, Exec. Dir.

Nebraska Parent's Information &
  Training Center
3610 Dodge St.
Omaha, NE 68131
402/346–0525
Contact: Dixie Nickel, Project Director

Pilot Parents
3610 Dodge St.
Omaha, NE 68131
402/346–5220
Contact: Arretta Johnson, Coordinator

Easter Seal Society of Nebraska
3015 N. 90th Street
Suite 6
Omaha, NE 68134
402/571–2162
Contact: Letitia Simmons, Pres.

NEVADA

Director of Special Education
Dept. of Education

400 W. King St., Capitol Complex
Carson City, NV 89710–0004
702/885–3140
Contact: Jane Early, Dir.

Rehabilitation Division
Dept. of Human Resources
State Capitol Complex
505 E. King St.
Carson City, NV 89710
702/885–4440
Contact: Stephen Shaw, Administrator

Mental Hygiene
Mental Retardation Division
Kinkead Bldg., Rm. 403
505 E. King St.
Carson City, NV 89710
702/885–5943
Contact: Brian Lahren, Administrator

DD Council/Dept. of Rehab.
505 E. King St., Rm. 502
Carson City, NV 89710
702/885–4440
Contact: Paul Haugen, Dir.

Office of Protection & Advocacy
2105 Capurro Way, Ste. B
Sparks, NV 89431
702/789–0233; 800/992–5715
Contact: Holli Elder, Project Dir.

UCP of Southern Nevada
1050 E. Sahara, Ste. 412
Las Vegas, NV 89104
Contact: Lonnie James, Exec. Dir.

Assn. for Retarded Citizens/NV
680 S. Bailey St.
Fallon, NV 89406
702/423–4760
Contact: Frank Weinrauch, Exec. Dir.

Project ASSIST
CHANCE Parent Project
3015 Heights Dr.
Reno, NV 89503
702/747–0669 (in Reno); 702/486–6262
  (in Las Vegas)
Contact: Debby Davis, Dir.

Nevada Easter Seal Society
1455 E. Tropicana
Suite 660
Las Vegas, NV 89119
702/739–7771
Contact: Linda Knobloch, Exec. Dir.

NEW HAMPSHIRE

Special Education Bureau
Dept. of Education
101 Pleasant St.
Concord, New Hampshire 03301–3860
603/271–3741
Contact: Robert T. Kennedy, Dir.

Div. of Vocational Rehab.
Dept. of Education
78 Regional Dr., Bldg. JB
Concord, NH 03301
603/271–3471
Contact: Bruce Archambault, Dir.

Div. of Mental Health & Dev. Svcs.
State Office Park South
105 Pleasant St.
Concord, NH 03301
603/271–5013
Contact: Richard Lepore, Asst. Dir.

NH Council on Dev. Disabilities
Concord Center
10 Ferry St., Box 315
Concord, NH 03301
603/271–3236
Contact: Edward Burke, Exec. Dir.

Disabilities Rights Center
P.O. Box 19
Concord, NH 03302–0019
603/228–0432
Contact: Donna Woodfin, Dir.

Assn. for Retarded Citizens/NH
10 Ferry St., Box 4
Concord Center
Concord, NH 03301
603/228–9092
Contact: Christine Nicolleta, Dir.

Parent Information Center
155 Manchester St.
P.O. Box 1422
Concord, NH 03301
603/224–6299
Contact: Judith Raskin, Dir.

Easter Seal Foundation of New
   Hampshire
555 Auburn Street
Manchester, NH 03103
603/623–8863
Contact: Larry Gammon, Pres.

NEW JERSEY

Div. of Special Education
Dept. of Education
225 W. State St.
P.O. Box CN 500
Trenton, NJ 08625–0001
609/633–6833
Contact: Jeffrey Osowski, Dir.

Div. of Vocational Rehab.
Dept. of Labor and Industry
1005 Labor & Industry Bldg., CN 398
John Fitch Plaza
Trenton, NJ 08625
609/292–5987
Contact: Stephen Janick, III, Dir.

Div. of Dev. Disabilities
Dept. of Human Services
2–98 E. State St.
CN 726
Trenton, NJ 08625
609/292–3742
Contact: Robert Nicholas, Dir.

New Jersey DD Council
108–110 N. Broad St., CN 700
Trenton, NJ 08625
609/292–3745
Contact: Catherine Rowan, Exec. Dir.

Dept. of Public Advocate
Office of Advocacy for the DD
Hughes Justice Complex CN 850
Trenton, NJ 08625

609/292–9742; 800/792–8600 (in NJ)
Contact Sarah Mitchell, Dir.

UCP of New Jersey
354 S. Broad St.
Trenton, NJ 08608
609/392–4004
Contact: Myra Ryan, Exec. Dir.

Assn. for Retarded Citizens/NJ
985 Livingston Ave.
North Brunswick, NJ 08902
201/246–2525
Contact: John Scagnelli, Exec. Dir.

Statewide Parent Advocacy Network
(SPAN)
516 North Ave., East
Westfield, NJ 07090
201/654–7726
Contact: Diana Cuthbertson, Exec. Dir.

NJ Self-Help Clearinghouse
St. Clare-Riverside Medical Ctr.
Pocono Rd.
Denville, NJ 07834
201/625–9565; 800/367–6274 (in NJ)
Contact Edward Madara, Dir.

Easter Seal Society of New Jersey
32 Ford Avenue
P.O. Box 155
Milltown, NJ 08850
201/247–8353
Contact: Brain Fitzgerald, Pres.

NEW MEXICO

Special Education
Dept. of Education
300 Don Gaspar Ave.
Santa Fe, NM 87501–2786
505/827–6541
Contact: Jim Newby, State Director

Div. of Vocational Rehab.
Dept. of Education
604 W. San Mateo
Santa Fe, NM 87503
505/827–3511
Contact: Ross Sweat, Dir.

Developmental Disabilities Bureau
Health & Environment Dept.
1190 St. Francis Dr.
Santa Fe, NM 87501
505/827–2578
Contact: Steve Dossey, Chief

New Mexico DD Planning Council
2025 Pacheco St., Ste. 200-B
Santa Fe, NM 87505
505/827–2707
Contact: Chris Isengard, Dir.

Protection & Advocacy System
1720 Louisiana Blvd., NE, Ste. 204
Albuquerque, NM 87110
505/256–3100; 800/432–4682 (in NM)
Contact James Jackson, Exec. Dir.

Assn. for Retarded Citizens/NM
8210 La Mirada, NE, Ste. 500
Albuquerque, NM 87109
505/298–6796
Contact: John Foley, Exec. Dir.

Project Adobe
Parents Reaching Out (PRO)
1127 University Blvd., NE
Albuquerque, NM 87102
505/842–9045; 800/524–5176 (in NM)
Contact: Sallie Van Curie, Exec. Dir.

Education for Parents of Indian
    Children with Special Needs
P.O. Box 788
Bernalillo, NM 87004
505/867–3396
Contact: Randi Malach, Dir.

Easter Seal Society of New Mexico
2819 Richmond Drive, NE
Albuquerque, NM 87107
505/888–3811
Contact: Tim Taschwer, Pres.

NEW YORK

Dept. of Education
Education of Children with Handicap-
    ping Conditions
Education Bldg. Annex, Rm. 1073

Albany, NY 12234–0001
518/474–5548
Contact: Tom Neveldine, Acting Dir.

Office of Vocational Rehab.
Dept. of Education
99 Washington Ave.
Albany, NY 12230
518/474–2714
Contact: Richard Switzer, Deputy
Comm.

Office of MR/DD
44 Holland Ave.
Albany, NY 12229
518/473–1997
Contact: Arthur Webb, Commissioner

Dev. Disabilities Planning Council
One Empire State Plaza, 10th Fl.
Albany, NY 12223–0001
518/474–3655
Contact: Isabel Mills, Exec. Dir.

NY Comm. on Quality of Care for the
Mentally Disabled
99 Washington Ave.
Albany, NY 12210
518/473–4057
Contact: Clarence Sundram, Commissioner

UCP of New York State
330 W. 34th St.
New York, NY 10001
212/947–5770
Contact: Robert Schonhorn, Exec. Dir.

212/947–5770
NY State Assn. for Retarded Children
393 Delaware Ave.
Delmar, NY 12054
518/439–8311

Parent Network Center
1443 Main St.
Buffalo, NY 14209
716/885–1004
Contact: Joan Watkins, Dir.

Advocates for Children of NY
24–16 Bridge Plaza, South
Long Island, NY 11101
718/729–8866
Contact: Nancy Nevarez

Family Support Project for the DD
North Central Bronx Hospital
3424 Kossuth Ave., Rm. 15A20
Bronx, NY 10467
212/519–4796

New York Easter Seal Society
845 Central Ave.
Albany, NY 12206
518/438-8785

NORTH CAROLINA

Div. for Exceptional Children
Dept. of Public Instruction
Education Bldg., Rm. 442
116 W. Edenton
Raleigh, NC 27603–1712
919/733–3921
Contact: E. Lowell Harris, Dir.

Div. of Vocational Rehab. Svcs.
Dept. of Human Resources
620 N. West St.
P.O. Box 26053
Raleigh, NC 27611
919/733–3364
Contact: Claude Myer, Dir.

Div. of Mental Health/MR Svcs.
Dept. of Human Resources
Albemarle Bldg.
325 N. Salisbury St.
Raleigh, NC 27611
919/733–3654
Contact: Patricia Porter

NC Council on Dev. Disabilities
1508 Western Blvd.
Raleigh, NC 27606–1359
919/733–6566
Contact: James Keene, Exec. Dir.

Governor's Advocacy Council for Persons with Disabilities
1318 Dale St., Ste. 100
Raleigh, NC 27605
919/733–9250
Contact: Lockhart Follin-Mace, Dir.

UCP of North Carolina
P.O. Box 12728
Raleigh, NC 27605
919/832–3787
Contact: James Everest, Exec. Dir.

Assn. for Retarded Citizens/NC
16 Rowan St.
P.O. Box 20545
Raleigh, NC 27619
919/782–4632
Contact: Dave Richard, Exec. Dir.

Exceptional Children's Assistance Ctr.
(ECAC)
P.O. Box 16
Davidson, NC 28036
704/892–1321
Contact: Connie Hawkins, Dir.

Family Support Network
CB #7340 Trailer 31, Daniels Rd.
University of NC at Chapel Hill
Chapel Hill, NC 27599–7340
919/966–2841
Contact: Michael Sharp

Easter Seal Society of North Carolina
2315 Myron Dr.
Raleigh, NC 27607
919/783–8898
Contact: Adele Foschia, Pres.

NORTH DAKOTA

Director of Special Education
Dept. of Public Instruction
State Capitol
Bismarck, ND 58505–0440
701/224–2277
Contact: Gary W. Gronberg

Dept. of Vocational Rehab.
Dept. of Human Services
State Capitol Bldg.
Bismarck, ND 58505
701/224–2907
Contact: Gene Hysjulien, Dir.

Dev. Disabilities Division
Dept. of Human Services
600 E. Boulevard Ave.
State Capitol Bldg., Judicial Wing
Bismarck, ND 58505
701/224–3242
Contact: Sandra Noble, Dir.

Developmental Disabilities Council
Dept. of Human Services
State Capitol
Bismarck, ND 58505
701/224–2970
Contact: Tom Wallner, Dir.

Protection & Advocacy Project
State Capitol
600 E. Blvd.
Judicial Wing, 1st Fl.
Bismarck, ND 58505
701/224–2972; 800/472–2670 (in ND)
Contact: Barbara C. Braun, Dir.

Assn. for Retarded Citizens/ND
417 ½ E. Broadway, No. 9
P.O. Box 2776
Bismarck, ND 58502
701/223–5349
Contact: Jac L. Bye, Exec. Dir.

Pathfinder Parent Ctr.
16th St. & 2nd Ave., SW
Arrowhead Shopping Center
Minot, ND 58701
701/852–9426
Contact: Kathryn Erickson, Dir.

Easter Seal Society of North Dakota
Box 1206
Bismark, ND 58554
701/663–6828
Contact: Dan Ulmer, Exec. Dir.

OHIO

Division of Special Education
State Dept. of Education
933 High St.
Worthington, OH 43085–4017
614/466–2650
Contact: Frank E. New, Director

Rehab. Services Commission
400 E. Campus View Blvd.
Columbus, OH 43235
614/438–1210
Contact: Robert Rabe, Administrator

Dept. of Mental Retardation/Dev. Disabilities
State Office Tower
30 E. Broad St., Rm. 1280
Columbus, OH 43224
614/466–5214
Contact: Robert E. Brown, Dir.

Ohio DD Planning Council
Dept. of MR/DD
8 E. Long St.
Atlas Bldg., 6th Fl.
Columbus, OH 43215
614–466–5205
Contact: Ken Campbell, Exec. Dir.

Ohio Legal Rights Service
8 E. Long St., 6th Fl.
Columbus, OH 43215
614/466–7264; 800/282–9181 (in OH)
Contact: Carolyn Knight, Exec. Dir.

UCP of Ohio
P.O. Box 14780
Columbus, OH 43214
614–262–0289
Contact: Francis McCaffrey, Exec. Dir.

Ohio Assn. for Retarded Citizens
360 S. 3rd St., Ste. 101
Columbus, OH 43215
614/228–4412
Contact: Carolyn Sidwell, Exec. Dir.

Ohio Coalition for the Education of Handicapped Children
933 High St., Ste. 106
Worthington, OH 43085
614/431–1307
Contact: Margaret Burley, Exec. Dir.

Tri-State Organized Coalition for Persons with Disabilities
106 Wellington Place, Lower Level
Cincinnati, OH 45219
Contact: Cathy Heizman, Exec. Dir.

Ohio Easter Seal Society
2204 S. Hamilton Rd.
P.O. Box 32462
Columbus, OH 4323–0462
614/868–9126
Contact: Sheila Dunn, Exec. Dir.

OKLAHOMA

Special Education Division
Dept. of Education
Oliver Hodge Memorial Bldg., Rm. 215
Oklahoma City, OK 73105–4599
405/521–3352
Contact: Connie Siler, State Director

Dept. of Human Services
Div. of Rehab. & Visual Services
P.O. Box 25352
Oklahoma City, OK 73125
405/424–4311, ex. 2873
Contact: Jerry Dunlap, Asst. Dir.

Developmental Disabilities Svcs.
Dept. of Human Services
P.O. Box 25352
Oklahoma City, OK 73125
405/521–3571
Contact: Eranell McIntosh-Wilson, Administrator

Oklahoma Planning Council/DD
Will Rogers Bldg., Rm. 307
P.O. Box 25352
Oklahoma City, OK 73125
405/521–4985
Contact: Ms. Pat Burns, Dir.

Protection & Advocacy Agency for DD
9726 E. 42nd St.
Osage Building, Room 133
Tulsa, OK 74146
918/664–5883
Contact: Bob M. VanOsdol, Dir.

UCP of Oklahoma
1917 S. Harvard Ave.
Oklahoma City, OK 73128
405/681–9611
Contact: Director

Parents Reaching Out in OK (PRO-Oklahoma)
1917 S. Harvard Ave.
Oklahoma City, OK 73128
405/681–9710; 800/PL94–142 (in OK)
Contact: Connie Motsinger, Dir.

Positive Reflections
6141 NW Grand, Ste. 103
Oklahoma City, OK 73116
405/843–9114
Contact: Dana Baldridge, Nancy Thompson

OK Areawide Service Info. System (OASIS) for the Handicapped
Children's Hospital of OK
Nicholson Tower, Rm. 360
940 NE 13th St.
Oklahoma City, OK 73104
800/24–OASIS (in OK)

Oklahoma Easter Seal Society
2100 NW 63rd St.
Oklahoma City, OK 73116
405/848–7603
Contact: Wallace Bonifield, Exec. Dir.

OREGON

Special Education & Student Services Div.
Dept. of Education
700 Pringle Parkway, SE
Salem, OR 97310–0290
503/378–3591
Contact: Karen Brazeau, Assoc. Supt.

Vocational Rehab. Div.
Dept. of Human Resources
2045 Silverton Rd., NE
Salem, OR 97310
503/378–3850
Contact: Joil A. Southwell, Administrator

Program for Mental Retardation & DD
Div. of Mental Health
2575 Bittern St., NE
Salem, OR 97310
503/378–2429
Contact: James D. Toews, Asst. Administrator

Oregon Dev. Disabilities Planning Council
540 24th Place, NE
Salem, OR 97301
503/373–7555
Contact: Russ Gurley, Dir.

Oregon Advocacy Center
Board of Trade Bldg.
310 SW 4th Ave., Ste. 625
Portland, OR 97204–2309
503/243–2081
Contact: Elam Lantz, Jr., Exec. Dir.

UCP of OR
7830 SE Foster Rd.
Portland, OR 97206
503/777–4167
Contact: Bud Thoune, Exec. Dir.

Assn. for Retarded Citizens/OR
1745 State St.
Salem, OR 97301
503/581–2726
Contact: Janna Starr, Exec. Dir.

Oregon COPE Project
999 Locust St., NE, Box B
Salem, OR 97303
503/373–7477
Contact: Cheron Mayhall, Dir.

Easter Seal Society of Oregon
5757 S.W. Macadam Ave.
Portland, OR 97201

503/228–5109
Contact: William Hamilton, Pres.

PENNSYLVANIA

Bureau of Special Education
Dept. of Education
333 Market St.
Harrisburg, PA 17126–0333
717/783–6913
Contact: James Tucker, State Dir.

Bureau of Vocational Rehab.
Dept. of Labor and Industry
Labor and Industry Bldg., Rm. 1300
7th and Forester Sts.
Harrisburg, PA 17120
717/787–5244
Contact: Jay Snyder, Exec. Dir.

Deputy Secretary for Mental Retardation
Dept. of Public Welfare
Health & Welfare Bldg., Rm. 302
Harrisburg, PA 17120
717/787–3700
Contact: Steve Eidelman

Dev. Disabilities Planning Council
Forum Bldg., Rm. 569
Commonwealth Ave.
Harrisburg, PA 17120–0001
717/787–6057
Contact: David B. Schwartz, Exec. Dir.

PA Protection & Advocacy
116 Pine St.
Harrisburg, PA 17101
717/236–8110; 800/692–7443 (in PA)
Contact: Kevin Casey, Exec. Dir.

UCP of PA
925 Linda Lane
Camp Hill, PA 17011
717/761–5656
Contact: Ellen Liversidge, Exec. Dir.

Assn. for Retarded Citizens/PA
123 Forester Place
Harrisburg, PA 17102

717/234–2621
Contact: W.A. West, Exec. Dir.

Parents Union for Public Schools
311 S. Juniper St., Ste. 602
Philadelphia, PA 19107
215/546–1212
Contact: Christine Davis, Dir.

Mentor Parent Program
Rte. 257, Salina Rd.
P.O. Box 718
Seneca, PA 16346
814/676–8615; 800/447–1431
Contact: Gail Walker, Dir.

Parent Education Network
J.F. Kennedy Center
240 Haymeadow Dr.
York, PA 17402
717/845–9722; 800/522–5827 (in PA)

Pennsylvania Easter Seal Society
P.O. Box 497
Middletown, PA 17057-0497
717/939–7801
Contact: Richard Sibert, Dir.

PUERTO RICO

Assistant Secretary of Special Education
Dept. of Education
P.O. Box 759
Hato Rey, PR 00919–0759
809/764–8059
Contact: Lucila Torres Martinez

Div. de Rehabilitacion Vocacional
Departmento de Servicios Sociales
Apartado 1118
Hato Rey, PR 00919
809/725–1792
Contact: Angel Jimenez

Asst. Secretary for Family Services
Dept. of Mental Health
P.O. Box 11398
Santurce, PR 00910
809/723–2127
Contact: Eva Alvarez de Orama

Puerto Rico DD Council
P.O. Box 9543
Santurce, PR 00908–0543
809/722–0595
Contact: Maria Luisa Mendia, Staff Dir.

Ombudsman for the Disabled
Governor's Office, D-A Team Tower
70 Ponce de Leon Ave.
Hato Rey, PR 00918
809/766–2333
Contact: Norma Perez

Asociacion De Padres Pro Bienstar/
Ninos Impedidos de FR
Box 21301
Rio Piedras, PR 00928
809/763–4665
Contact: Carmen Selles Vila, Project
Dir.

Easter Seal Society of Puerto Rico
G.P.O. Box 325
San Juan, PR 00936
809/767–6718
Contact: Nilda Gonzalez, Exec. Dir.

RHODE ISLAND

Special Education Programs
Dept. of Education
Roger Williams Bldg., Rm. 209
22 Hayes St.
Providence, RI 02908–5025
401/277–3505
Contact: Robert Pryhoda, Coordinator

Vocational Rehabilitation
Dept. of Human Services
40 Fountain St.
Providence, RI 02903
401/421–7005
Contact: Sherri Campanelli, Administrator

Div. of Retardation
Dept. of Mental Health, Mental Retar-
dation & Hospitals
Aime J. Forand Bldg.
600 New London Ave.
Cranston, RI 02920

401/464–3234
Contact: Robert Carl, Jr., Exec. Dir.

RI DD Council
600 New London Ave.
Cranston, RI 02920–3028
401/464–3191
Contact: Marie Citrone, Exec. Dir.

Rhode Island P&A System
55 Bradford St., 2nd Fl.
Providence, RI 02903
401/831–3150
Contact: Linda Katz, Exec. Dir.

UCP of RI
500 Prospect St.
Pawtucket, RI 02860
401/728–7800
Contact: Jennifer Ondrejka, Exec. Dir.

Assn. for Retarded Citizens/RI
99 Bald Hill Rd.
Cranston, RI 02920
401/463–9191
Contact: James Healey, Exec. Dir.

Parent to Parent
Rhode Island Dept. of Education
22 Hayes St., Rm. 209
Providence, RI 02908
401/277–3505
Contact: Connie Susa, Parent Training
Spec.

Easter Seal Society of Rhode Island
667 Waterman Avenue
E. Providence, RI 02914
401/438–9500
Contact: Nancy D'Wolf, Exec. Dir.

SOUTH CAROLINA

Office of Programs for the Handicapped
Dept. of Education
100 Executive Center Dr., A–24
Columbia, SC 29201
803/737–8710
Contact: Robert Black, Director

Vocational Rehabilitation Dept.
1410 Boston Ave.

P.O. Box 15
W. Columbia, SC 29171
803/822–4300

Dept. of Mental Retardation
2712 Middleburg Dr., Box 4706
Columbia, SC 29240
803/737–6444
Contact: Philip Massey, Commissioner

SC Dev. Disabilities Planning Council
Edgar Brown Bldg., Rm. 372
1205 Pendleton St.
Columbia, SC 29201
803/758–8016
Contact: LaNelle DuRant, Exec. Dir.

SC P&A System for the Handicapped
3710 Landmark Dr., Ste. 208
Columbia, SC 29204
803/782–0639; 800/933–5225 (in SC)
Contact: Louise Ravenel, Exec. Dir.

Assn. for Retarded Citizens/SC
7412 Fairfield Rd.
Columbia, SC 29203
803/754–4763
Contact: John Beckley, Exec. Dir.

Parents Reaching Out to Parents
220 Great North Rd.
Columbia, SC 29223
803/736–4595
Contact: Sue Slater, Director

Easter Seal Society of SC
3020 Farrow Rd.
Columbia, SC 29203
803/256–0735
Contact: Herman Shealy, Exec. Dir.

SOUTH DAKOTA

Section for Special Education
Richard F. Kneip Bldg.
700 N. Illinois St.
Pierre, SD 57501–2293
605/773–3315
Contact: Dean Myers, State Director

Div. of Rehabilitation Services
700 N. Governors Dr.
Pierre, SD 57501
605/773–3125
Contact: Tim Kuehn, Acting Dir.

Office of Dev. Disabilities and Mental
  Health
Dept. of Social Services
700 Governors Dr.
Pierre, SD 57501
605/773–3438
Contact: Thomas Scheinost, Prog.
  Admin.

South Dakota Advocacy Project
221 S. Central Ave.
Pierre, SD 57501
605/224–8294; 800/742–8108 (in SD)
Contact: Robert J. Kean, Exec. Dir.

UCP of South Dakota
3600 S. Duluth Ave.
Sioux Falls, SD 57105
605/334–4220
Contact: Harvey DeJager, Exec. Dir.

Assn. for Retarded Citizens/SD
P.O. Box 502
Pierre, SD 57501
605/224–8211
Contact: John Stengle, Exec. Dir.

Parent to Parent
Center for Dev. Disabilities
Univ. of SD School of Medicine
414 E. Clark
Vermillion, SD 57069
605/677–5311
Contact: Cecilia Rohusek, Exec. Dir.

Easter Seal Society of SD
106 W. Capitol
Pierre, SD 57501
605/224–5879
Contact: Rose Wendell, Exec. Dir.

TENNESSEE

Special Education Program
Dept. of Education

132 Cordell Hull Bldg.
Nashville, TN 37219
615/741–2851
Contact: Joseph Fisher, Asst. Commissioner

Div. of Vocational Rehab.
Dept. of Human Services
400 Deaderick St., 15th Fl.
Nashville, TN 37219
615/741–2019
Contact: Patsy Mathews, Asst. Commissioner

Dept. of Mental Health & Mental Retardation
The Doctor's Building
706 Church St.
Nashville, TN 37219–5393
615/741–3803
Contact: James G. Foshee

Developmental Disabilities Planning Council
The Doctor's Building, 3rd Fl.
706 Church St.
Nashville, TN 37219–5610
615/741–3807
Contact: Wanda Willis, Director

Effective Advocacy for Citizens with Handicaps (EACH)
P.O. Box 121257
Nashville, TN 37212
615/298–1080; 800/342–1660 (in TN)
Contact: Harriette Derryberry

UCP of the Mid-South
2670 Union Ave., Ste. 500
Memphis, TN 38112
901/323–0190
Contact: Diana Reid, Exec. Dir.

Assn. for Retarded Citizens/TN
1805 Hayes, Ste. 100
Nashville, TN 37203
615/327–0294
Contact: Roger Blue, Exec. Dir.

Support and Training for Exceptional Parents (STEP)
1805 Hayes St., Ste. 100
Nashville, TN 37203
615/327–0294
Contact: Carol Westlake, Dir.

Parents Offering Support to Other Parents (POSTOP)
801 A Teaberry Lane
Knoxville, TN 37912
615/691–2418
Contact: Ann Farr

Easter Seal Society of TN
2001 Woodmont Blvd.
P.O. Box 158145
Nashville, TN 37215
615/29–6639
Contact: Jayne Sutton, Pres.

TEXAS

Texas Education Agency
William B. Travis Bldg., Rm. 5–120
1701 N. Congress Ave.
Austin, TX 78701–2486
512/463–9414
Contact: Jill Gray, Director

Texas Rehab. Commission
4900 N. Lamar
Austin, TX 78751
512/483–4001
Contact: Vernon M. Arrell, Commissioner

Mental Retardation Services
Dept. of Mental Health & MR
P.O. Box 12668, Capitol Station
Austin, TX 78711
512/465–4520
Contact: Jaylon Fincannon, Deputy Commissioner

Texas Planning Council for Dev. Disabilities
4900 N. Lamar Blvd.

Austin, TX 78751–2316
512–483-4099
Contact: Roger Webb, Exec. Dir.

Advocacy, Inc.
7800 Shoal Creek Blvd.
Suite 171–E
Austin, TX 78757
512/454–4816; 800/252–9108 (in TX)
Contact: James Comstock-Galagan,
    Exec. Dir.

UCP of Texas
900 Congress Ave., Ste. 220
Austin, TX 78701
512/472–8696
Contact: Patty Anderson, Exec. Dir.

Assn. for Retarded Citizens/TX
833 Houston St.
Austin, TX 78756
512/454–6694
Contact: Libby Doggett, Exec. Dir.

Partnerships for Assisting Texans with
    Handicaps (PATH)
6465 Calder Ave.
Suite 202
Beaumont, TX 77707
409/866–4726; 800/866–4726
Contact: Janice Foreman, Dir.

Texas Easter Seal Society
800 West Ave., Bldg. C
Suite 100
Austin, TX 78701
512/474–1272
Contact: Georgia Jarvis, Pres.

UTAH

Special Education
State Office of Education
250 E. 500 South
Salt Lake City, UT 84111–3204
801/538–7706
Contact: Steven Kukic, Coordinator

Office of Rehabilitation
State Office of Education
250 E. 500 South

Salt Lake City, UT 84111
801/538–7530
Contact: Judy Ann Buffmire, Dir.

Div. of Svcs. to the Handicapped
Dept. of Social Services
150 W. Temple, Ste. 234
P.O. Box 45500
Salt Lake City, UT 84145
801/538–4199
Contact: Theron Olsen, Dir.

Utah Council for Handicapped & DD
    Persons
120 N. 200 West, 3rd. Fl.
P.O. Box 1958
Salt Lake City, UT 84110–1958
801/538–4184
Contact: Frances Morse, Exec. Dir.

Legal Center for the Handicapped
455 E. 400 South, Ste. 201
Salt Lake City, UT 84111
801/363–1347; 800/662–9080 (in UT)
Contact: Phyllis Geldzahler, Exec. Dir.

UCP of UT
P.O. Box 812
Midvale, UT 84047
801/255–8965
Contact: Alan Robinson

Assn. for Retarded Citizens/Utah
455 E. 400 South, Ste. 300
Salt Lake City, UT 84111
801/364–5060; 800/662–4058 (in UT)
Contact: Ray Behle, Exec. Dir.

Utah Parent Center
2290 E. 4500 South, No. 110
Salt Lake City, UT 84117
801/272–1051; 800/468–1160 (in UT)
Contact: Helen Post

Parent to Parent
455 E. 400 South, Ste. 300
Salt Lake City, UT 84111
801/364–5060; 800/662–4058 (in UT)

Easter Seal Society of Utah
331 S. Rio Grande Street

Suite 206
Salt Lake City, UT 84101
801/531–0522
Contact: John Pinter, Pres.

VERMONT

Division of Special Education
120 State St.
State Office Bldg.
Montpelier, VT 05602–3403
802/828–3141
Contact: Marc Hull, Director

Vocational Rehab. Division
Dept. of Social & Rehab. Svcs.
Agency of Human Resources
103 S. Main St.
Waterbury, VT 05676
802/241–2196
Contact: Richard Douglas, Dir.

Division of Mental Retardation
  Programs
Dept. of Mental Health
103 S. Main St.
Waterbury, VT 05676
802/241–2636
Contact: Charles Moseley, Dir.

Vermont Dev. Disabilities Council
Waterbury Office Complex
103 S. Main St.
Waterbury, VT 05676–1534
802/241–2612
Contact: Thomas Pombar, Exec.
  Secretary

Vermont Dev. Disabilities Law Project
12 North St.
Burlington, VT 05401
802/863–2881
Contact: Judy Dickson, Director

Citizen Advocacy, Inc.
Champlain Mill, Box 37
Winooski, VT 05404
802/655–0329
Contact: Katherine Lenk, Dir.

UCP of Vermont
P.O. Box 6292
Montpelier, VT 05702
802/223–5161
Contact: Lee Viets, Exec. Dir.

Vermont Assn. for Retarded Citizens
Champlain Mill, No. 37
Winooski, VT 05404
802/655–4014
Contact: Joan Sylvester, Exec. Dir.

VT Information and Training Network
  (VITN)
37 Champlain Mill
Winooski, VT 05404
802/655–4016
Contact: Connie Curtin, Director

Parent to Parent
37 Champlain Mill
1 Main St.
Winooski, VT 05404
802/655–5290
Contact: Nancy DiVenere

VIRGINIA

Special & Compensatory Education
Dept. of Education
P.O. Box 6Q
Richmond, VA 23216–2060
804/225–2402
Contact: William L. Helton, State Dir.

Dept. of Rehabilitative Svcs.
State Board of Vocational Rehab.
P.O. Box 11045
Richmond, VA 23230
804/367–0318
Contact: Susan Urofsky, Commissioner

Office of Mental Retardation Svcs.
P.O. Box 1797
Richmond, VA 23214
804/786–1746
Contact: Stanley Butkus, Director

Dev. Dis. Planning Council
101 N. 14th St., 17th Fl.
Richmond, VA 23219

804/225–2042; 800/552–3962 (in VA)
Contact Sarah Liddle, Acting Dir.

Dept. for Rights of the Disabled
James Monroe Bldg.
101 N. 14th St., 17th Fl.
Richmond, VA 23219–3641
804/225–2042; 800/552–3962 (in VA)
Contact: Sandra Reen, Acting Director

UCP of Virginia
1308 Sherwood Ave.
Richmond, VA 23220
804/321–6666
Contact: Stephen Conley, Exec. Dir.

Assn. for Retarded Citizens/VA
6 North 6th St.
Richmond, VA 23219
804/649–8481
Contact: Chris Rowe, Exec. Dir.

Parent Education Advocacy Training
  Center (PEATC)
228 S. Pitt St., Rm. 300
Alexandria, VA 22314
703/836–2953; 800/869–6782
Contact: Winifred Anderson, Dir.

Parent to Parent of Virginia
VA Inst. for Dev. Disabilities
VA Commonwealth University
301 W. Franklin St., Box 3020
Richmond, VA 23284
804/225–3875; 800/344–0012 (in VA)
Contact: Mary Cunningham, Coor-
  dinator

Easter Seal Society of Virginia
4841 Williamson Rd.
P.O. Box 5496
Roanoke, VA 24012
703/362–1656; 800/54–5900 (in VA)
Contact: Robert Knight, Pres.

VIRGIN ISLANDS

State Director of Special Education
P.O. Box 6640
Charlotte Amalie
St. Thomas, VI 00801

809/776–5802
Contact: Priscilla Stridiron

Div. of Vocational Rehabilitation
Dept. of Human Resources
Barbel Plaza South
Charlotte Amalie
St. Thomas, VI 00801
809/774–2835
Contact: Sedonie Halbert, Dir.

VI Dev. Disabilities Council
P.O. Box 2671, Kingshill
St. Croix, VI 00850–9999
809/772–2133
Contact: Mark Vinzant, Dir.

VI Coalition of Citizens with Dis-
  abilities
St. Thomas Chapter
P.O. Box 9500
St. Thomas, VI 00801
809/776–1277

VI Coalition of Citizens with Dis-
  abilities
St. Croix Chapter
P.O. Box 5156 Sunny Isles
St. Croix, VI 00820
809/778–7370

VI Parent Support Group
P.O. Box 11868
St. Thomas, VI 00801
809/776–4303
Contact: Don Laird, Dir.

WASHINGTON

Special Education Section
Supt. of Public Instruction
Old Capital Bldg.
Olympia, WA 98504–6733
Contact: Robert Lagarde, Interim Dir.

Division of Vocational Rehab.
Dept. of Social & Health Svcs.
State Office Bldg. No. 2
MS: OB–21C
Olympia, WA 98504

206/753–2544
Contact: Jeanne Munro, Dir.

Div. of Dev. Disabilities
Dept. of Social & Health Svcs.
P.O. Box 1788, OB–42C
Olympia, WA 98504
206/753–3900
Contact: Susan Elliot, Director

Dev. Disabilities Planning Council
9th & Columbia Bldg., MS: GH–52
Olympia, WA 98504–4151
206/753–3908
Contact: Sharon Hansen, Exec. Dir.

WA Protection & Advocacy System
1401 E. Jefferson
Seattle, WA 98122
206/324–1521
Contact: Mark Stroh, Exec. Dir.

UCP of Washington
4409 Interlake Ave., North
Seattle, WA 98103
206/632–6191
Contact: Ervin Larsen, Exec. Dir.

Assn. for Retarded Citizens/WA
1703 E. State St.
Olympia, WA 98506
206/357–5596

Parents Advocating Vocational Education (PAVE)
6316 S. 12th St.
Tacoma, WA 98465
206/565–2266; 800/572–7368
Contact: Kathy Babel, Project Coordinator

Pierce County Parent to Parent
12208 Pacific Highway, S.W.
Tacoma, WA 98499
206/588–1741
Contact: Betty Johnston, Coordinator

Easter Seal Society of Washington
521 2nd Ave., West
Seattle, WA 98119

206/281–5700
Contact: Paul Sorensen, Exec. Dir.

WEST VIRGINIA

Office of Special Education
Dept. of Education
Bldg. 6, Room B–304, Capitol Complex
Charleston, WV 25305
304/348–2696
Contact: Nancy Thabet, Director

Div. of Rehabilitation Svcs.
State Board of Rehabilitation
State Capitol
Charleston, WV 25305
304/766–4601
Contact: John Panza, Director

Developmental Disabilities Svcs.
Division of Behavioral Health
Dept. of Health
1800 Washington St., East
Charleston, WV 25305
304/348–0627
Contact: Jim Green, Acting Director

Dev. Disabilities Planning Council
625 D St.
South Charleston, WV 25303–3111
304/348–0416
Contact: Julie Pratt, Director

West Virginia Advocates
1524 Kanawha Blvd., East
Charleston, WV 25311
304/346–0847; 800/950–5250 (in WV)
Contact: Vicki Smith, Exec. Dir.

UCP of North Central West Virginia
450 W. Pike St.
Clarksburg, WV 26301
304/622–8845
Contact: Anne Alkire, Exec. Dir.

Assn. for Retarded Citizens/WV
Market Square Bldg., Rm. 400
700 Market St.
Parkersburg, WV 26101
304/485–5283
Contact: Nancy Lipphardt, Exec. Dir.

Project STEP
116 E. King St.
Martinsburg, WV 25401
304/263–HELP
Contact: Carol Tamara, Dir.

WV Easter Seal Society
1305 National Rd.
Wheeling, WV 26003
304/242–1390
Contact: Rosemary Front, Exec. Dir.

WISCONSIN

Div. of Handicapped Children and
  Pupil Services
125 S. Webster St.
P.O. Box 7841
Madison, WI 53707–7841
608/266–1649
Contact: Victor J. Contrucci, Asst. State
  Superintendant

Div. of Vocational Rehabilitation
Dept. of Health and Social Services
1 West Wilson St., Rm. 830
P.O. Box 7852
Madison, WI 53707
608/266–5466
Contact: Judy Norman-Nunnery, Ad-
ministrator

Developmental Disabilities Office
Dept. of Health and Social Svcs.
P.O. Box 7851
Madison, WI 53707
608/266–9329
Contact: Dennis Harkins, Director

Council on Dev. Disabilities
P.O. Box 7851, Rm. 344
Madison, WI 53707–7851
608/266–7826
Contact: Jayne Wittenmyer, Exec. Dir.

Wisconsin Coalition for Advocacy
16 N. Carroll, Ste. 400
Madison, WI 53703
608/267–0214
Contact: Lynn Breedlove, Exec. Dir.

UCP of Wisconsin
P.O. Box 1605
Madison, WI 53701
608/251–6533
Contact: Exec. Director

Assn. for Retarded Citizens/WI
6120 University Ave.
Middleton, WI 53560
608/231–3335
Contact: Jon Nelson, Exec. Director

Parent Education Project (PEP)
UCP of SE Wisconsin
230 W. Wells St., Ste. 502
Milwaukee, WI 53203
414/272–4500; 800/472–5525 (in WI)
Contact: Liz Irwin, Project Director

Parent to Parent
ARC
121 S. Hancock St.
Madison, WI 53703
608/251–9272
Contact: Jon Nelson

Easter Seal Society of Wisconsin
1409 Emil Street
Madison, WI 53713
608/257–3411
Contact: Roy Campbell, Exec. Dir.

WYOMING

Special Programs Unit
Dept. of Education
Hathaway Building, 2nd Fl.
2300 Capitol Ave.
Cheyenne, WY 82002
307/777–7414
Contact: Margie Simineo, Director

Div. of Vocational Rehabilitation
Dept. of Health and Social Services
Hathaway Building, Rm. 327
Cheyenne, WY 82002
307/777–7389
Contact: Joan Watson, Director

Div. of Community Programs
355 Hathaway Bldg.

Cheyenne, WY 8200–0170
307/777–7094
Contact: Steve Zimmerman, Administrator

Planning Council on DD
122 W. 25th St.
Hersch Bldg., 1st Fl. East
Cheyenne, WY 82002
307/777–7230
Contact: Sharon Kelsey, Exec. Director

Wyoming Protection and Advocacy System
2424 Pioneer Ave., No. 101
Cheyenne, WY 82001
307/632–3496; 800/328–1110
Contact: Jeanne Kawcak, Exec. Dir.

Assn. for Retarded Citizens/WY
P.O. Box 1205
Cheyenne, WY 82003
307/632–7105
Contact: Scott Bergey, Exec. Dir.

Parent-to-Parent
Council on Dev. Disabilities
Barrett Building, Rm. 408
301 Central Ave.
Cheyenne, WY 82002
307/777–7230
Contact: Rose Kor, Program Manager

Index